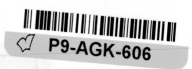

Toxicological Risk Assessment

Volume I

Biological and Statistical Criteria

Editors

D. B. Clayson
Chief, Toxicological Research Division
Bureau of Chemical Safety
Sir Frederick G. Banting Research Centre
Ottawa, Canada

D. Krewski
Chief, Biostatistics and Computer Applications
Environmental Health Directorate
Health Protection Branch
Health and Welfare Canada
Ottawa, Canada

I. Munro
Director, Canadian Center for Toxicology
Guelph, Ontario
Canada

CRC Press, Inc.
Boca Raton, Florida

Library of Congress Cataloging in Publication Data
Main entry under title:

Toxicological risk assessment.

  Bibliography: p.
  Includes index.
  Contents: v. 1. Biological and statistical
criteria -- v. 2. General criteria and case studies.
3. Environmental health--Evaluation.   4. Environmental
health--Government policy--Decision making.
5. Environmental health--Government policy--United
States--Decision making.   I. Clayson, D. B.
II. Krewski, D.   III. Munro, Ian C.   IV. Title: Risk assessment.
RA1199.T68   1985   615.9   84-12679
ISBN 0-8493-5976-7 (v. 1)
ISBN 0-8493-5977-5 (v. 2)

Direct all inquiries to CRC Press, Inc., 2000 Corporate Blvd., N.W., Boca Raton, Florida, 33431.

© 1985 by CRC Press, Inc.
Second Printing, 1986
Third Printing, 1986

International Standard Book Number 0-8493-5976-7 (Volume I)
International Standard Book Number 0-8493-5977-5 (Volume II)

Library of Congress Card Number 84-12679
Printed in the United States

FOREWORD

The rise of the modern pharmaceutical and chemical industry during the first half of this century has resulted in a dramatic enhancement in the quality of life and life expectancy, particularly in the industrialized nations. Modern treatment methods have substantially influenced the pattern of human disease. Mortality has changed from many deaths at younger ages due to microbial diseases to many deaths being attributable to cancer, heart disease, or other degenerative diseases which occur usually, but not always, in older people. Although the number of cases of the latter diseases have increased, it is noteworthy that for most types of cancer (excluding those of the bronchus and lung and of the stomach and pancreas), age-adjusted rates of mortality have been relatively constant for the last 50 years.

Our society, instead of lauding the chemical and pharmaceutical industries for their major contribution to the control of disease, seemingly holds industry responsible as a perceived major cause of the increased number of cancer cases. This reaction has been fuelled by sensational public reports that certain individual substances may induce cancer in laboratory animals and, by extension, in humans as well. Concern is further heightened by discoveries that extremely toxic chemicals, such as dioxin and aflatoxin, contaminate our environment.

This is the frenetic background against which modern toxicological science is developing. Society-mediated political pressure has led to the adoption and use of toxicological tests to protect the public health, sometimes before these tests are validated and before their significance to the species of primary concern, *Homo sapiens*, has been evaluated. Thus, we find ourselves with an elaborate battery of whole animal, microorganism, cell or tissue culture tests for various aspects of toxicology that are routinely carried out by highly competent and able scientists. Often, confusion arises first about how these tests should be applied to the protection of humanity and, second, of the part science on the one hand, or political considerations on the other, should play in controlling environmental risks. The latter difficulty can only be overcome if risk assessment, the scientific estimate of risk, is clearly separated from risk management, the regulatory decision making procedure that balances the scientific data on risk against the overall significance of regulation to the whole community. This is a highly judgmental process.

The editors of the present book recognized the cardinal importance of risk assessment to reasonable regulation. They have sought contributions from scientists, statisticians, and regulators with a broad experience in this area and have assembled the work in a form that they believe will be valuable to toxicologists, statisticians, regulators, and legislators who wish to obtain a deeper understanding of the difficulties and pitfalls that may befall the unwary in this area. Additionally, authors have been asked to suggest how particular areas of toxicological science may develop in future years.

The book is presented in two volumes. The first is concerned with the biological and statistical criteria that must be regarded as the foundations of any regulatory decision. These are presented separately: Section A is concerned with the experimental findings and Section B with statistical analysis. The second volume considers more general criteria and case studies. Section A is concerned with the interpretation of the scientific data base extrapolated to likely human exposure levels. Consideration is also given to assessing the benefits of chemical usage as well as other regulatory issues. In Section B, a number of specific examples are considered in detail as illustrations of the care needed and the difficulties that can be met in the use of the data. The emphasis of these two volumes is directed mainly towards the induction of cancer, as this is the most active area of toxicological risk assessment at this time. However, the issue of how to best increase the safety of individual members of our community without at the same time destroying the apparent benefits of our current lifestyle is common to all aspects of toxicology and regulation.

In Volume I, Chapter 1, Hart and Fishbein discuss biological factors that may lead to species differences in response to particular toxic agents. The importance of xenobiotic metabolism to such differences is considered in greater detail in the following two chapters. Withey, in Chapter 2, discusses the importance of pharmacokinetic studies on the test agent and its metabolites. In Chapter 3, O'Flaherty indicates how metabolism may vary quantitatively or even qualitatively with the dose level of the agent. The concluding two chapters address the induction of cancer by chemicals. In Chapter 4, Shank and Barrows discuss what is known about the mechanisms of chemical carcinogenesis and how they may ultimately be found to be more diverse than hitherto imagined, a conclusion firmly based on these authors' observations. Clayson, in Chapter 5, concludes this section with a discussion of a possible means of deriving the strength or potency of a carcinogen from bioassay data. He speculates on whether a compatible value for potency could be derived for humans using in vitro studies.

The statistical methodology discussed in Section B serves two functions. First, methods for the design and analysis of toxicological experiments which are both valid and efficient are discussed. Second, statistical models are identified to permit the extrapolation from the high doses fed to animals to the much lower doses to which humans may be exposed. The first two chapters in this section are devoted to carcinogenesis bioassay in small rodents. Bickis and Krewski (Chapter 6) discuss the many complex design issues involved in such tests and provide an overview of currently used methods of analysis. Lagakos and Louis (Chapter 7) treat the IARC method for analyzing time to tumor data in detail. Seilken (Chapter 8) discusses the one extrapolation model that appeared to fit the data of the massive ED01 experiment on mouse carcinogenicity induced by N, 2-fluorenylacetamide. This model differs from others in considering both dose and time on test and, if sufficient data is available, may prove of great value for low dose extrapolation of carcinogenicity bioassay results. In Chapter 9, Crump and Howe review other methods for low dose extrapolation and consider the most promising avenues for future development. Hoel, in Chapter 10, emphasizes the importance of attempting to make low dose extrapolations compatible with the results of pharmacokinetic studies, a valuable approach to the consolidation of more than one type of toxicological test within the statistical data base.

Volume II is concerned with the practical implications of toxicity data. It opens with a consideration by Day of the utility and sensitivity of epidemiological methodology to identify chemicals or mixtures that may adversely affect people (Chapter 1). Without the information provided by epidemiology, toxicology would appear to be an esoteric academic exercise rather than the major practical endeavor that it is today. Kraybill (Chapter 2) outlines the immense body of knowledge we presently have on human exposures to foreign chemicals with a major emphasis on the drinking water supply as an example of possible sources of human contamination. Newberne (Chapter 3), on the other hand, discusses the difficult area of nutrition in respect to toxic response and clearly shows how different levels and types of nutrition may markedly affect the responses in man and animals. Section A concludes with three chapters discussing how the body of information on human exposure and toxic effects may be reconciled with demands for a safe environment, and with the clear need for our society to continue. In Chapter 4, Darby points out that many of the chemicals with which we as a society are most concerned pose benefits as well as risks. Thompson, Chapter 5, considers health benefits as a way to balance the apparent health hazards associated with the continued use of chemicals. In Chapter 6, Miller addresses the specific issues to food regulation in which regulatory decisions may affect each and every member of our community.

Finally, an attempt is made in Section B to determine how our societal efforts at chemical regulation are working out in practice. This is achieved by considering five chemicals in considerable depth. All of these are well known either because of their widespread use or because of recent discussions in the media. They are asbestos discussed by Meek, Shannon, and Toft (Chapter 7); formaldehyde by Starr, Gibson, and Swenberg (Chapter 9); poly-chlorinated biphenyls by Cordle, Locke, and Springer (Chapter 10); and finally the very controversial artificial sweetening agent, saccharin, by Arnold and Clayson (Chapter 11).

It is hoped that this work will be of use in helping society, including the regulators, toxicologists, consumers, and industrialists, to arrive at a more unified view of where we should be going in order to achieve a safer but still satisfying environment for society as a whole. The editors would each like to pay tribute to each individual author for a substantial contribution achieved at the cost of personal effort and time. The problems that remain to be solved are immense, but, if we can learn where we are presently situated, we have a far better chance of deciding where we need to go and thereafter to choose the correct path.

D. B. Clayson
D. Krewski
I. C. Munro

THE EDITORS

Dr. David B. Clayson Ph.D., is Chief, Toxicology Research Division, Bureau of Chemical Safety of the Canadian Food Directorate. He trained in Natural Sciences (Chemistry) at the University of Oxford, England and took his Ph.D. in Experimental Pathology and Cancer Research at the University of Leeds, England. Dr. Clayson's interests during the 26 years he was at the University of Leeds were in occupational bladder cancer, the mode of chemical induction of bladder tumors, the nature and mode of action of chemical carcinogens. In 1974, he was appointed Deputy Director of the Epply Institute for Cancer Research, University of Nebraska Medical Center in Omaha, and came to Ottawa in 1981. Dr. Clayson, in 1962, published *Chemical Carcinogenesis* the first comprehensive text on this subject, and has contributed over 120 publications to the Cancer Research literature ranging from the mode of action of occupational bladder carcinogens to possible approaches to the difficult problems of carcinogen regulation. Dr. Clayson was Founder Secretary of the Toxicology Forum and is a member of the Society of Toxicology and the American Association of Cancer Research. He has been a member of numerous scientific committees in the United Kingdom, the United States, and Canada, and has also served on international panels such as the International Commission for the Protection of the Environment against Mutagens and Carcinogens, and groups established by the World Health Organization and the International Agency for Research on Cancer.

Dr. Daniel Krewski Ph.D., is currently Chief of the Biostatistics and Computer Applications Division in the Environmental Health Directorate of Health and Welfare Canada and a member of the Laboratory for Research Statistics and Probability at Carleton University in Ottawa. Dr. Krewski has published over 40 articles on biostatistics and risk assessment and has participated in scientific committees established by the Toxicology Forum, International Life Sciences Institute, Institute for Environmental Studies, and International Agency for Research on Cancer. He is presently a member of the Board of Directors of the American Statistical Association and is an Associate Editor of the *Canadian Journal of Statistics* and *Risk Abstracts*.

Dr. Ian C. Munro, Ph.D., is the Director of the Canadian Centre for Toxicology. Immediately prior to accepting the position of Director of the Centre, Dr. Munro was the Director General of the Food Directorate, Health Protection Branch, Health and Welfare Canada from 1979 to 1983. He was past Chairman of the Tripartite Toxicology Committee (U.S., U.K., and Canada) and is Assistant Editor of the *Journal of the American College of Toxicology*. He has published over 60 articles in the field of toxicology.

CONTRIBUTORS

D. L. Arnold, Ph.D.
Research Scientist
Toxicology Research Division
Food Directorate
Health and Welfare Canada
Ontario, Canada

L. R. Barrows, Ph. D.
Department of Pharmacology
George Washington University
Washington, D.C.

M. Bickis
Senior Consulting Statistician
Environmental Health Directorate
Health and Welfare Canada
Ontario, Canada

F. Cordle
Chief
Epidemiology and Clinical Toxicology
Center for Food Safety and Applied
  Nutrition
Food and Drug Administration
Washington, D.C.

K. S. Crump, Ph.D.
President
K. S. Crump and Co.,
Ruston, Louisiana

W. J. Darby, M.D., Ph.D.
Professor Emeritus of Biochemistry
  (Nutrition)
Vanderbilt University School of Medicine
Nashville, Tennessee

N. E. Day, Ph.D.
Chief, Unit of Biostatistics and Field
  Studies
International Agency for Research on
  Cancer
Lyon, France

L. Fishbein
Associate Director for Scientific
  Coordination
National Center for Toxicological
  Research
Jefferson, Arkansas

J. E. Gibson, Ph.D.
Vice President and Director of Research
Chemical Industry Institute of Toxicology
Research Triangle Park, North Carolina

R. W. Hart, Ph.D.
Director, National Center for
  Toxicological Research
National Center for Toxicological
  Research
Jefferson, Arkansas

D. G. Hoel, Ph.D.
Director, Biometry and Risk Assessment
  Program
National Institute of Environmental
  Health Sciences
Research Triangle Park, North Carolina

R. B. Howe, Ph.D.
Professor of Mathematics and Statistics
Louisiana Tech University
Ruston, Louisiana

H. F. Kraybill, Ph.D.
Scientific Coordinator for Environmental
  Cancer
National Cancer Institute
Bethesda, Maryland

S. W. Lagakos, Ph.D.
Associate Professor, Biostatistics
Harvard School of Public Health
Boston, Massachusetts

R. Locke
Environmental Protection Agency
Washington, D.C.

T. A. Louis, Ph.D.
Associate Professor, Biostatistics
Harvard School of Public Health
Boston, Massachusetts

M. E. Meek, M.Sc.
Biologist
Monitoring and Criteria Division
Bureau of Chemical Hazards
Department of National Health and
  Welfare
Ottawa, Canada

S. A. Miller, Ph.D.
Director, Center for Food Safety and
  Applied Nutrition
Food and Drug Administration
Washington, D.C.

P. M. Newberne, D.V.M., Ph.D.
Professor of Nutritional Pathology
Massachusetts Institute of Technology
Cambridge, Massachusetts
  and Professor of Pathology
Boston University School of Medicine
Boston, Massachusetts

E. J. O'Flaherty, Ph.D.
Associate Professor of Environmental
  Health
Department of Environmental Health
University of Cincinnati College of
  Medicine
Cincinnati, Ohio

G. M. Paddle, Ph.D., D.I.C.
Biostatistician to Central Medical Group
Central Medical Group
Imperial Chemical Industries PLC
Cheshire, England

I. F. H. Purchase, Ph.D., FRC Path.
Director, Central Toxicology Laboratory
Imperial Chemical Industries PLC
Cheshire, England

R. C. Shank, Ph.D.
Professor, Community and Environmental
  Medicine and Pharmacology
College of Medicine
University of California
Irvine, California

H. S. Shannon, Ph.D.
Assistant Professor, Department of
  Clinical Epidemiology and Biostatistics
McMaster University
Hamilton, Canada

R. L. Sielken, Jr., Ph.D.
Professor of Statistics
Texas A and M University
College Station, Texas

K. J. Skinner, Ph.D.
Special Assistant, Center for Food Safety
  and Applied Nutrition
Food and Drug Administration
Washington, D.C.

J. Springer
Epidemiology Branch
Environmental Protection Agency
Washington, D.C.

J. Stafford, Ph.D.
Plastics and Petrochemicals Division
Imperial Chemical Industries PLC
Hertfordshire, England

T. B. Starr, Ph.D.
Scientist-Mathematician
Department of Epidemiology
Chemical Industry Institute of Toxicology
Research Triangle Park, North Carolina

J. A. Swenberg, Ph.D., DVM.
Head, Department of Biochemical
  Toxicology and Pathobiology
Chemical Industry Institute of Toxicology
Research Triangle Park, North Carolina

M. S. Thompson, Ph.D.
Associate Professor, Health Policy and
  Management
Harvard University
Boston, Massachusetts

P. Toft, D.Phil.
Chief
Monitoring and Criteria Division
Bureau of Chemical Hazards
Department of National Health and
  Welfare
Ottawa, Canada

J. R. Withey, Ph.D.
Research Scientist
Toxicology Research Division
Foods Directorate
Bureau of Chemical Safety
Health and Welfare Canada
Ontario, Canada

TABLE OF CONTENTS

Volume I

TABLE OF CONTENTS

Volume II

Section A—Biological Criteria

Chapter 1

INTERSPECIES EXTRAPOLATION OF DRUG AND GENETIC TOXICITY DATA

Ronald W. Hart and Lawrence Fishbein

TABLE OF CONTENTS

I. INTRODUCTION

Toxicology is the study of the spectrum of potentially harmful interactions between chemicals and living organisms. Included in this broad panoply are animal studies which measure the toxic effects resulting from both long-term exposures to low concentrations of agents as well as short-term exposures at high concentration. Integral to any meaningful assessment of risk and safety is the difficult problem of extrapolation of data obtained from these studies to other populations. Extrapolation may be either between species or between dose-response curves ranging from high doses to dosage levels far below the range of observation. The development of surrogate animal and non-animal systems is necessary for extrapolation purposes since human experimentation is obviously largely precluded and/or yields very limited data.

There are two basic paradigms for research on the action and effect of toxic substances. One, which can be referred to as the ontogenic, seeks to account for or describe the effect of a toxic substance on an organism as being a function of dose, time, or route of administration. This approach is basic to dose extrapolation. The other, which can be called the evolutionary-comparative approach, is concerned with the differences in the genetically determined constitutive characteristics of a species (or any genetically defined population) that may account for species differences in the effect of a toxic substance between species and between individuals within a species.[1,2] This approach is basic to interspecies extrapolation.

The former of these approaches dominates contemporary research in toxicology and will continue to do so, for it produces important descriptive information. However, it must be recognized that at present it cannot by itself solve the problem of risk assessment, since it currently does not provide adequate information required for extrapolation between species. A major reason for this is the fact that the ontogenic approach to toxicology focuses primarily on effect rather than on cause and differences in effects. An observed toxic effect, no matter how close it may be to the fundamental biosynthetic or operative processes remains a species-specific effect which must have been an antecedent cause or difference between species which would explain species differences in response. In order to obtain or attempt such extrapolations between species with a requisite degree of confidence, a significant amount of information is required concerning; (a) the species of interest, (b) the behavior and impact of the substance in the test species, (c) the similarities and differences between test species (generally rat or mouse) and man that influence the manifestation of adverse effects and the probability of their occurrence. In order to best accomplish this task, species differences in absorption, distribution, pharmacokinetics, storage, biotransformation, activation, interaction with target molecules and receptors, detoxification, repair and/or expression and excretion of either the toxicant or its metabolites and the resulting insult to the biological system(s) under investigation should be known. These factors represent biochemical and molecular modulators of toxicity. As the placental mammals evolved from small short-lived species to large long-lived species, better specific means to protect more cells for a longer period of time must also have evolved. Identification of these modulators and how they differ between species is basic to interspecies extrapolation of toxicity data.

A major problem encountered in attempting to anticipate the fate of a xenobiotic is not in predicting the possible routes of its metabolism but rather in predicting which of these potential routes will actually occur in a particular animal species. This can best be attempted when the fate of structurally related compounds have been studied in a number of animal species under standard conditions which keeps other variables to a minimum.[3,4]

Such standardized conditions are important since, in addition to the above biochemical and molecular modulators of toxicity, the extrapolation of data derived in non-animal systems to human health effects is also limited by higher order animal functions which are also known to modulate toxicity (e.g., diet, stress, sex, age, hormonal balance, stage of development, etc.). These latter factors, while somewhat species specific, can be better controlled for experimentally than can the former class of modulators.

The evolutionary comparative paradigm is based on two postulates; (1) a difference in the effect of a toxic substance between two basically similar organisms, under similar experimental conditions, is due to a difference between the physiochemical environments of the essential macromolecules of the two organisms and (2) the parameters of the molecular environment within an organism are the expression of its genome. Therefore, the eventual fate of the organism, in terms of its susceptibilities to toxic substances, is primarily determined by specific genetically determined constitutive properties (class one modulators), both molecular and organizational, which can be measured both in vitro and in vivo. Higher order functions (class two modulators), however, can only be determined in vivo and may to some extent be adjusted for experimentally. In extrapolation of cell and animal data to human health effects, the basic question which must be addressed is what one species does differently from another, if anything, by way of protection, stabilization, and repair or its essential molecules in order to maintain homeostasis in the face of environmental toxicants.

A number of methods have been developed to attempt to overcome the above limitations in interspecies extrapolation, but it is acknowledged that each of these methods is empirical in nature and hence limited as a model of nature. The comparative toxicology data available are limited in both amount and scope and normally represent studies from a number of laboratories and thus present the recognized intrinsic difficulties associated with comparison of such data. Nevertheless, comparative toxicology data on species differences in metabolism, activation and deactivation of compounds, induction of DNA damage, its repair, replication and expression do exist in a manner consistent with the evolution of the placental mammals. These data will thus be reviewed and species differences relative to extrapolation discussed.

II. USE OF EXPERIMENTAL ANIMALS IN PREDICTIVE TOXICITY AND CARCINOGENICITY BIOASSAYS

The choice of a suitable strain or species for toxicological study is generally decided on the basis of either the degree of sensitivity to the toxicant in question or the similarity of the metabolism to that in humans. The physiological and biochemical differences between the species are principally quantitative rather than qualitative, inasmuch as they deal with rates of growth, development and metabolic disposition, hematologic and biochemical composition, and the physical bases for interrelating dose levels between species. For example, the blood serum levels of enzymes, among other constituents, vary between the species and suggest differences in the biotransformation of foreign substances as well as of normal food constituents. The species of choice in toxicological studies, however, is often determined by considerations of economics and time rather than scientific desirability. Thus, generally rodent (rat or mouse) and, less often, non-rodent (dog or cat) models are used. Table 1 lists the advantages and disadvantages of the rat as an experimental model for humans.[5]

While there are many similarities between rodents and humans, marked differences also exist, including; (1) the structure and function of the placenta, (2) reproductive physiology, (3) the lack of an emetic reflex and the practice of coprophagy in the rodents, (4) lack of dependence in the rodent on dietary ascorbic acid and absence of a gallbladder, and (5) an altered ability of the rodent to oxidize uric acid enzymatically to allantoin as an end product of purine metabolism.[5,6] Additionally, while most values for chemical constituents in rat serum are in approximately the same range as those in human serum, bilirubin, cholesterol, crentinine, and uric acid levels are much lower in the rat.

Metabolic enzymes vary widely between rat and human (Table 2).[5,7] However, although many of these are not specifically involved in detoxification processes, such differences are

Table 1
ADVANTAGES AND DISADVANTAGES OF THE RAT AS AN EXPERIMENTAL MODEL FOR HUMANS[a]

Advantages	Disadvantages	
Widely studied	Anatomic:	Nutritional:
Small size (housing)	Lack of gallbladder	Mineral requirements
Prolific	Yolk-sac placenta	Vitamin requirements
Brief gestation/lactation	Multiple mammae	Ascorbic acid
Rapid growth to maturity	No emetic reflex	Histidine
Short life span	Fur-bearing	Behavioral:
Omnivorous	Physiological:	Nocturnal
Dry diet acceptable (food	Estrus cycle +	Coprophagy
consumption)	menstrual cycle	Cannibalism
Multiple dosage routes	multiparous	Strain variation:
Low initial and main-	Hematology	Intercurrent infections
tenance cost	Metabolic:	Spontaneous tumors
Docile	Purines to allantoin	Maintenance:
No better alternative	Clinical chemistry	Temperature
	Enzymatic biotrans-	Humidity
	formations	Noise
		Careful handling

[a] This includes both genders.

From Oser, B. L., Ed., *J. Toxicol. Environ. Hlth.*, Hemisphere Publishing, 8, 521, 1981. With permission.

Table 2
ENZYMES OF HUMAN AND RAT SERUM (BOTH SEXES)

Enzyme	Human	Rat	Rat/human
Alkaline phosphatase, IU/dℓ	25.0	87.7	3.51
Acid phosphatase, IU/dℓ	1.13	38.3	33.8
SGPT[a], IU/dℓ	9.71	23.9	2.46
SGOT[b], IU/dℓ	13.4	63.3	4.72
Lactate dehydrogenase, IU/dℓ	198	91.3	0.46
Creatine phosphokinase, IU/dℓ	50	6.2	0.12
Amylase, somogyiunits/dℓ	108	220	2.04

[a] Serum glutamic-pyruvic transaminase
[b] Serum glutamic-oxaloacetic transaminase

From Oser, B. L., Ed., *J. Toxicol. Environ. Hlth.*, Hemisphere Publishing, 8, 521, 1981. With permission.

compatible with the variation of other tissue enzymes normally present or induced that do affect the metabolism of drugs and xenobiotics.[5] Pathways of metabolism are often similar between rat and human, but there are marked differences in rates of metabolism (Table 3).[5] It should be stressed, however, regarding the above comparison of rates of metabolism, that in only a few cases has the same substance been studied under comparable test conditions in both species by a single investigator.

The mouse also has numerous well recognized advantages in toxicological studies. First used in cancer research 60 years ago,[8,9] it is relatively inexpensive, has a prolific rate of reproduction, is small in size and has a relatively short life span. Due to the long-term nature of carcinogenicity testing and the large numbers of animals required for statistically valid

Table 3
SPECIES DIFFERENCES IN BIOTRANSFORMATION RATES

Substance	Pathway (phase)[a]	Rat (%)	Human (%)
Butylated hydroxy-anisole (BHA)	Demethylation (I)	+	0
	Glucuronide (II)	72	27-77
	Sulfate (II)	14	Trace
Butylated hydroxy-toluene (BHT)	Methyl oxidation (I)	36	3
	Glucuronide (II)	4	35
	Sulfate (II)	14	ND[b]
Coumarin	Ring opening (I)	20	4
	Ring hydroxylation (I)	0.4	79
Limonane	Methyl (side chain) oxidation (I)	48	7
	C-C hydroxylation (I)	33	34
Phenol	Glucuronide (II)	40	12
	Sulfate (II)	45	80
Phenylacetic acid	Glycine (II)	40—90	ND
	Glutamine (II)	—	93
Benzo(d)isothiazoline (saccharin precursor)	Ring opening (I)	55	13-16

[a]   I, molecular change; II, conjugation.
[b]   Not detected.

From Oser, B. L., Ed., *J. Toxicol. Environ. Hlth.*, Hemisphere Publishing, 8, 521, 1981. With permission.

results, this species is generally the one of choice;[10] however, it also has many of the same limitations listed above for the rat.[10-12] The incidence of "spontaneous" tumors in the mouse can be modulated significantly by various environmental and genetic factors.[11,13] Grasso and Crampton[10] in their critical review of the value of the mouse in carcinogenicity testing suggested that in mice, the induction (sometimes sex-specifically) of pulmonary tumors and of hepatoma by a diversity of systemically acting agents can often be best explained as a co-carcinogenic rather than a direct carcinogenic effect. Additionally, the induction of mammary tumors can often be related to viral and endocrine influences, and lymphomas and leukemias, with or without evidence of a viral etiology, often depend on immunosuppression factors.[10,11] Although the mouse resembles other mammalian species in its response to carcinogenic agents, care should be taken to adjust for species, strain and colony differences which might exist. For example, data from control animals are particularly important in assessing the significance of rare tumors, a scattered dose-response, and wide incidence variations between groups in carcinogenicity bioassays.[14-19] False positive results may occur at sites with high and variable tumor rates[15] and are dependent on the rate of spontaneous tumor incidence. High incidence rates for certain tumor types may make the end points for carcinogenesis tests uncertain if a chemical causes only a slight or moderate increase in the incidence of these tumors.[18] A rare tumor has less chance of occurring than a common tumor and hence has less chance of causing a false positive.[16] This latter observation is based upon an extensive survey by Chu et al.[16] (Table 4) who evaluated the following six factors in 200 NCI bioassays; (1) the adequacy of the bioassay data, (2) the presence of a significantly increased incidence of tumors, (3) the adequacy of the number of animals at risk of developing tumors, (4) the adequacy of the dose of chemical treatment, (5) the etiology and pathogenesis of lesions, and (6) other factors that may influence an evaluation such as a shortened latency period for tumor formation in dosed animals or the stability of the chemical.

Table 4
PERCENT SPONTANEOUS PRIMARY TUMORS IN UNTREATED SPECIES USED AT NCI FOR CARCINOGEN BIOASSAYS

Organ/tissue	Mouse B6C3F1 Male 3543[a]	Mouse B6C3F1 Female 3617	Rat Fischer 344 Male 2960	Rat Fischer 344 Female 2924	Rat OSB-MNDL Male 270	Rat OSB-MNDL Female 270	Rat SPR.-DAW. Male 440	Rat SPR.-DAW. Female 205	Rat CHAR. RIV. CD Male 184	Rat CHAR. RIV. CD Female 184
Brain	<.1%	.1%	.8%	.6%	—	—	.7%	.5%	2.7%	1.6%
Skin	3.1	1.7	7.8	3.2	8.9	5.9	3.2	3.4	7.1	3.3
Mammary gland	—	1.3	1.5	20.9	3.7	28.5	1.4	39.0	.5	45.1
Circulatory system[b]	2.9	2.4	.7	.4	4.1	2.6	—	—	2.2	—
Lung/bronchi/trachea	13.7	5.2	3.0	1.9	1.5	.7	.2	.5	1.6	1.6
Liver	24.6	4.7	2.2	1.9	1.1	1.9	—	—	.5	2.2
Pancreas	<.1	<.1	.2	—	—	—	—	—	—	—
Stomach	.4	.4	.3	.2	—	.4	—	—	—	.5
Intestines[c]	.5	.2	.6	.3	.4	.4	.2	—	—	.5
Kidney	.3	<.1	.5	.2	3.3	2.6	—	1.0	1.6	—
Urinary bladder[d]	<.1	<.1	.1	.3	.4	—	.2	—	.5	—
Preputial gland[d]	—	—	2.4	1.8	1.6	1.2	—	—	—	—
Testes[e]	.4	NA	82.3	NA	.7	NA	2.0	NA	3.9	NA
Ovary	NA	.9	NA	.4	NA	1.5	NA	—	NA	.5
Uterus	NA	1.6	NA	17.0	NA	3.7	NA	4.4	NA	3.8
Pituitary	.3	3.6	14.7	34.9	7.4	20.0	5.9	40.0	33.2	57.6
Adrenal	1.4	.6	12.4	5.2	10.4	10.0	.7	2.9	7.6	4.3
Thyroid	1.0	1.7	8.2	6.8	9.6	11.1	.9	2.0	3.8	—
Pancreatic islets	.4	.2	3.9	.8	3.0	1.9	.5	.5	2.7	—
Body cavities	.4	.3	2.6	.4	1.9	.4	.5	1.9	2.2	—
Leukemia/lymphoma	10.3	20.6	19.9	13.4	3.3	1.8	4.8	0.5	3.3	3.3

a   Number necropsied. (Studies terminated at 21—25 months for mice and 23—25 months for rats).
b   Hemagioma and hemangiosarcoma.
c   Duodenum, jejunum, ileum, cecum and colon.
d   Clitoral gland in females.
d   Seminal vesicle and testis.

From Chu, K. C., Cueto, C., Jr., and Ward, J. M., *J. Toxicol. Environ Hlth.*, Hemisphere Publishing, 8, 251, 1981. With permission.

Differences in the expression of carcinogenic effects between mammalian species do occur, and these are due to critical differences between species as well as to details of experimental design. For example, a number of interspecies comparisons of carcinogenicity[20,21] and carcinogenic potency[21,22] have been reported. Purchase[20] compared the carcinogenicity of 250 chemicals in the rat and mouse from the published literature through three independent sources: NCI Bioassay Program; International Agency for Research on Cancer, Monograph Series, 1972 to 1978; and carcinogenicity studies obtained from U.S. Public Health Service Document No. 149. Of the 250 compounds listed, 38% were non-carcinogenic in both rats and mice, and 44% were carcinogenic in both species. A total of 43 compounds produced different results in the two species, 21 (8%) being carcinogenic in mice only, 17 (7%) in rats only and 5 (2%) having differing results from other species. A comparison of the major target organs affected by chemicals carcinogenic in both species revealed that 64% of the chemicals studied produced cancer at the same site. While these data have been used to justify interspecies extrapolation, it is important to note that both rat and mouse belong to the group of mytomorph rodents, have less than 1% difference in their DNA and similar species maximum achievable lifespans.

Purchase[20] points out that extrapolation from a single-animal study to man may be subject to substantial errors since "an accurate extrapolation to man requires an intimate knowledge of the metabolism and mode of action of the chemical in the species selected for laboratory tests and knowledge of whether the key features established in the laboratory animal are also present in man".[20] It must also be noted that the factors known to influence chemical carcinogenesis vary during the life of a test animal or man. For example, liver metabolism is not efficient in early gestation; the hormonal environment of the immature offspring and the adult varies, as does immunological competence.[22,23]

Tomatis et al.[24] evaluated a total of 368 chemicals which were reviewed in the Monograph Program of the International Agency for Research on Cancer (IARC) from 1971 to 1977. For 26 chemicals (or industrial processes), a positive association between the exposure and the occurrence of cancer in humans was observed and a comparison of target organs and main routes of exposure in animals and humans made (Table 5). For 221 chemicals some evidence of carcinogenicity was found in at least one species of experimental animals, but no evaluation of the carcinogenic risk of these chemicals to humans was made, either because no epidemiological studies or case reports were available or because the results of available human studies were inconclusive.

It has been suggested that data on animal carcinogenesis be used as a quantitative predictor of human risk especially if the animal's metabolism is similar to that of humans. Attempts to determine dose levels of several known or putative human carcinogens for certain populations and compare these levels with those known to produce neoplasms in animals were described by the Meselson Committee in 1975.[21] These data are summarized in Table 6 and suggests that the cumulative dose required per kg body weight for tumor induction in the human and in experimental animals is of the same order of activity. It should be noted that a more detailed comparison would have required a correction for the relatively short observation time in a number of the studies on humans, e.g., diethylstilbestrol and vinyl chloride, since many cancers in humans are not observed for 20 to 30 years following exposure. Additionally, it should be noted that in both the vinyl chloride and diethylstilbestrol studies only a rare tumor type was considered by the Meselson Committee.[21]

Crouch and Wilson[22] recently assessed experimental data on which such comparisons could be based and thus outlined an interspecies comparison of carcinogenic potency. The NCI series of Carcinogenicity Bioassay Reports describing experiments with similar experimental designs on rats and mice contained sufficient data to compile values of the carcinogenic potency (kg d/mg). It was demonstrated empirically that good correlations exist between different species (rat and mouse) for suitably defined carcinogenic potencies for

Table 5

CHEMICALS OR INDUSTRIAL PROCESSES ASSOCIATED WITH CANCER INDUCTION IN HUMANS: COMPARISION OF TARGET ORGANS AND MAIN ROUTES OF EXPOSURE IN ANIMALS AND HUMANS

Chemical or industrial process	Humans			Animals		
	Main type of exposure[a]	Target organ	Main route of exposure[b]	Animal	Target organ	Route of exposure
1. Aflatoxins	Environmental, occupational[c]	Liver	p.o., inhalation[c]	Rat	Liver, stomach, colon, kidney	p.o.
				Fish, duck, marmoset, tree shrew, monkey	Liver	p.o
				Rat	Liver, trachea	i.t.
					Liver	i.p.
				Mouse, rat	Local	s.c. injection
				Mouse	Lung	i.p.
2. 4-Aminobiphenyl	Occupational	Bladder	Inhalation, skin, p.o.	Mouse, rabbit, dog	Bladder	p.o.
				Newborn mouse	Liver	s.c. injection
				Rat	Mammary gland, intestine	s.c. injection
3. Arsenic compounds	Occupational, medicinal, and environmental	Skin, lung, liver[c]	Inhalation, p.o., skin	Mouse, rat, dog	Inadequate, negative	p.o.
				Mouse	Inadequate, negative	Topical, i.v.
4. Asbestos	Occupational	Lung, pleural cavity, gastrointestinal tract	Inhalation, p.o.	Mouse, rat, hamster, rabbit	Lung, pleura	Inhalation or i.t.
				Rat, hamster	Local	Intrapleural
				Rat	Local	i.p., s.c. injection
					Various sites[c]	p.o.
5. Auramine (manufacture of)	Occupational	Bladder	Inhalation, skin, p.o.	Mouse, rat	Liver	p.o.
				Rabbit, dog	Negative	p.o.
				Rat	Local, liver, intestine	s.c. injection
6. Benzene	Occupational	Hemopoietic system	Inhalation, skin	Mouse	Inadequate	Topical, s.c. injection

No.	Chemical	Exposure	Human target organ	Route of human exposure	Animal	Animal target site	Route
7.	Benzidine	Occupational	Bladder	Inhalation, skin, p.o.	Mouse	Liver	s.c. injection
					Rat	Liver	p.o.
					Rat	Zymbal gland, liver, colon	s.c. injection
					Hamster	Liver	p.o.
					Dog	Bladder	p.o.
8.	Bis(chloro-methyl)ether	Occupational	Lung	Inhalation	Mouse, rat	Lung, nasal cavity	Inhalation
					Mouse	Skin	Topical
9.	Cadmium-using industries (possibly cadmium oxide)	Occupational	Prostate, lung^c	Inhalation, p.o.	Rat	Local, lung	s.c. injection
					Rat	Local	s.c. injection
					Rat	Local, testis	s.c. or i.m. injection
10.	Chloramphenicol	Medicinal	Hemopoietic system	p.o., injection		(No adequate tests)	
11.	Chloromethyl methyl ether (possibly associated with bis(chloromethyl)ether	Occupational	Lung	Inhalation	Mouse	Initiator	Skin
						Lung^c	Inhalation
						Local, lung^c	s.c. injection
					Rat	Local^c	s.c. injection
12.	Chromium (chromate-producing industries	Occupational	Lung, nasal cavities^c	Inhalation	Mouse	Local	s.c., i.m. injection
					Rat	Lung	intrabronchial implantation
13.	Cyclophosphamide	Medicinal	Bladder	p.o., injection	Mouse	Hemopoietic system, lung	i.p., s.c. injection
					Rat	Various sites	p.o.
						Bladder^c	i.p.
						Mammary gland	i.p.
						Various sites	i.v.
14.	Diethylstilbestrol	Medicinal	Uterus, vagina	p.o.	Mouse	Mammary	p.o.
					Mouse	Mammary, lymphoreticular, testis, vagina	s.c. injection, s.c. implantation
					Rat	Mammary, hypophysis^c bladder	Local
							s.c. implantation
					Hamster	Kidney	s.c. injection, s.c. implantation
					Squirrel monkey	Uterine serosa	s.c. implantation

Table 5 (continued)
CHEMICALS OR INDUSTRIAL PROCESSES ASSOCIATED WITH CANCER INDUCTION IN HUMANS: COMPARISION OF TARGET ORGANS AND MAIN ROUTES OF EXPOSURE IN ANIMALS AND HUMANS

Chemical or industrial process	Main type of exposure[a]	Humans — Target organ	Main route of exposure[b]	Animal	Animals — Target organ	Route of exposure
15. Hematite mining (? radon)	Occupational	Lung	Inhalation	Mouse, hamster, guinea pig	Negative	Inhalation, i.t.
				Rat	Negative	s.c. injection
16. Isopropyl oils	Occupational	Nasal cavity, larynx	Inhalation		(No adequate tests)	
17. Melphalan	Medicinal	Hemopoietic system	p.o., injection	Mouse	Initiator	Skin
					Lung, lymphosarcomas	i.p.
18. Mustard gas	Occupational	Lung, larynx	Inhalation	Rat	Local	i.p.
				Mouse	Lung	Inhalation, i.v.
19. 2-Naphthylamine	Occupational	Bladder	Inhalation, skin, p.o.	Hamster, dog, monkey	Local, mammary	s.c. injection
				Mouse	Bladder	p.o.
				Rat, rabbit	Liver, lung	s.c. injection
					Inadequate	p.o.
20. Nickel (nickel refining)	Occupational	Nasal cavity, lung	Inhalation	Rat	Lung	inhalation
				Mouse, rat, hamster	Local	s.c., i.m. injection
				Mouse, rat	Local	i.m. implantation
21. N,N-Bis(2-chloroethyl)-2-naphthylamine	Medicinal	Bladder	p.o.	Mouse	Lung	i.p.
				Rat	Local	s.c. injection
22. Oxymetholone	Medicinal	Liver	p.o.		(No adequate tests)	
23. Phenacetin	Medicinal	Kidney	p.o.		(No adequate tests[a])	
24. Phenytoin	Medicinal	Lymphoreticular tissues	p.o., injection	Mouse	Lymphoreticular tissues	p.o., i.p.
25. Soot, tars, and oils	Occupational, environmental	Lung, skin (scrotum)	Inhalation, skin	Mouse, rabbit	Skin	Topical

| 26. Vinyl chloride | Occupational | Liver, brain[c], lung[c] | Inhalation, skin | Mouse, rat | Lung, liver, blood vessels, mammary, Zymbal gland, kidney | Inhalation |

[a] The main types of exposures mentioned are those by which the association has been demonstrated; exposures other than those mentioned may also occur.

[b] The main routes of exposure given may not be the only ones by which such effects could occur.

[c] Indicative evidence.

[d] The induction of tumors of the nasal cavities in rats given phenacetin has been reported recently (S. Odashima, personal communication, 1977).

From Tomatis, L., Agthe, C., Bartsch, H., Huff, J., Montesano, R., Saracci, R., Walker, E., and Wilbourne, J., *Cancer Res.*, 38, 877, 1978. With permission.

Table 6
A COMPARISON OF APPROXIMATE TOTAL DOSES FOR TUMOR INDUCTION IN HUMANS AND IN EXPERIMENTAL ANIMALS

	Human[a]	Incidence	Animal[a]	Incidence
Benzidine	50—200 mg/kg (av.) (bladder)	22—50%	10,000 mg/kg (mouse-liver)	67%
			50—100 mg/kg (rat-mammary gland)	50—80% (2%)[2]
Chlornaphazine	200 mg/kg (av.) (bladder)	16%	75—4800 mg/kg (mouse-lung)	40—100% (38%)[b]
Diethylstilbestrol	0.5—300 mg/kg (vaginal and cervical adenocarcinoma)	0.2%	2—13 mg/kg (male) (mouse-mammary gland)	4—27%
			400 mg/kg (newborn female mouse cervix and vagina)	33%
Aflatoxin B$_1$	0.1 mg/kg (liver)	0.5%	1.25—6.0 mg/kg (mouse-liver)	23—100% (3%)[b]
			0.3—1.5 mg/kg (rat-liver)	19—100%
Vinyl chloride	70,000 mg/kg (liver)	0.2%	30,000 mg/kg (mouse-lung and mammary gland)	25%, lung 13%, mammary
Cigarette smoke	from 1000 cigarettes/ kg (lung)	2.5%	40,000 mg/kg (rat-kidney and liver	9%, kidney 6%, liver
			From 400 cigarettes/kg (mouse-lung)	4.9%
			6000 cigarettes/kg (hamster-larynx)	6%

[a]   The average dose of the group(s). The tumor type and species (for the animals) are noted in parentheses below the dose.

[b]   Tumor incidence in control groups of animals. If not designated, control incidence was 0 or not given.

From Meselson, M. S., in Contemporary Test Control Practices and Prospects. The Report of the Executive Committee, National Academy of Sciences, Washington, D. C., 1, 75, 1975.

various chemicals. It was suggested that this permitted sufficient accuracy in extrapolating from animal data to human risk to support a logical scheme for evaluating such risks. Based upon this study, Table 7 depicts a comparison of potencies for 13 chemical agents (in addition to radiation and smoking) in the mouse, rat, dog, and human. The interspecies sensitivities appear to be ≤ 5:1 for both human:mouse and human: rat.[22]

Various agencies have included multiplicative factors to account for differing sensitivities in different species in attempting to derive carcinogenic potencies in humans from potencies in animals. For example, the NAS[25] report assumes that animals and humans are equally sensitive when they have the same total intake (as a fraction of body weight) which attempts to adjust for species differences in total number of cells at risk during a lifetime (which attempts to adjust for species differences in lifespans). The FDA assumes that animals and humans are equally sensitive when they have the same fraction of pollutant in their food or water intake. EPA makes a correction for surface area by the factor $(M_{human}/M_{animal})1/3$ where M is the mass. Table 8 lists the relative sensitivities between species using the Crouch and Wilson[22] definition of potency (kg d/mg) and Table 9 lists values used in calculating potencies.[25] All methodologies for extrapolation of cell and animal data to human health effects are limited to one degree or another by the lack of quantitative data on how different species modulate the toxic effects of various classes of chemical agents. Ideally, one would want

Table 7
COMPARISON OF POTENCIES: ANIMAL AND HUMAN

Chemical	Potency[a]			
	Mouse	**Rat**	**Dog**	**Human[b]**
AN	—	0.06	—	<0.3
Aflatoxin B₁	130[c]	500—1300	—	200 (3)
As	1.5—30	<0.01	—	15 (3)
Benzene	~0.0008	~0.0008	—	0.001 (3)
Benzidine	0.08	130—2500[d]	0.2	34 (10)
Chlornaphazine	20	—	—	2 (10)
Chloroform	0.01	0.002	—	<0.001
DCB	0.006	0.025	0.14	≤5
Diethylstilbestrol	14	—	—	1[e] (10)
EDB	6	6	—	0.8 (10)
Lead acetate	0.001	0.007	—	<2.5
Saccharin	—	0.0003[c]	—	<0.04
Vinyl chloride	0.004	0.01	—	0.02 (3)
Radiation, $(rem/yr)^{-1}$	0.01	—	—	0.02 (3)
Smoking, $(no./d \cdot kg)^{-1}$	0.06	—	—	0.6(3)

[a] Values are kg·d/mg except where noted.
[b] Number in parentheses next to human potency is our estimate of the accuracy of the number.
[c] Includes intrauterine exposure.
[d] Oral administration. Value for sc injection is 0.06 in rat and 0.08 in mouse.
[e] Women ingesting pills in pregnancy, resulting in cancer in their daughters.

From Crouch, E. and Wilson, R., *J. Toxicol. Environ. Hlth.*, 5, 1095, 1979. With permission.

Table 8
RELATIVE SENSITIVITIES BETWEEN SPECIES

Agency	Rat	Mouse	Human
National Academy of Sciences	~1.5	1	~35
Food and Drug Administration (% in diet)	1	0.35	4
Environmental Protection Agency (corrected for surface area)	1	0.43	4.7
Crouch and Wilson	~⅓—3	1	≤5

From Crouch, E. and Wilson, R., *J. Toxicol. Environ. Hlth.*, 5, 1095, 1979. With permission.

to develop a smooth mathematical function which would be based upon experimental data and permit extrapolation from a single species of placental mammal to any other species within this same class. Alternatively, however, in the absence of the ideal, knowing what differences exist in the modulation of toxicity between the few species used as model systems in toxicology will nevertheless permit a more rational extrapolation between these few species (primarily rodents and humans). The following sections attempt to evaluate a few of what are believed to be the key modulators of toxicity within the placental mammals and how they appear to differ between species. Unfortunately, in only a few instances does sufficient data exist to make any quantitative extrapolation or projections.

Table 9
VALUES USED IN CALCULATING POTENCIES

Species	Weight (kg)	Lifetime (yr)	Food consumption (g/d)	Water consumption (mℓ/d)	Air breathed (ℓ/d)
Mouse	0.025	1.75	5	5	40
Rat	0.25	2	15	25	200
Dog	10	10	250	500	15,000
Human	70	70	1500	2500	15,000

From Crouch, E. and Wilson, R., *J. Toxicol. Environ. Hlth.*, 5, 1095, 1979. With permission.

Table 10
TRANSFORMATIONS OF ANUTRIENT COMPOUNDS BY INTESTINAL MICROFLORA[34,35]

1. Hydrolysis of:
   - (a) Glucuronides
   - (b) Esters
   - (c) Amides
   - (d) Etheral sulphates
   - (e) Sulphamates
   - (f) Glycosides

2. Reduction of:
   - (a) Carbon-carbon double bonds
   - (b) Nitro- and azo-compounds
   - (c) N-oxides, N-hydroxy compounds
   - (d) Carbonyl compounds
   - (e) Alcohols, phenols (dehydroxylations)
   - (f) Arsonic acids

3. Degradation by:
   - (a) Decarboxylation
   - (b) Dealkylation (0- and N-alkyl)
   - (c) Deamination
   - (d) Dehalogenation

4. Synthesis by:
   - (a) Esterification
   - (b) Acetylation
   - (c) Formation of nitrosamines

5. Miscellaneous: Aromatization

III. TYPES OF MOLECULAR TRANSFORMATION OF NUTRIENT COMPOUNDS BY INTESTINAL MICROFLORA

Most foreign compounds are ingested via the gastrointestinal tract and after adsorption are transported to the liver where they tend to accumulate and undergo metabolism.[25-31] Initial metabolism of these compounds, however, occurs in the gut microflora.[32-36] It has been suggested that the metabolic potential of the intestine is comparable to that of the liver.[32,34,36] The types of molecular transformations resulting from the activity of intestinal microflora have been reviewed by Scheline[34,35] and are shown in Table 10. It can be seen that these reactions are mainly hydrolytic or other degradations and reductions. This contrasts with hepatic metabolism of anutrients where oxidations and syntheses (conjugations) predominate. Hence, this can give rise to many possibilities of competition between mammalian

Table 11
FACTORS AFFECTING INTESTINAL
METABOLISM OF ANUTRIENTS

1. Nature of anutrient
   (a) Polarity
   (b) Formulation and dose
   (c) Structure and stability

2. Nature of exposure
   (a) Time and method of administration
   (b) Chronic dosing and adaptation

3. Nature of animal
   (a) Species differences in structure of the gastrointestinal tract
   (b) Gut motility
   (c) Pathological conditions (enteropathies, diarrhea)

4. Nature and distribution of gut flora
   (a) Influence of diet
   (b) Exposure to infection (germ-free, specific pathogen-free)
   (c) Modification by drugs
   (d) Coprophagy

and microbial metabolism, as well as sequential reactions and enterohepatic circulation.[32] The factors which might influence the intestinal metabolism of anutrients is shown in Table 11. In general, intestinal metabolism is most important for polar compounds which are not well absorbed from the gut and for those compounds which are excreted, free, or conjugated, in the bile.[32] Interspecies comparisons of microflora metabolism are rare. The few studies which have been performed examined the range of microflora in a single strain of animal or individual. From these studies, it appears that while most placental mammals have similar microflora, there are differences both in the ratio between microflora species and in their metabolic activity. Further, studies in this area, especially between carnivores, herbivores, and omnivores would be of interest regarding their susceptibility to certain classes of carcinogens.

IV. METABOLISM

A. Overview

The basic pattern of metabolism of xenobiotics is considered to be essentially the same in all species in that most foreign compounds are metabolized in two phases.[3,37-42] In Phase I, the compound may be oxidized, reduced, or hydrolyzed; and in Phase II the products of the first phase may undergo a synthesis or conjugation to yield polar excretory products. However, it is well recognized that differences can occur within this pattern since the enzymes which catalyze the reaction of these phases can be influenced by many factors. One of the most important of these factors is the species itself. Species variations in the nature and extent of the biotransformation of foreign compounds are complex and sometimes unexpected.[37] At present, three major reasons underlie interspecies differences in compound metabolism; (1) defectiveness of a species in its ability to carry out common metabolic reactions, (2) variations in the relative extent of two or more competing reactions which a compound may undergo, and (3) restriction in the occurrence of a reaction to a particular species.

Although the majority of species have the capacity to carry out reactions of drug metabolism, there exist recognizable combinations of substrate and species from which one of

Table 12
DEFECTIVENESS OF A SPECIES IN ITS ABILITY
TO CARRY OUT A COMMON METABOLIC
REACTION

Species	Defective reaction
Rat	N-Hydroxylation of aliphatic amines
Guinea pig	N-Hydroxylation of aromatic amides
Cat	Glucuronidation of small phenols and aromatic acids
Dog	Acetylation of many primary amino groups

From Caldwell, J., *Drug Metab. Revs.*, 12, 221, 1981. With permission of Marcel Dekker, Inc.

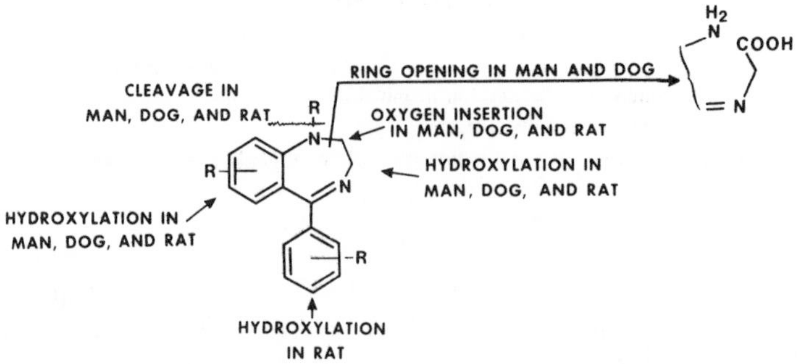

FIGURE 1.   Basic structure of the benzodiazepines and the major routes of their metabolism in man, dog, and rat. (From Caldwell, J., *Drug Metab. Revs.*, 12, 221, 1981. With permission of Marcel Dekker, Inc.)

these reactions is absent. Hence, such species are termed defective in this particular reaction[3,38,42] (Table 12). While most xenobiotics possess within their structure a number of possible sites for metabolic attack, most species have the capability for each of the various metabolic pathways.[3] However, it is very common to encounter considerable species variation regarding the relative extents of two or more competing reactions which a compound may undergo.[3] Figure 1 illustrates species differences in the various routes of metabolism of the multifunctional benzodiazepine skeleton.[3,41,43]

Although it has been suggested that for many groups of compounds the fates of individuals are essentially similar in a particular species, sufficient data are available for too few groups to permit a proper assessment of the possible existence of species patterns.[3] Amphetamines offer one of the best data bases for such an assessment.[3,41] The general structure of the amphetamines, together with the four major metabolic routes which these molecules can undergo are illustrated in Figure 2. Table 13 summarizes the major metabolic routes of these compounds in six species and demonstrates that the overall metabolic patterns of these compounds within each species show very definitive similarities.[3,41]

Figure 3 summarizes the metabolic processes that impact upon the expression of both beneficial and toxic effects. The numerous metabolic processes implicit in this figure are interdependent and proceed simultaneously.[44]

B. Biotransformation

Table 14 contains an abbreviated list of the major classes of enzymes involved in the transformation of molecular structures, usually, but not exclusively to less toxic metabolites (Phase I) and the conjugation reactions (Phase II) that facilitate solubilization and excretion

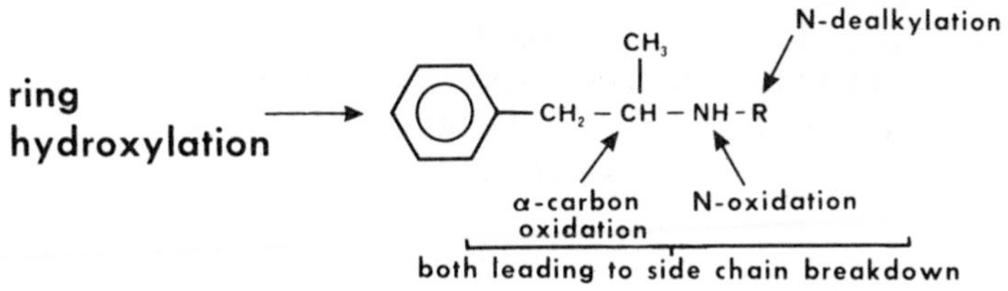

FIGURE 2. Basic structure of the amphetamines and their major routes of metabolism. (From Caldwell, J., *Drug Metab. Revs.*, 12, 221, 1981. With permission of Marcel Dekker, Inc.)

Table 13
SUMMARY OF SPECIES VARIATIONS IN THE METABOLISM OF AMPHETAMINES

Species	Number of compounds	Relative extent of pathway[a]			
		Aromatic hydroxylation	N-Dealkylation	Deamination	Excreted unchanged
Rat	11	+ + + +	+ + +	+	+ +
Guinea pig	6	0	+ +	+ + + +	+ +
Rabbit	8	+	+ +	+ + + +	+
Marmoset	4	+	—	+	+ + + +
Rhesus monkey	4	+ + +	—	+ + +	+ +
Man	13	+ +	+	+ + +	+ + +

[a] + to + + + + is an arbitrary quantitation (0 is absent, — is no data).

of toxicants. Included in this table are reactions types and examples. Phase I metabolites are the primary oxidation products. Since metabolites are somewhat more water soluble than the substrate, they are more easily transported through cells. Thus metabolites are formed through one or more reactions catalyzed by different specific enzymes and are subsequently conjugated with various soluble cellular components which make them more available for excretion from the body. The conjugated metabolites constitute the Phase II metabolites.[40,45] Table 15 lists the specific enzymes involved in both Phase I and Phase II reactions. When a chemical interacts with these metabolizing systems a large spectrum of Phase I and Phase II metabolites can be formed; however, the ratio between these metabolites varies as a function of species, strain, age, diet and physiological environment of the organism. Therefore, it can be considered that the first step in tumor induction by a chemical carcinogen in some instances is a misdirected by-product of the normal excretion process. While species and strain differences do exist, it is difficult to develop any scheme for extrapolation between species based upon these differences since most studies; (a) have been performed under induced conditions, (b) have been performed in different laboratories under different conditions, and (c) have not accounted for higher order functions which might modulate induction.

C. Cytochrome P-450 and Mixed-Function Oxidases

Most chemical carcinogens require metabolic activation to electrophiles in order to exert their tumor-induction properties.[46-48] A scheme for the metabolism of organic chemical carcinogens is illustrated in Figure 4, while Figure 5 depicts the interaction of ultimate carcinogens with biological nucleophiles and the resultant effects. The transformation of precarcinogens to electrophiles is accomplished metabolically within the endoplasmic reticulum[49] and the nucleus[50] of mammalian cells. Metabolic activation invariably involves

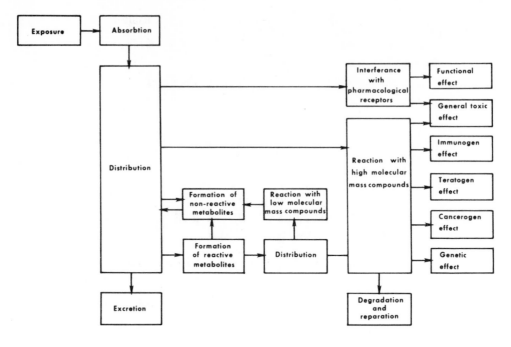

FIGURE 3.   Metabolic processes that impact upon the expression of both beneficial and toxic effects. (From DiCarlo, F. J., *Drug Metab. Revs.*, 13, 1, 1982. With permission of Marcel Dekker, Inc.)

Table 14
ENZYMATIC BIOTRANSFORMATIONS

Enzyme type	Reaction type[a]	Example
Oxidases	Carbinol	$RCH_2OH \rightarrow RCHO$
	Carbonyl	$RCHO \rightarrow RCO_2H$
	Aromatic hydroxylation	Coumarin $\rightarrow$ OH-coumarin
	Aliphatic ring	Camphor $\rightarrow$ 3- and 5-OH-camphor
	Aromatization	α-Phellandrene $\rightarrow$ p-cymene
	Alkyl oxidation	Toluene $\rightarrow$ benzoic acid
Reductases	Disulfide	$RS 60-SR' \rightarrow RSH + R'SH$
	Hydrogenation	$RR'CO \rightarrow RR'CHOH$
		$RCH = CHR' \rightarrow RCH_2CH_2R'$
		$R-N = N-R' \rightarrow RNH = NH-R'$
	Hydrazo	$RNH- NHR' \rightarrow RNH_2 + R'NH_2$
	Nitro	$RNO_2 \rightarrow RNH_2$
Hydrotases	Ester hydrolysis	$RCOR' \rightarrow RCO_2H + ROH$
	Amide hydrolysis	$RCONH_2 \rightarrow RCO_2H + NH_3$
	Peptide hydrolysis	$RCONH-R' \rightarrow RCO_2H + RNH_2$
		Protein $\rightarrow$ amino acids
	Epoxide hydrolysis	$RCHO-CHR' \rightarrow RCHOH-CHOH-R'$
Transferases	Transamination	Pyruvate $\rightarrow$ alanine
	Acetylation	$RNH-NH_2 \rightarrow R-NH-NHOCCH_3$
Conjugations	Glucuronide	$RNH_2 \rightarrow RNH$-glucuronide
		$RCO_2H \rightarrow RCO$-glucuronide
	Glycine	Benzoic acid $\rightarrow$ hippuric acid
	Mercapturic acid	Benzyl chloride $\rightarrow$ Benzylmercapturic acid
	Sulfate	Phenol $\rightarrow$ phenylsulfate

[a]   Also methylation, S-oxidation, etc.

Table 15

PHASE I

(1)   Cytochrome P-450 containing enzymes, and flavoprotein NADPH-cytochrome P-450 reductase catalyze epox-
        idation of aromatic rings or olefinic double bonds, produce hydroxylation of aromatic rings or alkyl chains,
        perform oxidative dealkylation, and N-oxidation.[41] This system occurs mainly in the endoplasmic reticulum
        of liver, kidney, lung, intestine, and many other tissues. These enzymes are in multiple forms which exhibit
        different or overlapping substrate-specificity.[41]
(2)   Epoxide hydrolase catalyzes the hydrolysis of arene oxide into the trans-dihydrodiol metabolite.
(3)   Dehydrogenase, microsomal flavoprotein mixed-function oxidase and xanthine oxidase.

PHASE II

(1)   Glutathione S-transferases catalyze the conjugation reaction between glutathione and a variety of electrophilic
        compounds such as arene oxide. These enzymes exist in multiple forms.[41]
(2)   UDP-glucuronyltransferases catalyze the conjugation reaction between glucuronic acid with substrates such as
        phenol and bilirubin. These enzymes are also found in multiple forms.[41]
(3)   Sulfotransferase catalyzes the sulfate formation.
(4)   Acyltransferases and other transferases.

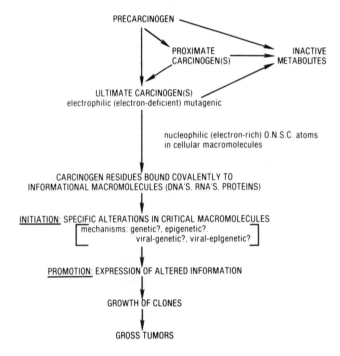

FIGURE 4.   Scheme for the metabolism of organic chemical carcinogens.

the action of a family of cytochrome P-450 isoenzymes and/or epoxide hydratase. The
resultant electrophilic species may subsequently interact with nucleophilic regions present
in any macromolecule.

Mixed-function oxidases (MFO) are a class of enzymes involved in the biotransformation
and oxidative activation of exogenous compounds including chemical carcinogens. These
enzymes are primarily located in the microsomal membrane and contain one or more of the
various forms of cytochrome P-450 and the associated electron transport enzymes, e.g.,
NADPH cytochrome P-450 reductase cytochrome b_5, and NADH cytochrome b_5 reductase.[51]
There is electrophoretic evidence indicating seven or more different cytochrome P-450
enzymes in the liver endoplasmic reticulum. The diversity of the reactions catalyzed by the

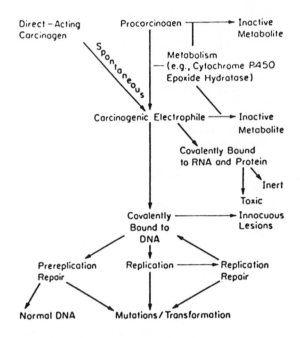

FIGURE 5.   Interaction of ultimate carcinogens with biological nucleophiles and the resultant effects. The term procarcinogen is defined as a potentially carcinogenic substance which requires metabolic activation.

various cytochrome P-450 systems in hepatic microsomes shown in Table 15 illustrates the versatility of these enzymes.[52] Quantitatively and qualitatively, the extent of induction of these enzymes varies as a function of chemical, species, and physiological environment.

The complexity of the metabolism of a particular carcinogen can be further illustrated by the multiple enzymatic pathways for the metabolism of benzo(a)pyrene to electrophilic metabolites (Figure 6). The scheme for the membrane-bound multicomponent monooxygenase system(s) and the various, possibly important, pathways for foreign compounds and endogenous substrates are shown in Figure 7. As shown in this figure, the reactive arene oxides or epoxides can rearrange nonenzymatically to form phenols (or alcohols), be hydrated to form trans-dihydrodiols, be conjugated with glutathione, or be reduced back to the parent compound. For any given substrate, the relative rates of k_1 to k_{10} are currently not known and most likely vary among different tissues, strains, and species. Age, nutrition, hormonal balance, diurnal variation, pH, and saturating versus non-saturating conditions of the substrates may all possibly be important factors in affecting these various rates.[53,54] Although the association between differences in enzymatic activity and variations in susceptibility to xenobiotics has been demonstrated in particular instances according to Walker,[55] little is known about major trends in these activities related to phylogenetic classification, habitat, or diet. Hodgson[56] has raised a key question, from the comparative point of view, on "whether cytochrome P-450 is an ancient enzyme of monophyletic origin which has been modified for many different functions or whether there is a class of heme pigments of polyphyletic origin with similar CO binding, but which vary considerably in other respects".

The presence of cytochrome P-450 associated mixed function oxidases in human tissues has been demonstrated indirectly by the presence of their enzyme-related activities such as aryl hydrocarbon hydroxylase (AHH), O-dealkylation, N-dealkylation and azo reductase in microsomal preparations.[51] The ability of human microsomal preparations to activate promutagens into DNA-damaging agents is yet another indirect indication of the existence of these enzymes.[51]

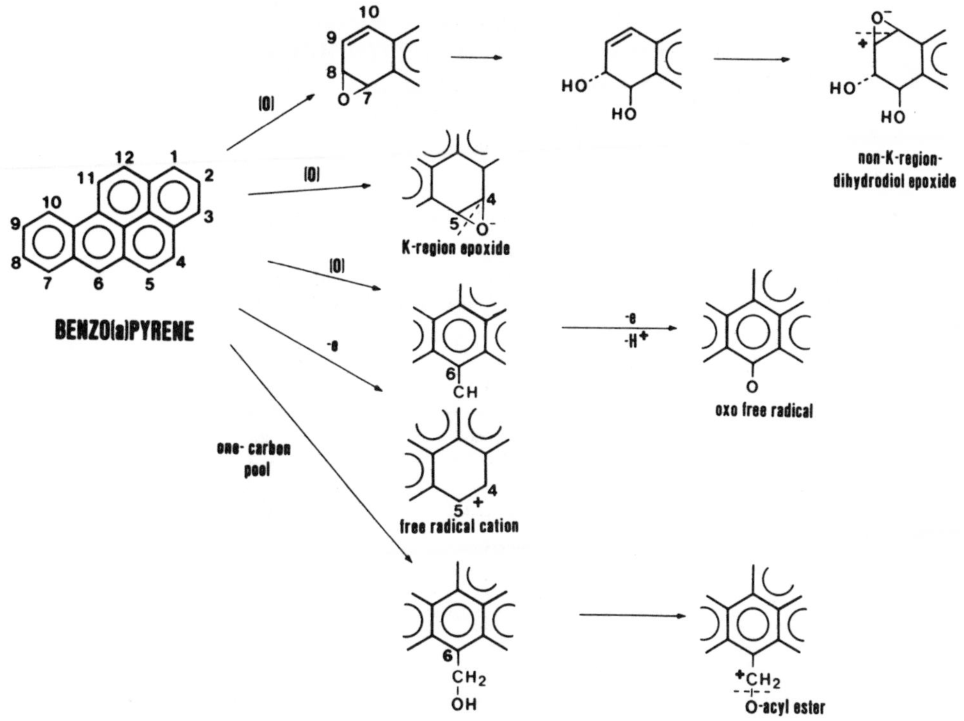

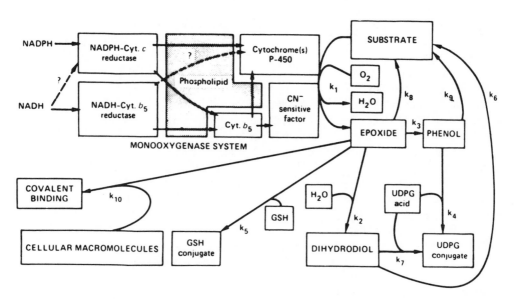

FIGURE 6. Multiple enzymatic pathways for the metabolism of benzo(a)pyrene to electrophilic reactants. (From Miller, E. C. and Miller, J. A., in *Chemical Carcinogens*, C. E. Searle, Ed., American Chemical Society Monograph No. 173, American Chemical Society, Washington, D.C., 1976, 762. With permission.)

FIGURE 7. Scheme for the membrane-bound multicomponent monooxygenase system(s) and the various possibly important pathways for foreign compounds and endogenous substrates.

Table 16

**METABOLISM OF DRUGS BY CYTOCHROME P-450
ENZYMES IN LIVER ENDOPLASMIA RETICULUM**

Type	Substrate	Product
Aromatic hydroxylation	Aniline	p-Aminophenol
Aliphatic hydroxylation	Hexobarbital	Hydroxyhexobarbital
Arene oxide formation	Bromobenzene	Bromobenzene epoxide
N-Dealkylation	Aminopyrene	4-Aminoantipyrine
N-Hydroxylation	2-Acetylaminofluorene	N-Hydroxy-2-acetyl amino fluorene
O-Dealkylation	p-Acetanisidine	p-Hydroxyacetanilide
S-Dealkylation	6-Methylthiopurine	6-Thiopurine
N-Oxidation	Dimethylaniline	Dimethylaniline N-oxide
S-Oxidation	Chloropromazine	Chloropromazine sulfoxide
Deamination	Amphetamine	Phenylacetone
Desulfuration	O-Ethyl-O-(4-nitro-phenyl)phenylphos-phonothionate	O-Ethyl-O-(p-nitrophenyl)-phenylphosphate
Dechlorination	Carbon tetrachloride	Chloroform
Dechlorination	Halothane	Trifluoroethanol
Dealkylation of metalloalkanes	Tetraethyl lead	Triethyl lead

From Gillette, J. R., *Drug Metab. Revs.*, 10, 59, 1979. With permission of Marcel Dekker, Inc.

V. VARIABLES AFFECTING DISPOSITION AND METABOLISM OF EXOGENOUS CHEMICALS IN EXPERIMENTAL ANIMALS

Numerous factors have long been recognized as capable of altering both qualitatively and quantitatively the metabolism of exogenous chemicals including both route of exposure and previous chemical exposure.[31,53] Among the major factors which affect metabolism are species, strain (genetic factors), age, sex, disease, stress, diet, and the administration of other foreign compounds.[48] Certain of these factors appear to exert effects on different individual steps in the conversion of precarcinogens to proximate and ultimate carcinogens (Figures 4 and 5) influencing reaction rates, and hence affecting both the concentration and duration of action of certain ultimate carcinogens.

One of the factors which most influences disposition of exogenous chemicals and their metabolism is nutrition. Recently, the influence of dietary factors on drug metabolism in animals[53,57-59] in relation to carcinogenesis[60-77] and mutagenesis[78,79] has been the subject of many reports. Various suggestions have been made that both pharmacological response and risk to toxic chemicals may be influenced by nutritional status (e.g., acute starvation, undernutrition, protein, mineral and vitamin deficiency, and dietary lipids).[57-59]

Diet should be considered a highly complex chemical mixture which includes such variables as (1) preformed exogenous carcinogens, e.g., aflatoxin and pyrolysates,(2) carcinogenic precursors, e.g., secondary amines and nitrates; (3) type and relative proportion of nutrients, e.g., ratio of saturated to nonsaturated fats and trace elements, (4) nonnutrient, not carcinogens per se, whether relatively inert, e.g., fiber, or biologically active, e.g., goitrogens, steroids, enzyme inducers, promoters, inhibitors, and antibiotics, and (5) nonspecific effects, e.g., calorie intake.[61-63] Numerous studies confirm the role of diet in modulating the induction of enzymes of potential significance in carcinogenesis.[53,65,67,71] However, despite the fact that the instinct diet of the placental mammals ranges considerably from carnivore to herbivore to omnivore, no comparative study as to spontaneous tumor occurrence, much less carcinogenic susceptibility, has yet been performed in a comparative fashion between species.

There is increasing literature which suggests that virtually every nutrient, when not ingested at optimum levels, tends to depress enzyme activities,[57-59] although there are important exceptions,[57] e.g., intakes of iron,[80] and thiamine[81] vary conversely with the rate of metabolism for certain mixed function oxidation (MFO) catalyzed reactions. Additionally, the activities of certain transferases[82,83] may be increased with a low dietary intake of protein. Campbell et al.[57] reviewed the in vitro and in vivo effects of dietary protein on drug metabolism in animals and concluded that its effect on MFO activities is striking both in terms of time required after protein ingestion and in terms of magnitude of response.

In situations where caloric intake influences tumor induction, animals fed diets with elevated protein levels have been found to have fewer tumors. Conversely, a diet restricted in protein has a lesser tumorigenic effect. In the case of the carcinogenic azo dyes, a protein restricted diet appears to increase the relative efficiency of the carcinogen. According to Weisburger and Williams,[77] diets completely devoid of protein (which can be administered only for limited periods of time), may decrease the effectiveness of certain carcinogens in specific target organs. Thus, protein restricted diets may result in a significant decrease in the number of enzymes bound to the endoplasmic reticulum resulting in a subsequent decrease in the biochemical activation of carcinogens.

Enzyme induction is a critical factor influencing carcinogenesis by many precarcinogens. Depending upon the nature of the inducer, the nature of the precarcinogen, the responsiveness of the target tissue and the nutritional adequacy of the diet, a number of variations in carcinogenic response can be possibly explained.[84] Organochlorine pesticides (e.g., DDT, DDE, DDD, chlordane, methoxychlor, endrin, aldrin, dieldrin, hexachlorocyclohexane, heptachlor and its epoxide) which have been found as trace contaminants in food and feed are very effective enzyme inducers.[85,86] Of the polycyclic hydrocarbons, methylcholanthrene and benz(a)anthracene were the most effective inducers while benzo(a)pyrene and chrysene were decidedly less; anthracene, fluoranthene, pyrene, perylene, phenanthrene, fluorene, and naphthalene required very large doses for a weak response or were entirely inactive.[87,88] Many of these compounds may have a differing effectiveness in inducing enzymes in different species; however, since few studies have been performed in a comparative fashion, it is impossible to interpret the impact of these compounds on enzyme interaction between species. Early observations on the effect of caloric intake of dietary fat and protein have been followed by an even broader appreciation of the enzyme inducers and toxicants that may act on the immune system.[13,89,90] Of additional importance is the consideration that when a chemical agent being tested is a promoter, the presence of carcinogenic contaminants in the diet may erroneously result in its classification as a carcinogen, with outcomes that may vary from species to species and from diet to diet.

VI. REPAIR

The metabolic activation of unreactive or precarcinogens in the host organism yields chemically highly reactive electrophiles[46-49] which subsequently either interact with a nucleophilic region present in a macromolecule, e.g., DNA, RNA or protein or decompose. The overall metabolic sequence and the resultant effects are shown in Figure 5. Replication of DNA and the subsequent proliferation of cells are prerequisites for the development of the neoplastic state.[1,22,77,91-98] As outlined in Figure 5 a carcinogen which is covalently bound to DNA (e.g., deoxyribonucleoside adducts) may be removed during prereplication repair which consists of either excision repair, DNA glycosylase, or an insertase reaction; thus the DNA-carcinogen adduct is removed and the appropriate base (as determined by Watson-Crick base-pairing) is inserted.[1,91-98] Thus, prereplicative DNA repair (repair occurring before semiconservative DNA synthesis) is thought to be a restorative process leaving the DNA in nearly its original state, while post-replicative DNA repair and semiconservative DNA synthesis are thought to lead to altered cells, some of which may be the progenitors of cancer.[22,99]

Induction of DNA damage and its repair have been studied in isolated DNA, bacteria, cell cultures, isolated cells, tissue slices, and in vivo. However, it is important to note that in vitro assays measuring DNA damage and repair neglect such whole animal factors as circulating hormones, blood constituents, mitotic rate, cell type differences, state of differentiation, temperature, pH, hypoxia, membrane transport, biological rhythms, and drug metabolites.[100,101]

Inducible repair systems and their implications for toxicology have been recently extensively evaluated by Schendel[96] and DNA repair assays as tests for environmental mutagens reviewed by Larsen et al.[102] Most recently, Setlow (Volume I) has reviewed differences in DNA repair between species.

VII. REPLICATIVE/NONREPLICATIVE CELLS

A. Fidelity/Infidelity

There may be a fundamental difference in the consequences of error accumulation in DNA in dividing and nondividing cells. In dividing cells, one is mainly concerned with replicative error propagation; that is, the transmission of mistakes in DNA replication from one generation to the next. Mechanisms which enhance the frequency of such mistakes could involve alterations in the DNA synthetic apparatus and have been referred to as intrinsic mutagenesis.[98] In nondividing cells, one is mainly concerned about the accumulation of unrepaired DNA damage. In the mechanism of carcinogenesis, consideration is normally limited to either dividing cells or to resting cells destined to undergo at least one further division cycle. If damaged DNA is repaired by a faithful, ''error-free'' mechanism, the damage is probably inconsequential with respect to cancer. Misrepair of DNA damage as a mechanism of cancer is possible since no system is entirely error-free and there is substantial evidence for the induction of an error-prone repair pathway (SOS) in bacteria and eukaryotes.[103-106] The underlying concept of this repair pathway is that it can alleviate potentially lethal damage, but only at the expense of inducing mutations. The induction of this pathway could be a programmed expression of cancer or could be permanently induced by damage to DNA at a site that regulates this pathway.

Of particular concern are errors in DNA that are not repaired or are inadequately repaired, so as to be present on the DNA template at the time of replication. Altered DNA need not always cause incorrect base substitutions during DNA replication. In such a situation, the parental cells containing the damaged DNA could be progressively diluted during cellular proliferation and may not be of consequence to tumor induction. It is common knowledge that, due to the redundancy of the genetic code, as well as other factors, approximately 25% of incorrect base substitutions may not result in amino acid substitutions. A number of modifications of the DNA template or of the DNA polymerases have also been shown to cause incorrect substitutions during copying by DNA polymerases in vitro.[107,108] If these modifications are not corrected by subsequent DNA repair, it is a reasonable expectation that these unrepaired lesions will result in mutations.[109]

B. Modifiers of DNA Synthesis

A list of changes (Table 17) in the reaction conditions that diminish the fidelity of DNA synthesis in vitro has recently been compiled by Loeb et al.[109] It should be stressed that the fidelity of DNA synthesis is altered by only a few types of changes in reaction conditions in this system using synthetic polynucleotide templates. The error rate of DNA polymerases

Table 17
CHANGING REACTION CONDITIONS THAT DIMINISH THE FIDELITY OF DNA SYNTHESIS

1. Ratio of incorrect to correct nucleotide substrates[117,118]

2. Type of incorrect nucleotide substrates[117]

3. Alkylation of DNA templates[121,122]

4. Irradiation of DNA templates[123]

5. Different metal activators for DNA polymerase[122]

6. Nonactivating metal mutagens and/or carcinogens[115]

7. Depurination of template[124]

has been shown to be dependent on the ratio of correct to incorrect nucleotides in vitro with both polynucleotide and natural DNA templates.[110,111] There is evidence that alterations in cellular nucleotide pool sizes and content are mutagenic,[112] and it is conceivable that cellular homeostatic mechanisms for precise maintenance of deoxynucleotide concentrations are altered by various chemical agents. Alkylating agents and carcinogens have been shown to induce misincorporation in vitro by modification of DNA templates and depurination.[108,113-115] Lindahl and Nyberg[116] calculated that the in vivo rate constant for depurination is approximately 1.8×10^{-9} min^{-1} suggesting that the production of apurinic sites on DNA may be as great as 200/cell/min. Furthermore, this rate constant may be increased by orders of magnitude after alteration of bases by alkylating agents. Even though there are efficient cellular mechanisms for correcting depurinated sites on DNA, they might not be adequate, and polymerases might encounter such sites during DNA replication. Lastly, mutagenic/carcinogenic metals, not reacting directly with DNA, have been shown to affect the fidelity of DNA synthesis in vitro.[108] Thus, various agents which do not directly damage DNA or enhance the production of metabolites which can induce such damage, may exert their effect by altering the fidelity of DNA replication. Methods to assess or screen for such agents are lacking except for the use of artificial templates. Newer methods which permit the use of natural templates are being developed, but have as yet to progress past the use of phage DNA.

C. DNA and Cellular Replication

There is a need for better models using more natural templates and conditions which mimic DNA replication in mammalian cells in vivo; however, few interspecies or interorgan studies have been performed. The importance of DNA replication per se, in the development of tumors, however, has been extensively studied. DNA replication is required for fixation of DNA damage and the beginning of the progression of a dormant, initiated cell to a clinically relevant mass.[117-119] Thus, the next stage of carcinogenesis has been postulated to involve a loss of response to normal control of cell proliferation[120,121] and a few rounds of DNA replication may be needed to amplify and stabilize errors introduced by chemical carcinogens.

In addition to the various compounds known to stimulate DNA replication without killing cells,[122] there is a proposed concept of a cytotoxic mechanism for tumor formation by toxic carcinogens based on a requirement for stimulation of DNA replication. For example, in mice, perchloroethylene, chloroform, or 1,4-dioxane, all of which have no or only minimal detectable genotoxicity in most bacterial tests, induce tumors while causing substantial necrosis in the target tissues of mice. The mechanism underlying this hypothesis is that the restorative hyperplasia from the cytotoxicity may increase the chance for errors in DNA replication and amplify the escape of the initiated cell from normal growth control during the DNA replication process. Manipulating the rate of cellular proliferation may thus modify the tumor incidence as has been demonstrated in the following: partial hepatectomy in animals treated with methylnitrosourea, dimethylnitrosourea and benzo(a)pyrene; chemical treatment combined with diet changes, drugs or natural physiological agents (hormones, bile acids); or the stimulated regenerative hyperplasia resulting from the toxic effect of carbon tetrachloride.[122] On the other hand, stabilizing the differentiated nondividing state of epithelial cells by retinoids has been used as a way of inhibiting mammary and colon carcinogenesis.[123,124] The degree of normal replication potential and the relative effect of various exogenous and endogenous agents on normal replication rate (and frequency between species, organs and tissues) may vary and should be considered in attempting quantitative interspecies extrapolation as to risk from carcinogens.

VIII. FACTORS WHICH MAY INFLUENCE STORAGE OR BODY BURDEN OF TOXICANTS

Marked variations in responsiveness to drugs are well recognized to occur in man. The variation in part is due to heritably determined factors. Environmental, occupational and dietary exposure and age to a spectrum of xenobiotics (e.g., chlorinated hydrocarbons such as DDT, lindane and PCBs, as well as lead) have been shown to alter the rates of drug biotransformation. Additionally, lifestyle, e.g., cigarette, alcohol, coffee, and tea consumptions, alterations in diet content of certain macromolecules (e.g., protein and carbohydrate), social use of drugs, and use of oral contraceptives by women can significantly alter biotransformation.[31-36,52,53,55-77,125-129]

Increasingly, pharmacologists and clinical biochemists have come to realize that a person's age affects how his or her body responds to therapeutic drugs. In the continuum from infancy to old age, the human body undergoes countless imperceptible changes in its biochemistry and physiology, and hence some of these changes impinge on its ability to absorb, distribute, metabolize, and eliminate drugs. With increasing age, a multitude of physiological and biochemical processes diminish, including metabolic rates. Thus, drugs and/or their metabolites persist in the body longer, due in part to less efficient excretion with the possibility of higher body accumulation leading to toxic effects. Hence, the elderly are more likely than younger people to experience adverse effects of drugs.[128] The prolonged lifetime of drugs such as diazepam in older people results, in part, from changes in the rate of specific metabolic pathways. For example, the oxidative metabolism of diazepam and related benzodiazepines is impaired markedly in old age particularly in men, when in contrast the conjugative transformation of these drugs is scarcely affected. Additionally, lipid-soluble drugs such as diazepam tend to accumulate in the elderly to a greater degree because their body tissues contain a higher percentage of fat.[128]

It is important to note additional factors that may influence storage (for body burden) of a toxicant. These include: its chemical structure and physical properties, intensity and duration of dosage, efficiency of absorption, sex, nutritional status, the integrity of organs, previous exposure, and/or concurrent doses of drugs, etc. Another factor that may play a role in the attainment of the storage level plateau is the induction of microsomal enzymes.

The multiplicity of either well-established or suspected host factors that may influence drug response in man is shown in Figure 8. In this representation of Vesell,[31,53] a line joins all such factors in the outer circle to indicate their close interrelationship. Many of these factors are interdependent. For example, age is often associated with changes that affect

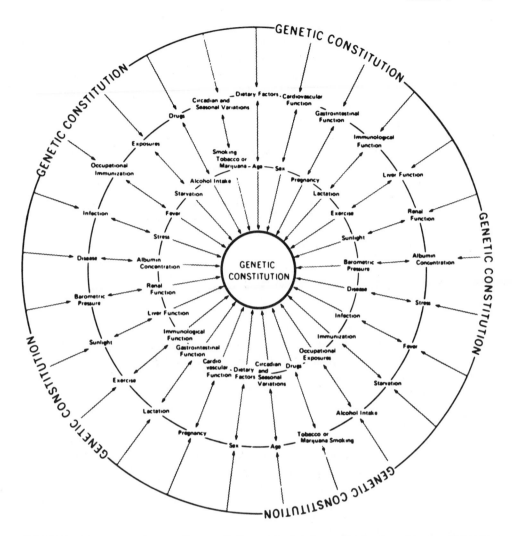

FIGURE 8. The concept of concentric outer circles was developed to emphasize the multiple possibilities that exist for interaction among host factors and to suggest that the magnitude of the impact of host factors on drug response may be modulated by genetic constitution. Because in most cases these specific interactions and modulations have not yet been investigated, much less firmly established, this design is largely speculative and intended to stimulate future research rather than to depict the current state of knowledge in the field. (From Vesell, E. S., *Clin. Pharmacol. Ther.*, 31, 1, 1982. With permission.)

diet, exercise, cigarette, alcohol and drug use, functional status of various organs, etc. Arrows from each factor in the outer circle of Figure 8 are wavy to indicate that effects of each host factor or drug response may occur at multiple sites and through different processes that include drug absorption, distribution, metabolism, excretion, receptor action and combinations thereof.

The interaction and interdependence among many host factors in the outer circle of Figure 8 and their modulation by genetic factors are emphasized further in Figure 9 through the device of concentric circles. A factor from one circle impinges on a factor beneath it, and vice versa. While the pattern illustrated in Figure 8 offers numerous opportunities for each host factor and for interactions among the various host factors to affect drug disposition, the design of Figure 9 serves to greatly extend this concept. Thus, when host factors are arranged in concentric circles, the potential for interrelationships among them is staggering. Not demonstrable in Figure 8 and suggested by Vesell[31,53] is the idea that the two circles

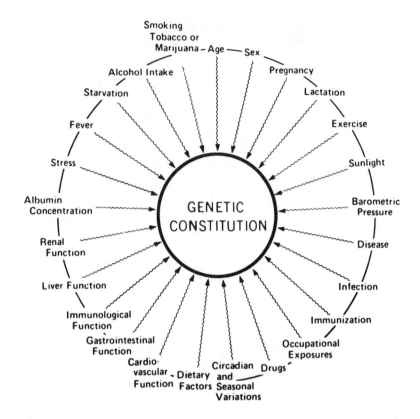

FIGURE 9.   This circular design suggests the multiplicity of either well-established or suspected host factors that may influence drug response in man. A line joins all such factors in the outer circle to indicate their close interrelationship. Arrows from each factor in the outer circle are wavy to indicate that effects of each host factor on drug response may occur at multiple sites and through different processes that include drug absorption, distribution, metabolism, excretion, receptor action, and combinations thereof. (From Vesell, E. S., *Clin. Pharmacol. Ther.*, 31, 1, 1982. With permission.)

representing host factors may turn at different rates thereby introducing a dynamic, temporal component. Temporal considerations could thus determine which factors interact at any given moment.

IX. THRESHOLD (NO-EFFECT) PHENOMENA

In the foregoing discussions we have noted that cellular formation of reactive and toxic species of chemicals is frequently counteracted by metabolic detoxification. As a consequence, according to Greim et al.[130] two threshold doses can be observed; (1) a no-effect level where no toxic or genotoxic effects become evident and (2) a disproportionate increase in the toxic effects when high concentrations of a chemical are present and inactivation can be overcome.

Nowhere is the general subject more hotly debated[131-134] than with regard to whether chemical carcinogens and mutagens exhibit thresholds, or doses below which there is either no effect or an effect considerably less than that predicted by linear extrapolation from responses at higher doses.

Falk[135] has reviewed the biological evidence for the existence of thresholds in chemical carcinogenesis and has particularly stressed that the role of absorption by the organism, metabolic change or deactivation of the proximate carcinogen by abundantly available en-

Table 18
MAJOR ARGUMENTS IN FAVOR OF "THRESHOLD DOSE"
(NO-EFFECT LEVEL)

1. Assumption of some critical level of exposure below which the carcinogenic process will not be initiated.

2. Chemical carcinogenesis is a multistage process involving: exposure, absorption, distribution, activation, deactivation, and elimination of the chemical per se or products formed from it. Interference with any of these processes may constitute a threshold. Possibility that activation of the system which leads to the carcinogenic products will not be initiated at low dose levels.

3. Small quantities of environmental chemicals may not reach their receptor because the rate of elimination or metabolic degradation is relatively more effective with smaller doses.

4. The possibility exists of a relatively greater effectiveness of repair mechanisms including DNA repair and immunosuppression at low doses.

5. Where effective repair processes are present, even if a substance interacts with the receptor, it need not necessarily produce an adverse effect.

6. Although carcinogenic and mutagenic chemicals may have special properties with regard to the nature and characteristics of their adverse effects, they are subject to the same physiochemical and biological interactions that are considered to result in a threshold dose for other chemicals.

7. Concept of proper detoxification and adequate repair systems including DNA repair and immunosuppression.

8. Possibility that activation of the system which leads to the carcinogenic products will not be initiated at low dose levels.

zymes such as epoxide hydrase or glutathione-S-transferase and reaction with molecules other than DNA have great bearing on thresholds because of their potential capacity to reduce the number of active molecules available for the carcinogenic process.

As noted earlier, those variables that affect DNA are especially critical. Thus, the extent to which DNA damage can be repaired depends to some degree on the site of alkylation.[1,91,135] For example, tumor production in some tissues is correlated with persistence of alkylation at specific locations in the base, particularly the O^6 guanine position. In contrast, alkylation of the N^7-guanine position was not associated with cancer formation since elimination of the N^7-alkylated guanine is far more efficient and enzymes are more readily available than for the elimination of an O^6-alkyl guanine base.[136]

The major arguments for and against threshold doses are summarized in Tables 18 and 19.

X. GENETIC POLYMORPHISMS OF DRUG METABOLISM

Genetically determined variation in blood groups, erythrocyte enzymes, plasma proteins, histocompatibility antigens, and other key components of cell function have been well documented. Additionally, corresponding variation at the chromosomal level as well as at the level of DNA sequences in genes has been revealed.[137]

Polymorphisms, by definition, are occurrences of more than one form of a particular gene and its gene product, usually a protein, with the less common variant having a frequency in the population of at least 1%, a frequency much too high to be accounted for by mutation alone.[137] The occurrence of genetic polymorphisms of drug metabolism means that populations contain subgroups (phenotypes) that greatly differ in their abilities to affect a number of metabolic substances.[138]

Table 19
MAJOR ARGUMENTS AGAINST "THRESHOLD DOSE"
(NO-EFFECT LEVELS)

1. For toxic effects such as neoplastic disease or mutations of genetic material, a single molecule of a chemical is sufficient to initiate a process that may progressively lead to an observed, irreversible, harmful effect so that it may not be possible to demonstrate a "threshold dose" for a carcinogen or a mutagen.

2. There are no known chemical carcinogens that can produce tumors that are not found to occur in the absence of that chemical. The threshold hypothesis requires the assumption that the carcinogen in question acts by some novel mechanism, independent of all ongoing processes on the target organ or site.

3. Experiments on radiation induced cancer have not revealed a threshold within the realm of statistical reliability.

4. Mathematically derived conclusions suggest that it is impossible to demonstrate no-effect levels experimentally. A "no-effect" level for a group of animals may occur because the dose is really below the theoretical no-effect level (e.g., below the threshold) or because the number of animals is too small or because the time of observation was too short (e.g., as in cancer with a long latent period between exposure and appearance of tumors).

5. Even if a threshold is postulated, there is presently no empirical or theoretical basis for determining the dose at which it may occur.

6. The human population is a very diverse, genetically heterogeneous group that is exposed in varying degrees to a large variety of toxicants. Assumption of one threshold is unrealistic. If thresholds to exist, not all members of the population have the same one.

Table 20
SOME HUMAN BLOOD PROTEINS WHICH
EXIST IN VARIANT FORMS

Protein	No. of variant forms
Catalase	3
Caeruloplasmin	3
Amylase	4
Pseudocholinesterase	5
Acid phosphatase	5
Carbonic anhydrase	5
6-Phosphate gluconate dehydrogenase	7
Hemoglobin: alpha-chain	26
beta-chain	46

From Ritchie, J. C., Sloan, T. P., Idle, J. R., and Smith, R. L.,
in *Environmental Chemicals, Enzyme Function and Human Disease*,
Ciba Foundation Symposium, 76, 219, 1980. With permission.

Genetic factors which appear at the center of Figure 8 tend to illustrate the fact that under carefully controlled environmental conditions, they exert a prominent role in the determination of a subject's capacity to metabolize certain drugs. However, numerous host factors can alter this capacity.[31,138-141]

Ritchie et al.[138] and Eichelbaum[140] recently reviewed the toxicological implications of polymorphic drug metabolism. The occurrence of genetic polymorphisms of drug metabolism means that populations contain subgroups (phenotypes) that differ sharply in their capabilities to effect a number of metabolic reactions. Hence, major inter-phenotype differences occur in responsiveness to drugs and toxic substances.[138] An indication of the prevalence of genetic polymorphism is shown by the large number of human blood proteins that exist in variant forms and is illustrated in Table 20.[138] It has been estimated that about 30% of human gene

Table 21
TYPES OF GENETIC CONTROL OF DRUG METABOLISM IN HUMANS

Type of control	Population distribution of the metabolic reaction	Reaction example
Polygenic	Unimodal	Glycine and glucuronic acid conjugation of salicylic acid
Monogenic	Polymodal	Acetylation of isoniazid Hydrolysis of succinylcholine Hydroxylation of debrisoquine

From Ritchie, J. C., Sloan, T. P., Idle, J. R., and Smith, R. L., in *Environmental Chemicals, Enzyme Function and Human Disease*, Ciba Foundation Symposium, 76, 219, 1980. With permission.

Table 22
POLYMORPHIC DRUG METABOLISM IN HUMANS

Metabolic reaction exhibiting polymorphism	Example of substrates
Acetylation	Sulfonamides (sulfamethazine), arylamines (dapsone), hydrazines (isoniazid)
Hydrolysis	Succinylcholine, paraoxon
Hydroxylation of carbon centers	Debrisoquine, guanosan, phenacetin
Oxidation at nitrogen centers	Sparteine
Glucuronidation	Paracetamol (acetaminophen)

From Ritchie, J. C., Sloan, T. P., Idle, J. R., and Smith, R. L., in *Environmental Chemicals, Enzyme Function and Human Disease*, Ciba Foundation Symposium, 76, 219, 1980. With permission.

products exhibit polymorphic variation.[142] Genetic polymorphisms and variant protein structure could be of significance in responsiveness to toxic substances in two major ways. First, they could influence dispositional events such as absorption, distribution, metabolism and excretion; secondly, they could also affect receptor events.[138,143-148]

The widely varying ability to metabolize drugs and toxic substances which is commonly encountered in the human population is due to variations in the nature and amounts of the enzymes that metabolize drugs.[138-147] These enzymes are controlled by a complex interplay of both genetic and environmental factors. The two types of genetic control (polygenic and monogenic) of metabolic reactions in humans are shown in Table 21.[138] The reaction examples for polygenic control are glycine and glucuronic acid conjugation of salicylic acid and for monogenic control, acetylation of isoniazid, hydrolysis of succinylcholine and hydroxylation of debrisoquine.

General metabolic reactions that exhibit genetic polymorphism have been studied in human populations, families and individuals and are depicted in Table 22.[138] The best known polymorphic reactions are acetylation of various sulfonamide drugs and hydrolysis of succinylcholine. Table 23 shows the alleles responsible for three genetic polymorphisms of drug metabolism: acetylation, hydrolysis and hydroxylation.

Variations in metabolism can be a major influence on interindividual differences in responsiveness to toxic substances. The case of acetylation, polymorphism and cholinesterase variants in terms of toxic responses and susceptible phenotypes is shown in Table 24.[138]

Table 23
ALLELES RESPONSIBLE FOR GENETIC POLYMORPHISMS OF DRUG METABOLISM

Metabolic reaction	Alleles controlling the reaction	Effect
Acetylation	Slow	Slow acetylation; rapid acetylation
	Rapid	
Hydrolysis	Various alleles at E_1 locus	Impaired hydrolysis of succinylcholine
Hydroxylation	D^H	Extensive hydroxylation of debrisoquine; impaired hydroxylation of debrisoquine
	D^L	

From Ritchie, J. C., Sloan, T. P., Idle, J. R., and Smith, R. L., in *Environmental Chemicals, Enzyme Function and Human Disease,* Ciba Foundation Symposium, 76, 219, 1980. With permission.

Table 24
GENETIC POLYMORPHISMS OF METABOLISM AND DRUG TOXICITY

Acetylation polymorphism

Drug	Toxic effect	Susceptible phenotype
Isoniazid	{peripheral neuritis	Slow acetylator
	{SLE[a] syndrome	Slow acetylator
	{hepatitis	Rapid acetylator
Hydralazine	SLE[a] syndrome	Slow acetylator
Salicylazosulfapyridine	Cyanosis and hemolysis	Slow acetylator

Plasma cholinesterase variants

Type of enzyme	Genotype (E_1 locus)	Response to normal doses of succinylcholine
Normal	$E_1^u E_1^u$	Rapid hydrolysis
Atypical	$E_1^u E_1^a$	Prolonged apnoea
Silent gene	$E_1^s E_1^s$	Prolonged apnoea
Fluoride-resistant	{$E_1^u E_1^f$	Rapid hydrolysis
	{$E_1^f E_1^f$	Prolonged apnoea

[a]   SLE, systemic lupus erythematosus.

From Ritchie, J. C., Sloan, T. P., Idle, J. R., and Smith, R. L., in *Environmental Chemicals, Enzyme Function and Human Disease,* Ciba Foundation Symposium, 76, 219, 1980. With permission.

Thus, in the case of acetylation polymorphism individuals who are slow acetylators are more likely to develop peripheral neuritis[148] and the systemic lupus erythematous (SLE) syndrome[149] as toxic reactions to isoniazid, than are those who are rapid acetylators.[138] Conversely, in isoniazid induced hepatitis rapid acetylators constitute the susceptible phenotype.[150]

Table 25
MONOGENICALLY DETERMINED PHARMACOGENETIC DEFECTS IN OXIDATIVE DRUG METABOLISM

Slow or defective condition	Inheritance	Frequency (%)	Response and side effects at standard doses	Impaired metabolism of other drugs in this condition
Benzylic hydroxylation of debrisoquine	ar	1.5—9[a]	Hypotension	Phenacetin, phenformin, phenytoin, nortriptyline, guanoxan
N-Oxidation of sparteine	ar	5	Diplopia, blurred vision, overstimulated uterus	Debrisoquine, nortriptyline
O-De-ethylation of phenacetin	? ar	?	Increased methae-moglobinemia	...[b]
Hydroxymethylation of tolbutamide	ar	25	Higher incidence of cardiovascular death	...[b]
p-Hydroxylation of phenytoin	?ad	?	Phenytoin intoxication	...[b]
mephenytoin	?ad	?	Mephenytoin intoxication	...[b]
N-Glucosidation of amylobarbitone (amobarbital)	ar	2	None observed	...[b]

Note: Abbreviations: ar = autosomal recessive; ad = autosomal dominant; ? unknown; a = large interethnic differences; b = not investigated.

From Eichelbaum, M., *Clin. Pharmacokinetic*, 7, 1, 1982. With permission.

Table 25 lists six monogenically determined pharmacogenetic defects in oxidative drug metabolism.[140] These are: benzylic hydroxylation of debrisoquine, N-oxidation of sparteine, O-de-ethylation of phenacetin, hydroxymethylation of tolbutamide, p-hydroxylation of phenytoin and mephenytoin and N-glucosidation of amylobarbitone. The incidence of these various pharmacogenetic conditions varies between 2 and 9% of the population. Among these conditions, the best studied examples are the polymorphic oxidation of debrisoquine and sparteine.[140,149-152]

REFERENCES

1. **Hart, R.,** Present limitations and fugure directions for molecular methodologies in risk assessment, in *Health Risk Analysis,* Walsh, P. J., and Copenhaver, E. D., Eds., Franklin Institute Press, Philadelphia, PA, 1981, 461.
2. **Sacher, G. A. and Hart, R. W.,** in *Birth Defects, Original Article Series,* Bergsma, D., and Harrison, E., Eds., New York, 1978, 14.
3. **Caldwell, J.,** The current status of attempts to predict species differences in drug metabolism, *Drug Metab. Revs.,* 12, 221, Marcel Dekker, N.Y., 1981.
4. **Glocklin, V. G.,** General considerations for the study of the metabolism of drugs and other chemicals, *Federation of American Societies for Experimental Biology, Symposium on Drug Metabolism in the Design and Implementation of Pathology and Toxicology Studies,* Atlanta, GA, 1981.
5. **Oser, B. L.,** The rat as a model for human toxicological evaluation, *J. Toxicol. Environ. Hlth.,* 8, 521, 1981.
6. **Oser, B. L., Ed.,** *Hawk's Physiological Chemistry,* 14th ed., Blakerton, New York, 1965.
7. **Mitruka, B. M. and Rawnsley, H. M.,** *Clinical, Biochemical and Hematological Reference Values in Normal Experimental Animals,* Masson Press, New York, 1977, 123.

8. **Passey, R. D.**, Experimental soot cancer, *Brit. Med. J.*, 2, 1112, 1922.
9. **Leitch, A.**, Paraffin cancer and its experimental production, *Brit. Med. J.*, 2, 1104, 1922.
10. **Grasso, P. and Crampton, P. F.**, The value of the mouse in carcinogenicity testing, *Food Cosmet. Toxicol.*, 10, 418, 1972.
11. **Faccini, J. M., Irisarri, E., and Monro, A. M.**, A carcinogenicity study in mice of a beta-adrenergic antagonist, primidolol; increased total tumour incidence without tissue specificity, *Toxicology*, 21, 279, 1981.
12. **Sher, S. P.**, Tumors in control hamsters, rats and mice: literature tabulation, *CRC Crit. Rev. Toxicol.*, 10, 4, 1982.
13. **Roe, F. J. C. and Tucker, M. J.**, Recent developments in the design of carcinogenicity tests on laboratory animals, *Proc. Eur. Soc. Tox.*, 15, 171, 1974.
14. IRLG, Scientific bases for identification of potential carcinogens and estimation of risk, *J. Natl. Cancer Inst.*, 63, 241, 1979.
15. **Fears, T. R., Tarone, R. E., and Chu, K. C.**, False-positive and false-negative rates for carcinogenicity screens, *Cancer Res.*, 37, 1941, 1977.
16. **Chu, K. C., Cueto, C., Jr., and Ward, J. M.**, Factors in the evaluation of 200 National Cancer Institute Carcinogen Bioassays, *J. Toxicol. Environ. Hlth.*, 8, 251, 1981.
17. **Ward, J. H., Goodman, D. G., Squire, R. A., Chu, K. C., and Linhart, M. S.**, Neoplastic and nonneoplastic lesions in aging (C56BL/6NHC3H/HeN)F$_1$ (B6C3F1 mice), *J. Natl. Cancer Inst.*, 63, 849, 1979.
18. **Goodman, D. G., Ward, J. M., Squire, R. A., Chu, K. C., and Linhart, M. S.**, Neoplastic and non-neoplastic lesions in ageing F344 rats, *Toxicol. Appl. Pharmacol.*, 48, 237, 1979.
19. **Gart, J. J., Chu, K. C., and Tarone, R. E.**, Statistical issues in interpretation of chronic bioassay tests for carcinogenicity, *J. Natl. Cancer Inst.*, 62, 957 1979.
20. **Purchase, I. F. H.**, Inter-species comparisons of carcinogenicity, *Brit. J. Cancer*, 41, 454, 1980.
21. **Meselson, M. S.**, in Contemporary Test Control Practices and Prospects. The Report of the Executive Committee, National Academy of Sciences, Washington, DC, 1, 75, 1975.
22. **Crouch, E. and Wilson, R.**, Interspecies comparison of carcinogenic potency, *J. Toxicol. Environ. Hlth*, 5, 1095, 1979.
23. **Clayson, D. B.**, Relationships between laboratory and human studies, *J. Environ. Pathol. Toxicol.*, 1, 31, 1977.
24. **Tomatis, L., Agthe, C., Bartsch, H., Huff, J., Montesano, R., Saracci, R., Walker, E., and Wilbourn, J.**, Evaluation of the carcinogenicity of chemicals: a review Research on Cancer (1971—1977), *Cancer Res.*, 38, 877, 1978.
25. National Academy of Sciences, Health Effects of Chemical Pesticides, *Report of the Consultative Panel on Health Hazards of Chemical Pesticides*, National Academy of Sciences, Washington, DC, 1, 7, 1975.
26. **Parke, D. V. and Williams, R. T.**, Metabolism of toxic substances, *Brit. Med. Bull.*, 25, 256, 1969.
27. **Watanabe, P. G., Hefner, R. E., Jr., and Gehring, P. J.**, Vinyl chloride induced depression of hepatic non-protein sulfhydryl content and effects on bromosulphalein (BSP) clearance in rats, *Toxicology*, 6, 1, 1976.
28. **Jaeger, R. J., Conolly, R. B., and Murphy, S. D.**, Diurnal variation of hepatic glutathione concentration and its correlation with 1,1-dichloroethylene inhalation toxicity in rats, *Res. Commun. Chem. Pathol. Pharmacol.*, 6, 465, 1973.
29. **McKenna, M. J., Zempel, J. A., Madrid, E. O., Braun, W. H., and Gehring, P. J.**, Metabolism and pharmacokinetic profile of vinylidene chloride in rats following oral administration, *Toxicol. Appl. Pharmacol.*, 45, 821, 1978.
30. **McKenna, M. J., Watanabe, P. G., and Gehring, P. J.**, Pharmacokinetics of vinylidene chloride in the rat, *Environ. Hlth. Persp.*, 21, 99, 1977.
31. **Vesell, E. S.**, On the significance of host factors that affect drug disposition, *Clin. Pharmacol. Ther.*, 31,1,1982.
32. **Walker, R.**, Influence of gut microorganisms on metabolism of drugs and food additives, *Proc. Nutr. Soc.*, 32, 73, 1973.
33. **Draser, B. S., Hill, M. J., and Williams, R. E. O.**, in *Metabolic Aspects of Food Safety*, Roe, F. J. C., Ed., Blackwell Scientific Publ., Oxford, 1970, 245.
34. **Scheline, R. R.**, Drug metabolism by intestinal microorganisms, *J. Pharm. Sci.*, 57, 2021, 1968.
35. **Scheline, R. R.**, Metabolism of some aromatic aldehydes and alcohols by rat intestinal microflora, *Xenobiotica*, 2, 227, 1972.
36. **Williams, R. T.**, in *Metabolic Aspects of Food Safety*, Roe, F. J. C., Ed., Blackwell Scientific Publications, Oxford, 1970, 1255.
37. **Williams, R. T.**, Species variations in the metabolism of drug metabolism, *Environ. Hlth. Persp.*, 22, 133, 1978.

38. **Williams, R. T.,** Interspecies variations in the metabolism of xenobiotics, *Biochem. Soc. Trans.,* 2, 359, 1974.
39. **Williams, R. T.,** Interspecies scaling, in *Pharmacology and Pharmacokinetics,* Teorell, T., Dedrick, R. L., and Condliffe, P. G., Eds., Plenum Press, New York, 1974, 105.
40. **Williams, R. T.,** *Detoxification Mechanisms,* 2nd ed., Chapman and Hall, London, 1959.
41. **Caldwell, J.,** in *Enzymatic Basis of Detoxification,* Jakoby, W., Ed., Academic Press, New York, 1974, 927.
42. **Caldwell, J., Williams, R. T., Bassir, O., and French, M. R.,** Drug metabolism in exotic animals, *Eur. J. Drug. Metab. Pharmacokin.,* 3, 61, 1977.
43. **Dring, L. G.,** in *Drug Metabolism from Microbe to Man,* Parke, D. V., and Smith, R. L., Eds., Taylor and Francis, London, 1976, 281.
44. **DiCarlo, F. J.,** Metabolism, pharmacokinetics, and toxicokinetics defined, *Drug Metab. Revs.,* 13, 1, 1982.
45. **Sims, P. and Grover, P. L.,** Epoxides in polycyclic aromatic hydrocarbon metabolism and carcinogenesis, *Adv. Cancer Res.,* 20, 165, 1974.
46. **Miller, J. A.,** Carcinogenesis by chemicals: an overview — G.H.A. Clowes memorial lecture, *Cancer Res.,* 30, 559, 1970.
47. **Miller, E. C. and Miller, J. A.,** in *Chemical Carcinogens,* C. E. Searle, Ed., American Chemical Society Monograph No. 173, American Chemical Society, Washington, DC, 1976, 762.
48. **Miller, J. A. and Miller, E. C.,** in *Origins of Human Cancer, Vol. B,* Hiatti, H. H., Watson, J. D., and Winsten, J. A., Cold Spring Harbor Laboratories, Cold Spring Harbor, NY, 1977, 627.
49. **Heidelberger, C.,** Chemical carcinogenesis, *Ann. Rev. Biochem.,* 44, 79, 1975.
50. **Bresnick, E.,** Nuclear metabolism of polycyclic hydrocarbons and interaction of polycyclic hydrocarbons with nuclear components, *Adv. Enz. Reg.,* 16, 347, 1978.
51. **Autrup, H.,** Carcinogen metabolism in human tissues and cells, *Drug Metab. Revs.,* 13, 603, 1982.
52. **Gillette, J. R.,** Effects of induction of cytochrome P-450 enzymes on the concentration of foreign compounds and metabolites and on the toxicological effects of these compounds, *Drug Metab. Revs.,* 10, 59, Marcel Dekker, N.Y., 1979.
53. **Vesell, E. S.,** in *Molecular and Cellular Aspects of Carcinogen Screening,* Montesano, R., Bartsch, H., and Tomatis, L., IARC Scientific Publication No. 27, The International Agency Research on Cancer, Lyon, 1980, 40.
54. **Nebert, D. W. and Atlas, J. A.,** The Ah locus: aromatic hydrocarbon responsiveness of mice and men, *Human Genet.,* 1, 149, 1978.
55. **Walker, C. H.,** Species differences in microsomal monooxygenase activity and their relationships to biological half-lives, *Drug Metab. Rev.,* 7, 295, 1978.
56. **Hodgson, E.,** Comparative aspects of the distribution of cytochrome P-450 dependent mono-oxygenase systems: an overview, *Drug Metab. Rev.,* 10, 15, 1979.
57. **Campbell, T. C., Hayes, J. R., Merrill, A. H., Jr., Maso, M., and Goetschius,** The influence of dietary factors on drug metabolism in animals, *Drug Metab. Rev.,* 9, 173, 1979.
58. **Campbell, T. C., and Hayes, J. R.,** Role of nutrition in the drug-metabolizing enzyme system, *Pharmacol. Rev.,* 26, 171, 1974.
59. **Basu, T. K. and Dickerson, J. W. T.,** Inter-relationships of nutrition and the metabolism of drugs, *Chem. Biol. Interactions,* 8, 193, 1974.
60. **Campbell, T. C.,** Influence of nutrition on metabolism of carcinogens, *Adv. Nutr. Revs.,* 2, 1977.
61. **Higginson, J.,** Rethinking the environmental causation of human cancer, *Food Cosmet. Toxicol.,* 19, 539, 1981.
62. **Higginson, J. and Muir, C. S.,** Environmental carcinogenesis: misconceptions and limitations to cancer control, *J. Natl. Cancer Inst.,* 63, 1291, 1979.
63. **Higginson, J.,** Importance of environmental and occupational factors in cancer, *J. Toxicol. Environ. Hlth.,* 6, 941, 1980.
64. **Gori, G. B.,** Diet and nutrition in cancer causation, *Nutr. Cancer,* 1, 5, 1978.
65. CIBA Foundation Symposium 76, Environmental Chemicals, Enzyme Function and Human Disease, *Excerpta Medica,* Amsterdam, 1980.
66. **Conney, A. J., Pantuck, E. J., Pantuck, C. B., Buening, M., Jerina, D. M., et al.,** Role of environment and diet in the regulation of human drug metabolism, in *The Induction of Drug Metabolism,* Eastbrook, R. W. and Lindenbaub, E., Eds., F. K. Schattauer Verlag, Stuttgart, New York, 1978, 583.
67. **Kalamegham, R., Krishnaswamy, K., Krishnamurthy, S., and Bhargava, R. N. K.,** Metabolism of drugs and carcinogens in man: antipyrine elimination as an indicator, *Clin. Pharm. Ther.,* 25, 67, 1979.
68. **Hirayama, T.,** Diet and cancer, *Nutr. Cancer,* 1, 67, 1979.
69. **Hoehn, S. K. and Carroll, K. K.,** Effects of dietary carbohydrate on the incidence of mammary tumors induced by rats by 7,12-dimethylbenz(a)-anthracene, *Nutr. Cancer,* 1, 27, 1979.

70. **Nerberne, P. L. M. and McConnell, R. G.,** Nutrient deficiencies in cancer causation, *J. Env. Path. Toxicol.,* 3, 323, 1980.

71. IARC Microecology Group, Dietary fiber, transit-time, fecal bacteria, steroids and colon cancer in Scandinavian populations, *Lancet,* 2, 207, 1977.

72. **Newberne, P. M., Weigert, J., and Kula, N.,** Effects of dietary fat on hepatic mixed-function oxidases and hepatocellular carcinoma induced by aflatoxin B_1 in rats, *Cancer Res.,* 39, 3986, 1979.

73. **Dion, P. W., Brighht-See, E. B., Furrer, R., Eng, V. W. S., and Bruce, W. R.,** The effects of dietary fat, ascorbic acid and alpha-tocopherol on fecal mutagens, in *Clinical Investigations, Proceeding of AACR and ASCO, AACR Abstracts,* 1980, 171.

74. **Wattenberg, L. W.,** Inhibition of chemical carcinogenesis, *J. Natl. Cancer Inst.,* 60, 11, 1978.

75. **Modan, B.,** Role of diet in cancer etiology, *Cancer,* 40, 1887, 1977.

76. **Tannenbaum, S. R. and Young, V. R.,** Endogenous nitrite formation in man, *J. Environ. Pathol. Toxicol.,* 3, 357, 1980.

77. **Weisburger, J. H. and Williams, G. M.,** Chemical carcinogens, in *Toxicology: The Basic Science of Poisons,* 2nd ed., Klassen, C. and Amdur, M., Eds., McMillan, New York, 1980, 138.

78. **Kawachi, T., Nagao, M., Yahagi, T., Takahashi, Y., Sugimura, T., Takayama, S., Kosuge, T., and Shudo, T.,** Mutagens and carcinogens in food, in *Advances in Medical Oncology Research and Education, Vol. 1, Carcinogenesis,* Margison, G. P., Ed., Pergamon Press, Oxford and New York, 1979, 199.

79. **Sugimura, T., Nagao, M., and Wakabayashi, K.,** Mutagenic heterocyclic amines in cooked food, in *Environmental Carcinogens Selected Methods of Analysis, Vol. 4,* Egan, H., Fishbein, L., O'Neill, I. K., Castegnaro, M., and Bartsch, H., Eds., International Agency for Research on Cancer, Lyon, 1981, 267.

80. **Wills, E. D.,** Effects of iron overload on lipid peroxide formation and oxidative demethylation by the liver endoplasmic reticulum, *Biochem. Pharmacol.,* 21, 239, 1972.

81. **Wade, A. E., Greene, F. E., Ciordia, R. H., Meadows, J. S., and Caster, W. O.,** Effects of dietary thiamine intake on hepatic drug metabolism in the male rat, *Biochem. Pharmacol.,* 18, 2288, 1969.

82. **Woodcock, B. G. and Wood, G. C.,** Effect of protein-free diet on UDP-glucuronyltransferase and sulphotransferase activities in rat liver, *Biochem. Pharmacol.,* 20, 2703, 1971.

83. **Erikson, M., Catz, C., and Yaffe, S. J.,** Effect of weanling malnutrition upon hepatic drug metabolism, *Biol. Neonate,* 27, 339, 1975.

84. **Falk, H. L.,** Possible mechanisms of combination effects in chemical carcinogenesis, *Oncology,* 33, 77, 1979.

85. **Fouts, J. R.,** Factors influencing the metabolism of drugs in liver microsomes, *Ann. N.Y. Acad. Sci.,* 104, 875, 1963.

86. **Hart, L. G. and Fouts, J. R.,** Further studies on stimulation of hepatic microsomal drug metabolizing enzymes by DDT and its analogs, *Arch. Exp. Path. Pharmakol.,* 249, 486, 1965.

87. **Welch, R. M., Harrison, Y. E., Gommi, B. W., Poppers, P. J., Finster, M., and Conney, A. H.,** Stimulatory effect of cigarette smoking on the hydroxylation of 3,4-benzpyrene and the N-demethylation of 3-methyl-4-monomethyl-aminoazobenzene by enzymes in human placenta, *Clin. Pharmacol. Ther.,* 10, 100, 1969.

88. **Miller, E. C., Miller, J. A., Brown, R. R., and MacDonald, J. C.,** On the protective action of certain polycyclic aromatic hydrocarbons against carcinogenesis by aminoazo dyes and 2-acetylaminofluorene, *Cancer Res.,* 18, 469, 1958.

89. **Gori, G. B.,** The regulation of carcinogenic hazards, *Science,* 208, 256, 1980.

90. **Kraybill, H. F.,** Symposium on chemical carcinogenesis. II. Carcinogenesis associated with foods, food additives, food degradation products, and related dietary factors, *Clin. Pharmacol. Ther.,* 4, 73, 1963.

91. **Bresnick, E. and Eastman, A.,** Alkylation of mammalian cell DNA persistence of adducts and relationship to carcinogenesis, *Drug Metab. Revs.,* 13, 189, 1982.

92. **Craddock, V. M.,** Cell proliferation and experimental liver cancer, in *Liver Cell Cancers,* Cameron, H. M., Linsell, D. S., and Warwick, G. P., Elsevier, Amsterdam, 1976, 153.

93. **Cayama, W., Tsuda, H., Sarma, D. S. R., and Farber, E.,** Initiation of chemical carcinogenesis requires cell proliferation, *Nature,* 275, 60, 1978.

94. **Hiatt, H. H., Watson, J. D., and Winsten, J. A., Eds.,** Origins of Human Cancer, *Proliferation, Vol. 4,* Cold Spring Harbor Laboratory, Cold Springs Harbor, New York, 1977.

95. **Van Lancker, J. L.,** DNA injuries, their repair and carcinogenesis, in *Current Topics in Pathology, Vol. 64,* Grundemann, E., and Kirsten, W. H., Eds., Springer-Verlag, Berlin, Heidelberg, 1977.

96. **Schendel, P. F.,** Inducible repair systems and their implications for toxicology, *CRC Crit. Revs. Toxicol.,* 8, 311, 1981.

97. **Hart, R. W.,** Current views on the mechanisms of cancer, in preparation.

98. **Santi, L., Parodi, S., Taningher, M., Cesarone, C. F., and Bolognesi, C.,** DNA alteration and repair, *Ecotoxicol. Environ. Safety,* 4, 85, 1980.

99. **Kakunaga, T.,** The role of cell division in the malignant transformation of mouse cells treated with 3-methyl cholanthrene, *Cancer Res.,* 35, 1637, 1975.

100. **Smith, R. L. and Williams, R. T.,** Comparative metabolism of drugs in man and monkeys, *J. Med. Primatol.,* 3, 138, 1974.
101. **Brash, D. E. and Hart, R. W.,** DNA damage and repair in vivo, *J. Environ. Pathol. Toxicol.,* 2, 78, 1978.
102. **Larsen, K. H., Brash, D., Cleaver, J. E., Hart, R. W., Maher, V. M., Painter, R. B., and Sega, G. A.,** DNA repair assays as tests for environmental mutagens: a report for the US EPA gene-tox program, *Mutat. Res.,* 98, 287, 1982.
103. **Radman, M., Villani, G., Bioteaux, S., Defais, M., Caillet-Fauquet, P. and Sapdari, S.,** in *Origins of Human Cancer: Mechanisms of Carcinogenesis,* Watson, J. D. and Hiatt, H., Eds., 4, 903, 1977.
104. **Witkin, E. M.,** Ultraviolet mutagenesis and inducible DNA repair in *Escherichia coli, Bacteriol. Rev.,* 40, 869, 1976.
105. **Sarasin, A. R. and Hanawalt, P. C.,** Carcinogens enhance survival of UV-irradiated simian virus 40 in treated monkey kidney cells: induction of a recovery pathway? *Proc. Natl. Acad. Sci., USA,* 75, 346, 1978.
106. **D'Ambrosio, S. M. and Setlow, R. B.,** Enhancement of postreplication repair in Chinese hamster cells, *Proc. Natl. Acad. Sci., USA,* 73, 2396, 1976.
107. **Loeb, L. A., Weymouth, L. A., Kunkel, T. A., Gopinathan, K. P., Beckman, R. A. and Dube, D. K.,** *Cold Spring Harbor Symposium in Quantitative Biology,* 43, 921, 1979.
108. **Sirover, M. A. and Loeb, L. A.,** Metal-induced infidelity during DNA synthesis, *Proc. Natl. Acad. Sci., USA,* 73, 2331, 1976.
109. **Loeb, L. A., Silber, J. R., and Fry, M.,** in *Biological Mechanisms in Aging Conference Proceedings,* June 1980, Schimke, R. T., Ed., 1981, 270.
110. **Battula, N. and Loeb, L. A.,** The infidelity of avian myeloblastosis virus deoxyribonucleic acid polymerase in polynucleotide replication, *J. Biol. Chem.,* 249, 4086, 1974.
111. **Kunkel, T. A. and Loeb, L. A.,** On the fidelity of DNA replication, *J. Biol. Chem.,* 254, 5718, 1979.
112. **Peterson, A. R., Landolph, J. R., Peterson, H., and Heidelberger, C.,** *Nature,* 276, 508, 1978.
113. **Kroger, M. and Singer, B.,** Ambiguity and transcriptional errors as a result of methylation of N-1 of purines and N-3 of pyrimidines, *Biochemistry,* 18, 3493, 1979.
114. **Mehta, J. R. and Ludlum, D. B.,** Synthesis and properties of O^6-methyldeoxyguanylic acid and its copolymers with deoxycytidylinic acid, *Biochem. Biophys. Acta.,* 521, 770, 1978.
115. **Dube, D. K. and Loeb, L. A.,** Manganese as a mutagenic agent during *in vitro* DNA synthesis, *Biochem. Biophys. Res. Commun.,* 67, 1041, 1975.
116. **Lindahl, T. and Nyberg, B.,** Rate of depurination of native deoxyribonucleic acid, *Biochemistry,* 11, 3610, 1972.
117. **Farber, E.,** Chemical carcinogenesis, *N. Engl. J. Med.,* 305, 1379, 1981.
118. **Chang, M. J. W., Hart, R. W., and Koestner, A.,** Retention of promutogenic O^6-ethylguanine in the DNA of various rat tissues following transplacental inoculation with ethylnitrosourea, *Cancer Lett.,* 9, 199, 1980.
119. **Solt, D. and Farber, E.,** New principle for the analysis of chemical carcinogenesis, *Nature,* 263, 701, 1976.
120. **Hull, L. A.,** Progress towards a unified theory of the mechanisms of carcinogenesis: role of cell cycle restriction points, *Med. Hypotheses,* 7, 187, 1981.
121. **Hull, L. A.,** Progress towards a unified theory of the mechanisms of carcinogenesis, Part III, Circumvention of proliferation controls, *Med. Hypotheses,* 8, 85, 1982.
122. **Stott, W. T., Reitz, R. H., Schumann, A. M., and Watanabe, P. G.,** Genetic and nongenetic events in neoplasia, *Food Cosmet. Toxicol.,* 19, 567, 1981.
123. **Mehta, R. G. and Moon, R. C.,** Inhibition of DNA synthesis by retinyl acetate during chemically induced mammary carcinogenesis, *Cancer Res.,* 40, 1109, 1980.
124. **Narisawa, T., Reddy, B. S., Wong, C. Q., and Weisburger, J. H.,** Effects of vitamin A deficiency on rat colon carcinogenesis by N-methyl-N'-nitro-N-nitrosoguanidine, *Cancer Res.,* 36, 1379, 1976.
125. **Alvares, A. P., Pantuck, E. J., Andersen, K. E., Kappas, A., and Conney, A. H.,** Regulation of drug metabolism in man by environmental factors, *Drug Metab. Rev.,* 9, 185, 1979.
126. **Dollery, C. T., Fraser, H. S., Mucklow, J. C., and Bulpitt, C. J.,** Contribution of environmental factors to variability in human drug metabolism, *Drug Metab. Rev.,* 9, 207, 1979.
127. **Jusko, W. J.,** Influence of cigarette smoking on drug metabolism in man, *Drug Metab. Rev.,* 9, 221, 1979.
128. **Dagani, R.,** Scientists explore drug metabolism/age tie, *Chem. Eng. News,* 23, 18, 1981.
129. **Gelboin, H. V. and Ts'O, P. O. P., Eds.,** *Polycyclic Hydrocarbons and Cancer, Vol. 1,* Academic Press, New York, 1978.
130. **Greim, H., Andrae, U., Goggelman, W., Hesse, S., Schwarz, L. R., and Summer, K. H .,** Threshold levels in toxicology: significance of inactivation mechanisms, *Adv. Exptl. Med. Biol.,* 136, 1389, 1982.
131. **Gehring, P. J. and Blau, G. E.,** Mechanisms of carcinogenesis: dose response, *J. Environ. Pathol. Toxicol.,* 1, 163, 1977.

132. **Gehring, P. J., Watanabe, P. G., Young, J. D., and Lebeau, J. E.,** Metabolic thresholds in assessing carcinogenic hazard, *Chem. Hum. Health Environ.*, 2, 57, 1977.

133. **Gehring, P. J., Watanabe, P. G., and Park, C. N.,** Risk of angiosarcoma in workers exposed to vinyl chloride as predicted from studies in rats, *Toxicol. Appl. Pharmacol.*, 49, 15, 1979.

134. **Jones, H.,** Dose-effect relationships in carcinogenesis and the matter of threshold of carcinogenesis, *Environ. Health Perspect.*, 22, 171, 1978.

135. **Falk, H. L.,** Biological evidence for the existence of thresholds in chemical carcinogenesis, *Environ. Hlth. Persp.*, 22, 167, 1978.

136. **Kleihues, P. and Cooper, H. K.,** Repair excision of alkylated bases from DNA in vivo, *Oncology*, 33, 86, 1976.

137. **Omenn, G. S.,** Predictive identification of hypersusceptible individuals, *J. Occup. Med.*, 24, 369, 1982.

138. **Ritchie, J. C., Sloan, T. P., Idle, J. R., and Smith, R. L.,** in *Environmental Chemicals, Enzyme Function and Human Disease*, Ciba Foundation Symposium, 76, 219, 1980.

139. **Vesell, E. S.,** in *Clinical Pharmacology and Therapeutics*, Turner, P., Ed., Proceedings of the First World Conference, Macmillan, London, 1980, 79.

140. **Eichelbaum, M.,** Defective oxidation of drugs-pharmacokinetic and therapeutic implications, *Clin. Pharmacokinetic*, 7, 1, 1982.

141. **Weber, W. W.,** Genetic variability and extrapolation from animals to man: some perspectives on susceptibility to chemical carcinogenesis from aromatic amines, *Env. Hlth. Persp.*, 22, 141, 1978.

142. **Harris, H.,** in *Frontiers of Biology: The Principles of Human Biochemical Genetics*, Vol. 19, Neuberger, A. and Tatum, E. L., Eds., Elsevier, New York, 1970.

143. **Atlas, S. A. and Nebert, D. W.,** in *Drug Metabolism from Microbe to Man*, Parke, D. V. and Smith, R. L., Eds., Taylor and Francis, London, 1977, 107.

144. **Doobis, A. R.,** in *Drug Toxicity*, Gorrod, J. W., Ed., Taylor and Francis, London, 1979, 51.

145. **Price-Evans, D. A.,** in *Drug Metabolism from Microbe to Man*, Parke, D. V. and Smith, R. L., Eds., Taylor and Francis, London, 1977, 369.

146. **Hughes, H. B., Biehl, J. P., Jones, A. P., and Schmidt, L. H.,** Metabolism of isoniazid in man as related to occurrence of peripheral neuritis, *Am. Rev. Tuberc. Pulm. Dis.*, 70, 266, 1954.

147. **Zingale, S. B., Minzer, L., Rosenberg, B., and Lee, S. L.,** Drug-induced lupus-like syndrome, *Arch. Intern. Med.*, 112, 63, 1963.

148. **Mitchell, J. R., Thorgiersson, W. D., Black, M. J., Timbrell, J. A., et al.,** Increased incidence of isoniazid hepatitis in rapid acetylators: possible relation to hydrazine metabolites, *Clin. Pharmacol. Ther.*, 18, 70, 1975.

149. **Eichelbaum, M., Spannbrucker, N., and Dengler, H. J.,** in *Biological Oxidation of Nitrogen*, Gorrod, J., Ed., Elsevier/North Holland Biomedical Press, Amsterdam, 1978, 118.

150. **Eichelbaum, M., Spannbrucher, N., Steincke, B., and Dengler, H. J.,** Defective N-oxidation of sparteine in man-new pharmacogenetic defect, *Eur. J. Clin. Pharm.*, 16, 183, 1979.

151. **Mahgoub, A., Idle, J. R., Dring, L. G., et al.,** Polymorphic hydroxylation of debrisoquine in man, *Lancet*, 2, 584, 1977.

152. **Tucker, G. T., Silas, J. H., Iyun, A. O., et al.,** Polymorphic hydroxylation of debrisiquine, *Lancet*, 2, 718, 1977.

Chapter 2

PHARMACOKINETIC DIFFERENCES BETWEEN SPECIES

J. R. Withey

TABLE OF CONTENTS

I. INTRODUCTION

By definition, a species is a group of animals with different characteristics which set them apart from others. These differences can vary from morphology, as in the case of mice and elephants, to more subtle biochemical variations where the metabolism of an ingested xenobiotic proceeds by different pathways. Toxicologic effects may, therefore, vary in both intensity and nature between species. The problem of extrapolating effects in highly inbred strains of genetically uniform animals to predict their magnitude and intensity in man has always been a challenge to the pharmacologist and toxicologist. Thus, the clinical testing of drugs and the toxicological assessment of xenobiotics has usually been carried out in animal species which closely resemble humans or in several species so that differences can be quantitatively estimated. Nevertheless, safety factors, often of several orders in magnitude, have been necessarily invoked to accomodate the requirements of regulatory organizations for the protection of human health.

More recently, as a consequence of the need to regulate environmental pollutants, and to assess acceptable risks for exposures to carcinogens, there has been a need to extrapolate data obtained in animal species to man with improved precision. This goal can be achieved only if a precise knowledge of the mechanism of toxic action and of the pharmacodynamics are available.[1] Indeed, a knowledge of the change in pharmacodynamics, including the variation in the amount or ratio of active metabolites, with dose, is of paramount importance in such extrapolation.[2]

II. EMPIRICAL METHODS

The traditional approach to dose equivalency between species is based on the body weight of the animal.[3] While many physiological constants in mammals, such as pulse and breathing rate, or the consumption of food, water, and oxygen,[4,5] are known to vary linearly with body weight the toxicity of some 15 to 20% of compounds do not vary linearly with this parameter. Other variants or power functions based on body weight fare little better.[6,7]

A quantitative comparison of antineoplastic drugs in various species based on the body surface area gives a reasonable correlation[8] and the activity of drugs in human infants and newborn is claimed to be related to body surface area.[9] The U.S. Environmental Protection Agency,[10] in developing a species conversion factor, relates the dose-effect to the two thirds power of the body weight. The conclusion, reached in these communications is that, unless there is a quantitative rationale, safety factors are necessary when applying these empirical relationships in the extrapolation of animal data to man.

In the light of the foregoing conclusion, it would therefore seem attractive to use a more rational approach which attempts to quantitate differences between animal species. A number of reports review those factors which affect the response to a given dose of a chemical and are known to vary across species.[11-17] A brief examination of the processes involved in the uptake, transport, distribution, metabolism, elimination, and the specific mechanisms involved at the site of action to elicit response would appear to be in order at this stage. A qualitative assessment of such processes is a part of the pharmacodynamics while their precise and quantitative evaluation is a part of the pharmacokinetics.[18]

III. PHARMACOKINETIC PROCESSES

Rall[17] suggests that absorption and distribution of compounds tends to be similar in vertebrate species. Similarly, excretion mechanisms for parent compounds and their metabolites, show few differences for animals and man. There is no doubt that metabolism is the most significant variable among species and it is this subject which has received the most attention in reviews.[13,14] The site of action and the mechanism of interaction is also comparable from species to species.[19]

It should be remembered that the metabolism of a compound can lead to the formation of active metabolites (activation) or inactive end products which are excreted (detoxification). Moreover, metabolites may be formed at different rates in different species, so that even if the metabolic patterns are similar the magnitude of the evoked response may be quite different. Some animal species have quite different metabolic pathways to man. Indeed, there may be an absence of some human metabolites in animal species altogether as was demonstrated in the case of amobarbital. In animals there was an absence of the N-glucoside conjugate of amobarbital known to be produced in humans while there was no evidence for the production of a diol metabolite in man although this is formed in several animal species.[20] As a consequence of this example, it is not inconceivable that man could react in a unique fashion to some compounds and any testing in any other animal species would be inappropriate. This may well be the case for the human carcinogens benzene and arsenic for which there appears to be no suitable animal model.

IV. ABSORPTION, DISTRIBUTION AND EXCRETION MECHANISMS

The mechanisms involved in absorption, by various routes, distribution to the tissues and site(s) of action and the elimination of xenobiotics is presented in two recent publications which also address the question of interactions affecting the response to a given dose of a chemical.[21,22] These include environmental factors, such as heat, cold, humidity, noise; altered nutrition (diet malnutrition, food intake, and vitamin deficiency); personal habits (alcohol intake, and smoking); strenuous exercise, and pregnancy. The altered response caused by these perturbations often confound the results of toxicological investigations both in man and in animals.[13]

A. Absorption

Few examples of large differences in the rate and extent of absorption of substances between species exist. Two β-blockers, nadolol[23] and atenolol,[24] having a similar chemical structure, show complete absorption after administration to the dog, *per os,* but are absorbed only to the extent of 25% after administration by the same route to mice, rats, hamsters, rabbits, rhesus monkey, and man. In this case, there is no evidence to suggest major differences in metabolism nor is there evidence of unusual mechanisms involved in the elimination of the drugs from the systemic circulation. For instance, biliary excretion is not observed so that the presence of large amounts of unchanged drug in the feces is indicative of poor absorption in all species tested, except for the dog.

Isoxepac, a non-steroidal anti-inflammatory agent is more slowly absorbed and eliminated in the rat and rabbit after oral dosing than in the dog, rhesus monkey and man.[25] A number of factors, which could account for these variations are discussed by the authors including biliary excretion of the parent compound and its metabolites and subsequent enterohepatic recycling which occurs only in the rat and dog. This might give rise to a prolongation of the absorption process but this should have been reflected in similar absorption rates for the rat and dog. In fact, the only common observation in the rat and the rabbit is a similar binding of isoxepac to erythrocytes. No clear rationale appears to explain these differences.

Rall[17] points out that the rate of absorption of an agent after intraperitoneal administration in the rat is so rapid as to be indistinguishable from an intravenous administration in man. Intraperitoneal administration of drugs in elasmobranch fish is also slow and erratic compared with mammalian species.[26] The absorption of nitrofuranes after *per os* administration varies from 70% of the dose in the pig, 50% in the rat and 0% in man.[27]

Several examples of species differences in absorption exist which are believed to be a consequence of the activity of microflora in the gastrointestinal tract, in particular with respect to the reduction of nitro groups to amines. In this respect, the LD_{50} of dinitrophenolic herbicides in the rat is about 10 mg/kg whereas, the lethal dose in bovines is greater than 50 mg/kg. Lead toxicity in dogs and man, due to the interaction with gastric hydrochloric acid and the formation of partially ionized lead chloride, contrasts with the increased toxicity of lead salts in ruminants as a consequence of interaction with the products of fermentation and the formation of lipid soluble lead acetate in the stomach.[27]

The percutaneous uptake of toxicants and the large variations due to the permeability of the skin of different species is also capable of producing altered toxic response. The rat, rabbit, and hare have skin which is very permeable and these species are notably sensitive to topically applied dinitrophenol herbicides.[28] These few examples serve to illustrate that while the diffusion of toxicants across epithelial barriers may be very similar in most species so that absorption is not usually a factor in considering species differences there are, nevertheless, good reasons to consider the variations due to differences in the physiology or environment of the absorption site. In respect of the latter, it might be particularly important to consider the interaction of an orally administered toxicant with the nature of the food intake in different species.

B. Distribution

The second stage in the pharmacokinetic processes is the distribution of the compound to various organs and to the target tissue and site of action. The apparent volume of distribution, V_d may well be indicative of extensive distribution although it is important to remember that this parameter is a hypothetical volume to which the dose would be distributed uniformly.[9,29] The fact that the dose will, frequently, be partitioned to physiological compartments at different concentrations, although they are a part of the central compartment, means that the volume of distribution can seldom have any meaning or relevance to a physical volume or the physiology of the animal. Indeed the calculated apparent volume of distribution can exceed the volume of the animal.

Multiphasic elimination curves, obtained after the administration and uptake of a dose and which fit multiexponential equations are usually indicative of multicompartment pharmacokinetic model behavior. In these instances, it is fair to assume that extensive distribution has taken place. It is therefore important to ascertain the nature of the pharmacokinetic model in preliminary experiments since this can vary from species to species as a consequence of such factors as binding to plasma proteins and differing physiological structure. The alkaloid pilocarpine, for example, is weakly bound in the plasma of the pig and more firmly bound in the cow, horse, sheep, and rabbit.[30] Saturation of the binding sites in the plasma of monkeys is observed at lower doses of the drug ciclazindol than in rats.[31]

Lipid soluble compounds like anaesthetic gases are particularly well absorbed and distributed to fat depots. Thus, animals with a high body fat/muscle ratio, like sheep and pigs, require higher doses of anaesthetic than lean species, like dogs and man, before steady state systemic circulation levels are achieved. Tissue binding in the lung is important in the assessment of the extent of toxic action of the pesticide paraquat and the specific, irreversible binding of this substance to lung tissue in man and dogs makes these species much more sensitive than the rat.[32]

Transplacental transport is extremely variable among species due, in part, to the very different placental physiology. The epitheliochorial structure of the placental membranes of the horse and pig contrasts with the syndesmo-chorial structure in ruminants, endotheliochorial structure in carnivores and the hemochorial structure in rodents and primates. Thus, the transplacental transfer of the sodium ion in the pig and ruminants varies from 0.028 to 0.43 mg g^{-1} hr^{-1} and for dogs and rodents from 0.79 to 9.2 mg g^{-1} hr^{-1}. Such variance could interfere with the assessment of embryotoxic and teratogenic substances and suggests that rodents are a good model for humans in teratogenic studies.

C. Excretion

After uptake to this systemic circulation and distribution to the major organs and tissues, most xenobiotic substances are excreted via the kidney into the urine. The original compound may well have been altered by anabolic and catabolic metabolism, particularly in the liver, although extrahepatic metabolism in organs, such as the kidney and lung, may occur and be the principal sites of metabolism.[33] The original compound and its metabolites may also be subject to conjugation with glucuronide, acetyl, sulfate, mercapturic acid, and amino acid (glycine and taurine). These conjugates are usually more water soluble than the parent compound or its primary metabolites and thus excretion via the kidney is facilitated.

Species differences are frequently associated with biliary excretion which can alter the pharmacokinetics significantly. Biliary excretion of drugs occurs more readily in the rat than in most other laboratory animals.[13] The importance of molecular size should not be omitted since it is known to affect the rate and extent of biliary excretion. It is suggested that the molecular weight threshold, for the parent compound, metabolites and conjugates is low in the rat and the dog (325 ± 50) and higher in the rhesus monkey and man (475 ± 50).[33] Thus, compounds with a molecular weight of between 350 to 450 would be subject to biliary excretion in the rat and dog, but not in primates.

A further consequence of biliary excretion is the phenomenon known as enterohepatic recycling in which the original compound; metabolites or conjugates may be reabsorbed from the gut. Gastrointestinal flora can often hydrolyze conjugates, excreted by the biliary route, prior to reabsorption. The impact of biliary excretion and enterohepatic recycling on the pharmacokinetics can range from a more rapid elimination rate when an absorbed substance is returned to the lower gastrointestinal tract and excreted in the feces to a prolonged elimination rate due to the successive reintroduction of fractions of the dose to the systemic circulation. Bromosulfonephthalein, procaine, and ouabaine are excreted much more slowly in the dog than in the rat or rabbit[34] due to enterohepatic recycling.

Baty[13,14] has presented numerous examples in which the disposition and pharmacokinetic rate coefficients have varied between species due to different excretory mechanisms. For example, the schistosomicide hycanthone was extensively excreted in the bile of dogs, cats, rabbits, and monkeys. Only in the case of monkeys and cats is there evidence of urinary excretion which may account for its high toxicity in the latter species.[36] Biliary excretion is considered to play an important role in the species differences as a consequence of differences in the routes of excretion noted with the drug danazol.[37] Indeed, it is suggested that both the route of administration and the dosage formulation of this compound causes differences in the excretion routes. Much more radiolabel was found in the bile of rats after i.v. administration than when it was given orally. A greater proportion of the drug was found in the urine of the rat after oral administration of a solution than when it was given by the same route as a powder. It is considered that Rose Bengal,[38] a dyestuff that is not apparently metabolized, is excreted via the bile in different species at widely different rates. In guinea pigs the excretion half-life is cited as 17 min, in rats and rabbits 30 min, while in the dog it was 46 min. There is a marked species difference in the route of excretion of benoxaprofen in that biliary excretion leading to fecal excretion was the only observed route in rats and dogs while excretion via the urine was extensive in man, rhesus monkeys and the rabbit.[39]

Although the author of major review articles on this subject notes that there is a change in emphasis in many papers towards a pharmacokinetic explanation to account for observations of species differences, it is unfortunate that many of the fundamental concepts in pharmacokinetics are ignored.[14] This is especially the case in reports of elimination and excretion data where comparative 'biological half-lives' are cited without reference to the nature of the pharmacokinetic model. Such citations can be misleading since the biological half-life (i.e., the half-life of elimination or excretion) for a one compartment model cannot be compared with the terminal half-life of elimination for a two compartment model. Unfortunately the term biological half-life has been defined in these terms.[24] It is the opinion of this author that the term biological half-life, or indeed half-life of elimination when used without reference to the pharmacokinetic model, has outlived its usefulness and its use should be discontinued.

V. METABOLISM

There is no doubt that the greatest difference between species in the pharmacokinetic handling of an administered dose is due to different routes, mechanisms and rates of metabolism. Not only do some species have enzyme activities which are different, as reflected in different responses to a given dose of a xenobiotic, but the differences in distribution and excretion rates between conjugates may be as important as their rates of formation.[14] As an illustration of the first point, Gillette cites the 50-fold species difference in the observed duration of the action of hexobarbital in animals receiving the same dose of the drug.[11] The plasma levels of this barbiturate are surprisingly similar when the animals recover and the duration of effect is due to different rates of metabolism rather than differences in the receptor sites. An example of the second kind is the observation of differences in the excretion rate of the metabolites of phenol.[41] Some 12% of the urinary metabolites of this compound in the sheep is conjugated with phosphate. This metabolite is not produced by the pig or rat, the principal metabolites being phenyl glucuronide and phenyl sulfate.

Metabolism is, in itself, usually a complex process. Baty has reviewed differences in conjugation and differences in enzyme activities.[13] In this review the author notes intraspecies differences, differences due to strain and sex, and effects due to circadian variations as well as pharmacogenetic and environmental factors like alcohol intake and smoking. The latter has been illustrated by significant differences in the metabolism of a single oral dose of ethanol (1.2 mℓ/kg body weight) in 19 identical and 21 fraternal healthy, adult, unselected male twin pairs.[42]

It should be remembered that first stage metabolism usually breaks down larger and more complex molecules (catabolism) into smaller units of lower molecular weight. This process can sometimes reduce or eliminate pharmacologic activity (detoxification) or result in the production of more reactive species (activation). These lower molecular weight metabolites will frequently increase the rate at which they can diffuse through tissue and membrane barriers so as to allow their excretion via the renal tubules or pulmonary alveoli. In cases where the primary metabolites are not water soluble secondary metabolism, involving the formation of covalent bonds to form water soluble conjugates (glucuronides, phosphates, sulfates, etc.) takes place which also facilitates their excretion. Enzymes are usually involved in both catabolism and conjugation reactions and these are capacity limited or saturable processes. The saturation limit for a particular enzymatic process can vary significantly from species to species and be responsible for different responses to the same dose.

Reitz and Ramsey have recently proposed methodology to calculate the concentration of 'active metabolite species' derived from different doses of a given toxicant.[43] Their treatment analyzes the effects of saturable kinetic phenomenon on observed pharmacokinetic rate coefficients and other parameters for specific compounds known to require metabolic activation. Essentially, the reversible formation of an enzyme-substrate intermediate species, in the simplest mechanism is

$$E + S \underset{k_2}{\overset{k_1}{\rightleftharpoons}} ES \tag{1}$$
$$\downarrow k_3$$
$$products$$

where k_1 and k_2 are the rate coefficients which describe the rates of the forward and reverse reactions for the formation of the enzyme-substrate intermediate. The ratio of k_1 to k_2, the equilibrium constant usually designated K_m, is termed the Michaelis constant. k_3 is the rate coefficient which determines the rate of breakdown of the complex to yield products. Thus, the overall rate of reaction is given by the expression:

$$Rate = \frac{V_{max} C}{K_m + C} \tag{2}$$

where V_{max} is the maximum velocity for the overall reaction, K_m is the Michaelis constant and C is the concentration of the transformed chemical species. At very high concentrations, it is clearly evident that the right hand side of equation 2 reduces to V_{max}, the maximum velocity:

$$Rate = V_{max}$$
$$(C \gg K_m) \tag{3}$$

Equation 3 is a rate equation of zeroth order.

At low concentrations of C, Equation 2 approximates to:

$$Rate = \frac{V_m}{K_m} C$$
$$(C \ll K_m) \tag{4}$$

Equation 4 is a first order rate equation.

Thus, at high concentrations of substrate where the enzyme receptor sites are saturated the zeroth order reaction proceeds at a constant rate characterized by V_{max}, the maximum velocity and at lower concentrations of substrate the rate is first order. It should be emphasized that the Michaelis-Menten Equation 2, is a model only and there are many variants which are more complex and specific for some enzyme reactions.[43]

It is plainly evident, from the foregoing conclusion, that both the rate and extent of metabolic activation, detoxification or conjugate formation will be dose dependent. It is also probable that metabolism, as a part of the elimination and excretion processes, will be the rate limiting step which determines the magnitude of a toxic effect in many cases. Thus, studies in different animal species at comparable doses could show large differences as a consequence of species difference in the values of K_m and V_{max}. Studies with supernatant fractions prepared from liver homogenates reveal a fourfold difference in values of K_m for the O-demethylation of harmine in the guinea-pig, rat, cow, rabbit, mouse, and cat.[44] The authors note a very large intra-species variation, except in the mouse, and conclude that it is important to define the statistical limits of mean values for K_m and V_{max} in experiments of this kind.

There is one other pharmacokinetic phenomenon, with respect to metabolic mechanisms, which deserves attention since it can also result in large species differences. This is known as the "first-pass" effect and arises as a consequence of absorption from the gastrointestinal tract and the transport of the total dose, via the portal circulation, through the liver. In cases where there is extensive hepatic metabolism, only a fraction of the unmetabolized dose will reach the systemic circulation after intragastric administration. The potent analgesic meptazinol is rapidly absorbed from the gastrointestinal tract after administration *per-os* and is extensively metabolized.[45] Only 6% of the drug is excreted unchanged in rats and monkeys, the principal metabolite being the glucuronide conjugate. However, administration of the same dose (25 mg/kg body weight) to these species resulted in peak plasma levels 17 times higher in the rat compared with the monkey. In addition, female rats lacked the capability to demethylate this drug and it is this metabolite which is more addictive, toxic, and more active as an analgesic in studies with mice.

There can be no doubt that the involvement of some or all of the foregoing mechanisms associated with metabolism provides adequate support for the need to perform acute and chronic toxicology studies in species which most closely resemble man. The use of non-human primates in this role, despite their expense and scarcity, is often justified on the grounds that they are the animal model which have similar metabolic pathways and enzyme activities resembling those in man. Inter-primate differences do, however, exist and must not be overlooked. The metabolism of meperidine, for example, is subject to oxidative metabolism, but a report of studies in the vervet, patas, mona, and mangabey monkeys showed wide variability in metabolic activity. The vervet is dissimilar to man while the mangabey is an acceptable animal model for this drug.[46]

On the available evidence it is apparent that the Old World Monkeys, in particular the rhesus, resemble man more closely with respect to metabolism.[47] It is considered that this judgement can be made on the basis of comparisons of competing reactions in 32 compounds. At least four metabolic reactions are known to occur in primates which do not take place in other species and there are no species defects in xenobiotic transformations.

VI. APPLICATION OF PHARMACOKINETIC PRINCIPLES

It would appear, from the variety of the numerous examples cited, that the pharmacokinetic processes involved in eliciting a toxic response present an impressively complicated scenario which would preclude the quantitative evaluation of all of the parameters needed to allow the precise extrapolation of toxicity data from one species to another. However, a very general and broad spectrum approach, which could accomodate all of the variables discussed in this review, is suggested in a communication by Gillette.[11]

It is suggested that, in the majority of examples so far examined, species differences are mainly due to the rate of elimination, which includes the rates of metabolism, distribution, and excretion together with the available pathways for metabolism. Gillette maintains that large species differences, which are apparent from single dose experiments, can be manipulated in multiple dosing experiments by adjusting the magnitude of the dose and the dosing interval so that they virtually disappear. This is especially true in cases where the elicited response is due to the administered compound *per se* and the effect is directly proportional to the plasma concentration, as in the case of hexobarbital and carisoprodol where a 50-fold species variation in the rate of elimination exists.[40,48] In fact, if all of the kinetic processes which contribute to the elimination rate are first order then the mean plasma concentration at steady state can be calculated from the relationship[9]

$$\overline{C}_\alpha = FD/V_d k_e T \tag{5}$$

where k_e is the elimination rate, V_d is the apparent volume of distribution, D is the dose, F the fraction of the dose absorbed and T is the dose interval. Thus, the same plasma

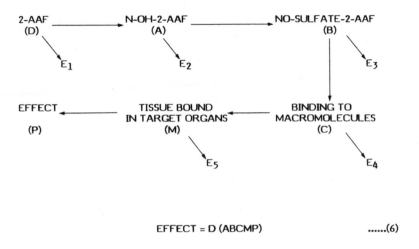

$$EFFECT = D (ABCMP) \qquad ......(6)$$

FIGURE 1. Consecutive reactions leading to effect for 2-acetylaminofluorene (2-AAF).

concentration at steady state can be achieved for animal species with different values of F, V_d and k_e by adjusting the dose or dose interval. If the first dose, sometimes termed the loading dose, is twice the maintenance dose then steady state levels are achieved after the first two or three doses.[49]

Where metabolic pathways are available in humans which do not exist in animal species, Gillette suggests that the co-administration of the human metabolites with the test compound could be useful in producing a suitable model for extrapolating animal data to humans. It is suggested, however, that caution be exercised if metabolites are subject to further reactions to form conjugates in humans prior to excretion or there is evidence of enhanced protein binding or other specific interaction in the human.

The ultimate goal in assessing the dose-response for a given toxicant depends, in most cases, on the determination of the fraction of a dose which is irreversibly bound to a reaction site. As Gillette points out, this may not always be related to the concentration of the toxicant or reactive metabolite in the systemic circulation especially if other factors, such as promotors (e.g., croton oil or phorbol esters in carcinogenesis mechanisms), co-enzymes, co-substrates or DNA repair mechanisms are involved. The calculation of the fraction of the administered dose which is available at a reaction site could be expressed as a function of the product of ratios of the original dose and its intermediates ($A \times B \times C.....$) leading to the ultimate reactive species. Another pair of factors will be needed to calculate the fraction of the available reactive species, M, which is bound to target molecules and a factor, P, representing the probability that the fraction of reactive species bound to a target molecule will evoke a toxic response in the target tissue. Gillette considers that the carcinogenic action of 2-acetylaminofluorene (2-AAF) is a good example to illustrate the multistage-multiproduct pharmacokinetics. The schema, shown in Figure 1, is believed to represent the stages that are involved in the production of tumors at the reaction sites.

A number of important conclusions can be drawn from an inspection of the pharmaco-kinetic coefficients which determine the relative concentrations for the metabolites and conjugates arising from the consecutive reactions depicted in Figure 1. Each factor in the product Equation 6 represents a ratio of the amounts formed to the amounts available for conversion (e.g., A = amount of N-OH-2-AAF divided by the dose, etc.). Only a fraction of the amount of product formed will be available for conversion to the next product in the series, the rest probably being excreted or eliminated. In the general case, if this fraction representing elimination is small and the step is the only route of metabolic elimination, then increases or decreases in the enzyme activity would alter the toxicity significantly although the elimination rate would not be affected. If the production of the metabolite represents a major elimination pathway then increases or decreases in enzyme concentration will have a pronounced effect on the toxicity without changing the elimination rate for the toxicant. It follows that when the ultimate reactive metabolite is converted to only one innoxious metabolite, changes in the enzyme activity may alter the toxicity markedly, yet leave the amounts and nature of urinary metabolites unchanged. Thus, toxicity may appear only in one species (which has a high concentration of the critical enzyme) even though all species have a similar pattern of urinary metabolites.

It should be noted that the kinetics of enzyme reactions, depicted in Equations 1 to 3, can lead to a variable kinetic order at high and low concentrations of substrate. At high concentrations of substrate, where the kinetics of the reaction are of zero order and the reaction velocity is constant and equal to V_{max}, no further increase in the dose will increase the amount of active metabolite produced. However, if the dose is divided into smaller doses which does not result in the saturation of the metabolizing enzyme, then the total amount of active metabolite will exceed that resulting from the larger single dose. It is not only enzyme catalyzed reactions which are saturable since diffusion processes, such as those which occur in the active transport systems in the kidneys, can also yield similar results to those discussed above. The depletion of co-substrates, like those involved in the formation of glutathione, sulfate, and phosphate conjugates, can also be depleted by a large single dose as opposed to the same dose given in divided amounts. As a further example to illustrate the variability and apparently incongruous results which can arise from a complex multi-stage consecutive series of reactions, Gillette also describes the complex interactions involved in the elicitation of the toxic response to bromobenzene. The rationale for a clearly established threshold for centrilobular necrosis caused by bromobenzene, at 1.2 mmoles/kg body weight in rats, is related to a saturation of the process leading to covalent binding in liver proteins. Gillete and his colleagues have demonstrated the importance of the principles considered above in relating pharmacokinetic mechanisms to dose-effect for a number of other processes including the limiting liver toxicity for isoniazid,[50] the threshold for the toxicity of furosemide[51] and the potentiation of acetaminophen toxicity in mice by pre-treatment with phenobarbital.[52,53]

It is evident that, even when different species metabolize a xenobiotic by the same metabolic pathways and all of the rate processes governing the response are known, caution must still be exercised in identifying a particular species as one which "most closely resembles man". The approach by Gillette to rationalize a calculation of the concentration or amount of ultimate reactive species which evokes the response and to reproduce these parameters to another species is a goal which is far from being achieved for the majority of compounds. In summary, pharmacokinetic studies have, as the examples in this chapter show, thrown light on the mechanisms known to be involved in eliciting toxic response. However, the majority of reports have given only semi-quantitative or qualitative information thus far. The prospect of providing the precise pharmacokinetic mechanism of action for a xenobiotic, the evaluation of the kinetic coefficients and their dependence on dose and the translation of these to physiological systems to allow a quantitative description of the molecular toxicology involved in every species, remains a challenge to investigators in the field of pharmacokinetics applied to toxicology.

REFERENCES

1. Food Safety Council, Proposed System for Food Safety Assessment, Columbia, Md., 1978, 7.
2. **Ramsey, J. C. and Reitz, R. H.,** Pharmacokinetics and threshold concepts, *Am. Chem. Soc. Symp. Ser.,* 160, 239, 1981.
3. **Goodman, L. S. and Gilman, A.,** *The Pharmacological Basis of Therapeutics,* 4th ed., Macmillan Co., London, Toronto, 1971.
4. **Krasovskii, G. N.,** Extrapolation of experimental data from animals to man, *Environ. Hlth. Perspect.,* 13, 51, 1976.
5. **Filov, V. A., Golubev, A. A., Liublina, E. I., and Tolokontsev, N. A.** *Quantitative Toxicology,* John Wiley & Sons, New York, 1979.
6. **Dixon, R. L.,** Problems in extrapolating toxicity data for laboratory animals to man, *Environ. Hlth. Perspect.,* 13, 43, 1976.
7. **Goldin, A., Carter, S., Homan, E., and Schein, P. S.,** Quantitative comparison of toxicity in animals and man, *Des. Clin. Trials Cancer Ther., Proc. Course Clin. Pharmacol.,* 58, 1973.
8. **Freireich, E. J., Gehan, E. A., Rall, D. P., Schmidt, L. H., and Skipper, H. E.,** Quantitative comparison of toxicity of anticancer agents in mouse, rat, hamster, dog, monkey, and man, *Cancer Chemotherap. Rep.,* 50, 219, 1966.
9. **Wagner, J. G.,** Biopharmaceutics and Relevant Pharmacokinetics, Drug Intelligence Publications, Hamilton, Ill., 1971, chap. 35.
10. U.S. Environmental Protection Agency, Fed. Regist., 44, 15926, 1979.
11. **Gillette, J. R.,** Application of pharmacokinetic principles in the extrapolation of animal data to humans, *Clin. Toxicol.,* 9, 709, 1976.
12. **Hilderbrandt, A. G., Roots, I., Heinemeyer, G., Nigam, S., and Helga, H.,** Aminopyrine as one of the parameters to measure the *in vivo* drug metabolism activity in man and animal, *Symp. Med. Hoechst.,* 14, 615, 1979.
13. **Baty, J. D.,** Species, strain and sex differences in metabolism, *Foreign C. Metab. Mammals,* 5, 159, 1979.
14. **Baty, J. D.,** Species, strain and sex differences in metabolism, *Foreign C. Metab. Mammals,* 6, 133, 1981.
15. **Caldwell, J.,** The current status of attempts to predict species differences in drug metabolism, *Drug Metab. Rev.,* 12, 221, 1981.
16. **Neale, R.,** Metabolism of toxic substances, in *Toxicology, The Basic Science of Poisons,* 2nd ed., Doull, J., Klaassen, C. D., and Amdur, M. O., Eds., MacMillan Publishing Co., New York, Toronto, 1980, 56.
17. **Rall, D. P.,** Difficulties in extrapolating the results of toxicity studies in laboratory animals to man, *Environ. Res.,* 2, 360, 1969.
18. **Young, J. F. and Holson, J. F.,** Utility of pharmacokinetics in designing toxicological protocols and improving interspecies extrapolation, *J. Environ. Pathol. Toxicol.,* 2, 169, 1978.
19. **Brodie, B. B., Cosmides, G. J., and Rall, D. P.,** Toxicology and the biomedical sciences, *Science,* 148, 1547, 1965.
20. **Tang, B. K., Grey, A. A., Reilly, P. A., and Kallow, W.,** Species differences in amobarbital metabolism, *Can. J. Physiol. Pharmacol.,* 58, 1167, 1980.
21. National Academy of Sciences, *Principles of Toxicological Interactions Associated with Multiple Chemical Exposures,* National Academy Press, Washington, D.C., 1980.
22. **Withey, J. R.,** Toxicodynamics and biotransformation in *Assessment of Multichemical Contamination,* Proceedings of an International Workshop, National Academy Press, Washington, D.C., 1982.
23. **Dreyfus, J., Shaw, J. M., and Ross, J. J.,** Absorption of the β-adrenergic agent, Nadolol, by mice, rats, hamsters, rabbits, dogs, monkeys, and man: an unusual species difference, *Xenobiotica,* 8, 503, 1978.
24. **Reeves, P. R., Barnfield, D. J., Longshaw, S., McIntosh, D. A. D., and Winrow, M. J.,** Disposition and metabolism of atenolol in animals, *Xenobiotica,* 8, 305, 1978.
25. **Illing, H. P. A. and Fromson, J. M.,** Species difference in the disposition and metabolism of 6,11-dihydro-11-oxodibenz(be)oxepin-2-acetic acid (Isoxepac) in rat, rabbit, dog, rhesus monkey and man, *Drug Metab. Disposit.,* 6, 510, 1978.
26. **Litchfield, J. T.,** The effects of sulfanilamide on the lower vertebrates, *J. Pharmacol.,* 67, 212, 1939.
27. **Keck, G.,** Species difference in the pharmacokinetics of chemicals: correlations with toxicity, *Toxicol. Eur. Res.,* 3, 207, 1981.
28. **Scala, J., McOsker, D. E., and Reller, H. H.,** The percutaneous absorption of ionic surfactants, *J. Invest. Dermatol.,* 50, 371, 1968.
29. **Gibaldi, M. and Perrier, D.,** *Pharmacokinetics,* Marcel Dekker, New York, 1975.
30. **Rückebüsch, Y.,** Physiologie, Pharmacologie Therapeutique Animale, Maloine, S. A., Paris, 1977 (cited by Keck, ref. 27).

31. **Swaisband, A. J., Pierce, D. M., and Franklin, R. A.,** The disposition of a novel pyrimidoindole, ciclazindol, in the rat and patas monkey, *Drug Metab. Disposit.,* 5, 419, 1977.

32. **Smalley, H. E. and Radelett, R. D.,** Comparative toxicity of the herbicide paraquat in laboratory and farm animals, *Toxicol. Appl. Pharmacol.,* 17, 305, 1970.

33. **LaDu, B. N., Mandel, H. G., and Way, E. L.,** *Fundamentals of Drug Metabolism and Drug Disposition,* Williams and Wilkins, Baltimore, Md., 1971.

34. **Klaassen, C. D.,** Absorption, distribution and excretion of toxicants, in *Toxicology, The Basic Science of Poisons,* 2nd ed., Doull, J., Klaassen, C. D., and Amdur, M. O., Eds., MacMillan Publishing Co., New York, Toronto, 1980, 28.

35. **Smith, R. L.,** *The Excretory Function of Bile,* Chapman and Hall, London, 1973.

36. **Davison, C., Scrime, M., and Edeloon, J.,** Species differences in the metabolism of hycanthone, *Arch. Int. Pharmacodyn.,* 230, 4, 1977.

37. **Davison, C., Banks, W., and Fritz, A.,** The absorption, distribution and metabolic fate of danazol in rats, monkeys and human volunteers, *Arch. Int. Pharmacodyn.,* 221, 294, 1976.

38. **Klaassen, C. D.,** Pharmacokinetics of rose bengal in the rat, rabbit, dog, and guinea pig, *Toxicol. Appl. Pharmacol.,* 38, 85, 1976.

39. **Chatfield, D. H. and Green, J. N.,** Disposition and metabolism of benoxyprofen in laboratory animals and man, *Xenobiotica,* 8, 133, 1978.

40. **Quinn, G. P., Axelrod, J., and Brodie, B. B.,** Species, strain and sex differences in metabolism of hexobarbitone, amidopyrine, antipyrine, and aniline, *Biochem. Pharmacol.,* 1, 152, 1958.

41. **Kao, J., Bridges, J. W., and Faulkner, J. K.,** Metabolism of (^{14}C) phenol by sheep, pig, and rat, *Xenobiotica,* 9, 141, 1979.

42. **Kopun, M. and Propping, P.,** The kinetics of ethanol absorption and elimination in twins and supplementary repetitive experiments in singleton subjects, *Eur. J. Clin. Pharmacol.,* 11, 337, 1977.

43. **Garfinkel, D.,** Computer modeling, complex biological systems, and their simplification, *Am. J. Physiol.,* 239, R-1, 1980.

44. **Burke, M. D. and Upshall, D. G.,** Species and phenobarbitone-induced differences in the kinetic constants of liver microsomal harmine O-demethylation, *Xenobiotica,* 6, 321, 1976.

45. **Franklin, R. A. and Aldridge, A.,** Pharmacokinetics and metabolism of the new analgesic meptazinol in rats and patas monkeys, *Xenobiotica,* 6, 499, 1976.

46. **Caldwell, J., Notarianni, L. J., Smith, R. L., Tafunso, M. A., French, M. R., Dawson, P., and Bossir, O.,** Non human primate species as metabolic models for the human situation: comparative studies on meperidine metabolism, *Toxicol. Appl. Pharmacol.,* 48, 273, 1979.

47. **Smith, R. L. and Caldwell, J.,** in *Drug Metabolism from Microbes to Man,* Parke, D. V. and Smith, R. L., Eds., Taylor and Francis, London, 1976, 331.

48. **Gillette, J. R.,** Drug toxicity as a result of interference with physiological control mechanism, *Ann. N.Y. Acad. Sci.,* 123, 1965, 42.

49. **Withey, J. R.,** Pharmacokinetic principles in *Proceedings of the First International Congress on Toxicology,* Plaa, G. L. and Duncan, W. A. M., Eds., Academic Press, New York, San Francisco, London, 1978, 97.

50. **Mitchell, J. R. and Jollow, D. J.,** Metabolic activation of drugs to toxic substances, *Gastroenterology,* 68, 1975, 390.

51. **Mitchell, J. R., Potter, W. Z., Hinson, J. A., and Jollow, D. J.,** Massive hepatic necrosis caused by furosemide, a furan-containing diuretic, *Nature,* 251, 1974, 508.

52. **Potter, W. Z., Thorgeirsson, S. S., Jollow, D. J., and Mitchell, J. R.,** Acetaminophen-induced hepatic necrosis. V. Correlation of hepatic necrosis, covalent binding and glutathione depletion in hamsters, *Pharmacology,* 12, 1974, 129.

53. **Jollow, D. J., Thorgeirsson, S. S., Potter, W. Z., Hashimoto, M., and Mitchell, J. R.,** Acetaminophen-induced hepatic necrosis, *Pharmacology,* 12, 1974, 251.

Chapter 3

DIFFERENCES IN METABOLISM AT DIFFERENT DOSE LEVELS

Ellen J. O'Flaherty

TABLE OF CONTENTS

I. INTRODUCTION

Construction of a dose-response curve within the dose range associated with a measurable response in human or animal populations of finite size is the first step in the process of risk estimation at low doses. Without at least one response measurement at a known dose, risk estimation is not possible. However, it is generally accepted that the more fully the dose-response curve can be defined and the better its nature understood, the more clearly the reliability of risk estimates based on that dose-response curve can be stated. Thus, in order to be meaningful, risk estimation should originate from a dose-response relationship made up of precise measurements of response over as broad a range of doses as reasonably possible.

Dose is most commonly expressed as external or administered dose. To express dose in this way is to imply that the total amount of active agent presented to receptor molecules is proportional to the administered dose; that is, to assume that all absorptive, distributive, and eliminative processes are first-order. However, as administered dose is extended upward into the toxic range, it becomes progressively more unlikely that first-order kinetics accurately describe all the individual processes that constitute the total absorption and disposition of a foreign compound. Metabolism, as well as certain absorptive and excretory mechanisms, is inherently saturable. Nearly all toxic and carcinogenic compounds are metabolized. The potential for dose-dependent metabolism, especially at the high or maximum tolerated doses characteristically employed in carcinogenicity studies, is becoming increasingly appreciated by the toxicology community.

Dose-dependent metabolism causes a shift in the relationship of external to internal dose of the administered compound, so that internal dose is no longer proportional to external dose. If the parent compound is toxic or carcinogenic and its metabolites are not, there will be a disproportionate increase in internal exposure to the active agent at absorbed doses approaching or exceeding the maximum capacity of metabolizing enzymes to transform the parent compound to its inactive metabolites.

Although metabolism generally results in production of more polar and therefore more water soluble and more readily excretable derivatives and can in this sense be viewed as a set of reactions whose primary function is to detoxify, the importance of many metabolites as toxic or carcinogenic agents in their own right has long been recognized. Certain of these metabolites, notably for example many of the epoxides, have very short mean lifetimes. Nonetheless, however fleeting their existence, their presence at critical sites at critical times may permit them to exert their characteristic toxic or carcinogenic effect.

In addition to shifting the relationship between administered and internal dose, dose-dependent metabolism alters the relationships between administered dose and magnitude and length of exposure to active metabolites. Furthermore, depending on the relative ease of saturation of enzymes catalyzing rate-limiting steps in parallel pathways of metabolism, saturation may modify the pattern of metabolism; that is, it may increase exposure to certain metabolites or to the parent compound at the expense of exposure to other metabolites. For example, the pattern of excretion of the four major urinary metabolites of 1,1-dichloroe-thylene in rats is dose-dependent.[1,2]

The chief metabolizing organ is the liver. Because of its large total metabolic capacity, the liver is also in a unique position with regard to first-pass metabolism. A first-pass effect is a reduction in systemic availability that results from metabolism or excretion during the absorption process. Although metabolizing enzymes are present in other first-pass organs such as lung and skin, the total metabolizing ability of these organs is much less than that of the liver. The lung exerts a significant first-pass effect with regard to excretion of volatile compounds, for example, the first-pass effect on inhaled chloroform discussed by Chiou.[3] However, this is a passive excretion process and therefore is not dose-dependent.

Little is known about the effect of first-pass metabolism in organs other than the liver on internal dose. However, saturable metabolism in lung or skin is unlikely to confer important dose dependency on the relationship between administered and internal dose of compounds absorbed by these routes, because of the limited total metabolic capacity of these organs. Dose-dependent first-pass metabolism in the liver, in contrast, is likely to cause significant disproportionalities in the relationship of administered dose to the magnitude and duration of exposure to both parent and metabolites. Dose-dependent first-pass metabolism in the lung could also become important in the case of induction of metabolizing enzymes, if hepatic metabolism is perfusion-limited but lung metabolism is capacity-limited. For an excellent review and discussion of the position of the lung relative to metabolism, see Roth and Wiersma.[4]

Elimination of a compound subject to first-pass metabolism in the liver is controlled by whichever of the two processes, liver blood flow or intrinsic hepatic clearance, is rate-limiting. Intrinsic clearance (Cl_{int}) is defined as the total ability of the liver to remove a particular compound from the blood irreversibly in the absence of any flow limitations. It is related to total metabolic capacity and its dimensions, like those of blood flow, are mℓ/min. If Cl_{int} is low relative to liver blood flow, then the first-pass effect will be only slight. Saturation of metabolizing enzymes will not significantly affect the systemic availability of an oral dose since this availability was high to begin with. Phenytoin (diphenylhydantoin), discussed in greater detail in Section III.a, is such a drug. Hepatic first-pass metabolism of phenytoin is negligible. Jusko et al.[5] calculated the bioavailability of phenytoin from oral doses to be 98%. Yet the elimination of half-life of phenytoin is dose-dependent as a direct result of the low hepatic capacity for its biotransformation. In a situation such as this, induction of metabolizing enzymes could shorten the elimination half-life without significantly altering the systemic availability of the orally administered compound.

At the other extreme are compounds whose Cl_{int} equals or exceeds liver blood flow. Such compounds will exhibit significant first-pass effects. Availability from the oral route will be low. There may even be a low dose range within which the rate of absorption does not approach the maximum metabolizing capacity of the liver and the absorbed compound does not reach the systemic circulation at all. In contrast, concentrations of stable metabolites in the plasma will be high and will reach a peak earlier than they would have had administration been intravenous. Both these points are illustrated in Figure 1.[6] Nortriptyline undergoes extensive first-pass metabolism. After oral doses of 40 mg of nortriptyline hydrochloride, plasma concentrations of its hydroxylated principal metabolite were much higher relative to plasma concentrations of nortriptyline itself than after intramuscular administration, and the metabolite concentration peak occurred much earlier.

First-pass saturation of metabolizing enzymes will have a significant effect on the systemic availability of a compound with high Cl_{int}. Paradoxically, however, elimination half-life may not be affected in the same dose range. Once the compound has reached the systemic circulation and been distributed into peripheral tissues, only a fraction of the total amount present in the body traverses the liver in a single pass. Thus, it is not surprising that concentrations (more precisely, absorption or delivery rates) may be sufficiently high to saturate the metabolizing enzymes on the first pass but not on subsequent passes. A good example is phenacetin, whose elimination in healthy humans is limited by hepatic blood flow. Raaflaub and Dubach[7] showed that while elimination of an intravenous dose of 250 mg of phenacetin was well described by a first-order kinetic model with a biological half-life of 37 to 74 minutes, bioavailability of oral doses was dose-dependent, being negligible in six subjects given a 250-mg dose and from 0 to 49% in four subjects given a 1-g dose. Induction of metabolism of compounds in this class will result in decreased systemic availability of an oral dose but may not affect elimination half-life. An analogy is capacity-limited acetylation, known to be bimodally distributed in the human population. Talseth[8]

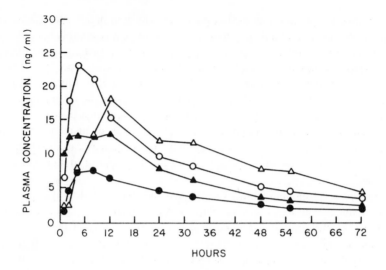

FIGURE 1. Mean plasma concentrations of nortriptyline (solid symbols) and its major metabolite 10-hydroxynortriptyline (open symbols) after oral (●,○) and intramuscular (▲,△) administration to 6 patients. (Reproduced from Alván, G., Lind, M., Mellström, B., and von Bahr, C., *J. Pharmacokinet. Biopharmaceut.,* 5, 193, 1977. With permission.)

demonstrated that systemic availability of oral doses of hydralazine was dose dependent in both slow and rapid acetylators. Saturation of first-pass hydralazine metabolism was observed in slow acetylators at doses of 25 to 50 mg and in rapid acetylators at doses of 100 to 150 mg, reflecting the difference in metabolic capacity between these two groups. Nonetheless, during the post-distributive phase following these oral doses, subjects in both groups had essentially the same hydralazine half-life. This half-life was not dose-dependent.

Saturation of metabolic processes is not the only explanation for dose-dependent metabolism. Stores of requisite cofactors for biotransformation processes will be depleted more rapidly at very high than at low doses, and may become rate-limiting after a short time. In one of the first reports of dose-dependent metabolism, it was observed that while small to moderate amounts of benzoic acid given to humans were excreted in the urine almost entirely as the glycine conjugate hippuric acid, larger amounts were excreted partly as the glucuronic acid conjugate.[9] The amount of hippuric acid formed is limited in this case by the supply of glycine. Hepatic stores of the tripeptide glutathione can be depleted by conjugation with reactive metabolites of a number of compounds when these are present in excess, and in some cases may be depleted to the point of becoming rate-limiting in elimination. Jollow et al.[10] showed that the epoxide metabolite of bromobenzene was detoxified by conjugation with glutathione, and demonstrated an inverse correlation between hepatic glutathione content and hepatic necrosis when bromobenzene was given to rats. Mitchell et al.[11] demonstrated a similar relationship in the case of acetaminophen exposure. Glutathione availability can also alter the pattern of metabolite formation, as has been demonstrated for metabolites of 1,1-dichloroethylene in rats.[1,2] It should be noted here, however, that not all compounds that deplete glutathione cause hepatotoxicity, and that detoxification by conjugation with glutathione is less important quantitatively in humans than in other species.[11,12]

Product or substrate inhibition may be postulated to occur at high doses, although such mechanisms have not been documented for toxicants or carcinogens. The compound may alter hepatic blood flow in a dose-dependent fashion, effectively altering the rate at which substrate is presented to metabolizing enzymes. Whether an alteration in blood flow alters the rate of metabolism depends upon whether metabolism is perfusion-rate-limited or metabolism-rate-limited (capacity-limited) in the dose range of interest. This point is discussed in Section III. Blood flow could be either increased or decreased by an active compound. For example, it has been speculated that a transient increase in glomerular blood flow in response to either prednisone or prednisolone may be partly responsible for the increase in clearance of these compounds with increasing dose in humans.[13] Other sources of dose-dependent metabolism, such as the influence of concentration-dependent plasma protein binding on rate of substrate delivery to metabolizing enzymes,[14] can readily be postulated.

It is apparent that no single model will suffice to explain all forms of dose-dependent metabolism. In this chapter, several examples will be developed in some detail. The compounds selected are those whose behavior most clearly illustrates the points to be made, and for which the relationship between dose-dependent metabolism and effect is best understood. No attempt is made to be comprehensive, or to provide a survey of toxicants and carcinogens whose metabolism is known or suspected to be dose dependent. A comprehensive review of saturable metabolism and its relationship to toxicity has appeared recently.[15]

The remainder of this chapter is divided into two parts. In the first (Section II), several ways of expressing dose are considered and compared. In the second (Section III), examples are given of how dose-dependent metabolism can affect the relationship between external exposure and effect, and wherever possible anomalous dose-effect curves are resolved by the application of models relating administered to internal dose.

II. EXPRESSION OF DOSE

In experimental studies of acute toxicity, the dose is an amount. Usually it is expressed either as the total amount or as an amount per unit body weight. As pointed out above to relate administered dose to effect or response is to assume that the total amount of active agent reaching the receptor sites is the same as, or at least directly proportional to, administered dose; that is, that integrated internal exposure (concentration × time) at the receptor sites is proportional to administered dose. If any of the kinetically significant parallel processes (distribution, metabolism, and excretion) responsible for disposition of the administered compound is dose-dependent, the assumption of proportionality between external and internal dose is violated. Since metabolism and excretion are especially likely to be dose dependent at the high exposures characteristic of toxicity and carcinogenicity studies, a more appropriate measure of exposure than administered dose must be sought.

If concentration at the receptor sites can safely be assumed to be proportional to concentration in the blood or blood plasma, then integrated effective internal exposure can be expressed as the integral of concentration in blood over time:

$$\int_{t=0}^{t=\infty} C(t)dt, \tag{1}$$

where $C(t)$ is the concentration at time t and the integration is carried out from time $t = 0$ to time $t = \infty$. The assumption of proportionality between blood or plasma concentration and concentration at receptor sites carries some risk; however, distribution processes are not as likely to be sources of dose-dependent kinetic behavior as are absorption or elimination processes.

The integral in Equation 1 represents the area under the plasma concentration vs. time curve, or AUC_∞. If disposition kinetics are not dose-dependent, $AUC\infty$ is proportional to administered dose. For example, the rate of change of concentration in the one-compartment model

$$\frac{dC(t)}{dt} = -k_e C(t), \tag{2}$$

from which

$$C(t) = C_o e^{-k_e t} \qquad (3)$$

and

$$AUC_\infty = \int_{t=0}^{t=\infty} C(t)dt \quad = \int_{t=0}^{t=\infty} C_o e - k_e t_{dt} \quad = \frac{C_o}{k_e} = \frac{D}{V_D k_e} \qquad (4)$$

where k_e is the overall rate constant of elimination, V_D is the volume of distribution (which is almost always an apparent volume), and the initial concentration $C_o = D/V_D$ where D is the dose administered instantaneously at $t=0$. In fact, $AUC_\infty = D/V_D k_e$ whether D is considered to be administered instantaneously (e.g., intravenously) or to be absorbed by a first-order mechanism (e.g., orally). In the latter case, D is replaced by the expression FD, where F is the fraction of the dose absorbed.

When elimination mechanisms are dose-dependent, AUC_∞ is still the appropriate measure of integrated internal dose. However, under these conditions it is no longer proportional to administered dose. For the simplest case of a single saturable pathway of elimination, the rate of loss of the compound from the plasma is

$$\frac{dC(t)}{dt} = - \frac{V_m C(t)}{K_m + C(t)} \qquad (5)$$

This is the familiar Michaelis-Menten equation, in which V_m is the maximum rate of elimination, achieved when all active elimination sites are occupied, and K_m is the half-saturation constant, or concentration at which $dC(t)/dt = V_m/2$. At very low $C(t)$ such that $K_m \gg C(t)$,

$$\frac{dC(t)}{dt} \approx - \left(\frac{V_m}{K_m}\right) C(t), \qquad (6)$$

so

$$(V_m/K_m) = k_e. \qquad (6A)$$

Compounds whose elimination follows equation (5) are said to exhibit Michaelis-Menten kinetics. The Michaelis-Menten equation can be integrated to give an expression for $C(t)$:

$$C(t) = C_o + K_m \ln(Co/C(t)) - V_m t. \qquad (7)$$

The AUC_∞ can be explicitly defined[16] (in this and all subsequent equations, D refers to the internal dose, or the total amount of the compound reaching the systemic circulation. When the compound is given by any route other than the intravenous route, internal dose may be only a fraction F of administered dose, as discussed above in connection with Equation (4)).

$$AUC_\infty = \frac{Co}{V_m} \left(\frac{Co}{2} + K_m\right) = \frac{D}{V_D V_m} \left(\frac{D}{2V_D} + K_m\right) \qquad (8)$$

It should be noted that when $C_o \ll K_m$, AUC_∞ reduces to $(K_m/V_m) C_o$ or $D/k_e V_D$, as it must; and when $C_o/2 \gg K_m$, AUC_∞ becomes $C_0^2/2 \, Vm$.

Clearance is a useful measure of elimination related to AUC_∞. The total clearance (Cl_{total}) of a compound given acutely is defined as

$$Cl_{total} = \frac{D}{AUC_\infty} \qquad (9)$$

Cl_{total} can be thought of as an average clearance taken over the entire time course of elimination. If all elimination processes are first-order, then from Equation (4),

$$Cl_{total} = k_e V_D. \qquad (10)$$

Thus, if all elimination processes are first-order, Cl_{total} is a constant, independent of concentration (e.g., of dose). First-order clearance by any specific route can conveniently be expressed in another way. For extraction and metabolism by the liver, with which we are principally concerned,

$$\frac{dH}{dt} = k_h\, C(t)\, V_D, \qquad (11)$$

where dH/dt is the rate of extraction and k_h is the first-order rate constant for the extraction process. (Equation (11) is written for extraction as the rate-limiting process because extraction is presumed to be first-order. In fact, either extraction or metabolism can be rate-limiting. In the latter case, hepatic elimination is saturable and the behavior of $Cl_{hepatic}$ is as described below.) From Equation (11),

$$Cl_{hepatic} = k_h V_D = dH/dt/C(t). \qquad (12)$$

Hepatic clearance, then, is calculable as the rate of extraction of the compound from blood perfusing the liver divided by its concentration in entering blood, provided that extraction is the rate-limiting step. If all elimination takes place by metabolism, then $Cl_{total} = Cl_{hepatic}$.

Irrespective of how it is calculated, clearance is expressed in units of volume per unit of time. Clearance therefore represents the volume of the compartment from which loss is occurring that is cleared of its content of the compound in the designated time unit. Clearance is most often expressed in units of $m\ell/min$.

If metabolism is the rate-limiting process and is saturable, substitution of Equation (8) into Equation (9) and simplification shows that

$$Cl_{total} = \frac{V_D V_m}{Co/2 + K_m}, \qquad (13)$$

from which it can be seen that Cl_{total} decreases as the dose is increased.

Chronic toxicity studies or environmental exposures present a different problem with regard to expression of dose. Although AUC_t to any time t can be defined and estimated (a sort of "integrated internal exposure" that increases continuously as length of exposure increases), there is considerable evidence that for most toxicants, exposure rates that have not been associated with untoward effects within 90 days may be continued indefinitely with little risk of appearance of an additional toxic effect.[17] An exception may be made for those effects that are slow in developing or appear later in life, such as lead-related nephropathy. However, often it is not certain whether the delay in onset of such effects is due to a requirement for continuing exposure to the precipitating agent or simply to a long induction period. For toxicants associated with effects that appear relatively promptly, steady-state plasma concentration is probably a better index of exposure than AUC during long-term exposure.

There is an interesting parallel between AUC_x and steady-state plasma concentration. When all elimination processes are first-order, steady-state plasma concentration

$$C_{ss} = \frac{DR}{k_e V_D} , \tag{14}$$

where DR is dose rate, expressed as the rate of absorption into the systemic circulation. Clearance under these conditions can be expressed as

$$Cl_{total} = \frac{DR}{C_{ss}} \tag{15}$$

This is equivalent to the definition of Cl_{total} given by equation (9).

For the case of a single saturable elimination mechanism,

$$C_{ss} = DR \left(\frac{K_m + C_{ss}}{V_D V_m} \right) \tag{16}$$

as long as DR does not exceed V_m. Thus,

$$\frac{DR}{C_{ss}} = \frac{V_D V_m}{K_m + C_{ss}} \tag{17}$$

Comparison of Equations 15 and 9, and of Equations 17 and 13, shows that clearance during chronic exposure is related to C_{ss} and DR in the same way in which total clearance after an acute exposure is related to AUC_x and D, irrespective of whether elimination kinetics are first-order throughout the entire concentration range of concern or reach saturation within that range.

During a continuous, constant exposure, as in an inhalation experiment, C_{ss} can be measured at any time in blood once steady state has been attained. Other experimental designs require that known doses of the test compound be given repeatedly; for example, by daily gavage. For the pattern of intermittent exposure at regular intervals τ, the average concentration $\overline{C}_n$ during the nth dosing interval can be defined as[18]

$$\overline{C}_n = \frac{1}{\tau} \int_{t_n}^{t_{n+1}} C(n,t) \, dt, \tag{18}$$

where t_n and t_{n+1} are the times at the beginning and end of the nth dosing interval, respectively. The integral is, of course, the AUC from t_n to t_{n+1}. It can be shown[19] that once steady state has been achieved, the value of this integral is $D/k_e V_D$, identical to the value of AUC_x after an acute dose D, so that the average concentration at steady state is

$$\overline{C}_n = \frac{D}{\tau k_e V_D} \text{ or } \frac{DR}{k_e V_D} \tag{19}$$

Thus, while C_{ss} is the appropriate measure of internal exposure during inhalation to steady state, in the case of a repeated-administration experimental design AUC from t_n to t_{n+1} at steady state may be used instead since it is directly proportional to C_{ss}.

For some toxicants or carcinogens it is not elimination of parent compound but production of an active metabolite that is of primary concern. If a metabolite is the active moiety, integrated internal exposure to metabolite could in principle be expressed as the area under the metabolite plasma concentration vs. time curve or $AUC_{m\infty}$. There is no exact solution for $AUC_{m\infty}$ as a function of dose of the parent compound when the process of metabolite formation is saturable. At very low exposures, where concentrations of the parent compound are much less than the K_m values of all the biotransformation enzymes acting on it, $AUC_{m\infty}$ will be proportional to the dose of parent compound. At very high exposures, where the rate of biotransformation is at its maximum during a major portion of the elimination period, $AUC_{m\infty}$ will be strongly influenced by V_m. Other factors, however, also act to influence total exposure to metabolite. The extent of metabolite formation will be affected by the degree to which the parent compound can be metabolized by other pathways, and by whether these pathways are saturable or are approaching saturation in the concentration range of interest. For example, a first-order elimination mechanism in parallel with saturable mechanisms will be responsible for elimination of increasingly greater fractions of the parent compound as concentrations approach and exceed the levels at which the other mechanisms are saturated. This behavior is characteristic of volatile compounds, which are eliminated unchanged in expired air in addition to being eliminated by metabolism. Since clearance from the lung is first-order, elimination by this route will account for increasingly larger fractions of the administered compound as the metabolic pathways approach saturation. Fasted rats exposed for 6 hr by inhalation to 1,1-dichloroethylene exhaled only 1.6% of their end-exposure body burden when the exposure atmosphere concentration was 10 ppm, but 8.4% when the concentration was 200 ppm.[20] Similarly, the percentage of vinyl chloride monomer body burden exhaled unchanged by rats increased from 1.6 to 12.3 as the concentration of vinyl chloride monomer in the inhaled air was increased from 10 to 1000 ppm.[21] Much larger percentages than these may be exhaled. In a recent study in which rats were exposed by inhalation to n-hexane, the authors reported that 88% of the amount taken up at an atmospheric n-hexane concentration of 500 ppm was metabolized, while only 38% of the amount taken up at 10,000 ppm was metabolized. Thus, 12% was eliminated unchanged by exhalation at 500 ppm but 62% was exhaled unchanged at 10,000 ppm.[22]

Nonvolatile chemicals may also be excreted by first-order pathways, of which glomerular filtration is an example. Biliary excretion may be first-order, but some chemicals are known to be excreted into the bile by saturable mechanisms.[23]

Measurement of $AUC_{m\infty}$ is straightforward in principle but often unachievable in practice. The identity of the active metabolite may not be known. Or the active metabolite may be a short-lived intermediate in a reaction sequence, so reactive or unstable that it does not leave the tissue in which it is formed to appear in the systemic circulation. If the metabolite is especially reactive, it may be quantitatively a very minor component of the metabolite mix whose behavior is not reflected in the overall kinetic behavior of the parent compound or of any of the other metabolites. Highly reactive compounds may bind covalently to cellular macromolecules and, by doing so, initiate carcinogenic or mutagenic sequences. Gillette[24,25] has discussed the kinetics and actions of reversibly acting (relatively unreactive) and irreversibly acting (reactive; capable of forming covalent bonds) compounds, and the difficulties associated particularly with estimation of total exposure to reactive metabolites.

One approach to estimation of exposure to metabolite when $AUC_{m\infty}$ cannot be measured directly has been to use the end products of metabolism; that is, the stable metabolites excreted in urine and possibly feces, as an index of total metabolite production. Provided that metabolite elimination is first-order, the "dose" of metabolite or total amount of metabolite produced should be proportional to $AUC_{m\infty}$. This is true of both single-dose and repeated-dose studies; see Equation 19. Thus, the amount and perhaps even the identity of the reactive precursor are inferred from the amounts and identities of the stable end products of metabolism.

Measurement of metabolic end products provides useful information (1) when there is only one stable end product, or (2) when all stable end products that are measured originate directly or indirectly from the toxic intermediate, or (3) in the unlikely event that all parallel metabolic pathways have the same V_m and K_m values. This technique has been used in a study of the metabolism and hepatotoxicity of perchloroethylene and trichlorethylene (see Section III).

A modification of the method of determining the total amounts of metabolites produced is to use the measured rate of metabolite production (or rate of loss of parent compound) as an index of the amount of metabolite formed. While this method may be experimentally somewhat simpler, it has certain drawbacks. The rate of metabolite production is not constant during the period of elimination of a single dose. At high doses of the parent compound, the rate of metabolite production may vary from a maximum of V_m downward to low rates proportional to terminal concentrations of parent compound during the course of elimination of a single dose. Furthermore, if virtually all of the parent compound is ultimately transformed to a single reactive metabolite, the rate at which that metabolite is formed may be of little or no importance. On the other hand, if the metabolite is relatively unreactive so that a substantial fraction is eliminated without having been combined with a receptor site, a very slow rate of formation relative to elimination may be of consequence in that plasma concentrations will remain low throughout the entire course of elimination and $AUC_{m\infty}$ may be determined by the rate of metabolite formation rather than by the rate of its elimination. This raises the related question whether AUC is necessarily always the most appropriate exposure index. Very slow formation of metabolite over a long period of time to produce prolonged low concentration in body fluids may not be equivalent in its effect to rapid production of metabolite with achievement of relatively high concentrations in body fluids, even though the areas under the two blood metabolite concentration-time curves are equal.

Other considerations also complicate estimation of exposure to metabolites. For example, transfer of parent to a storage tissue with slow postexposure release can greatly extend the period of first-order kinetics of metabolite formation. The apparent half-life of carbon monoxide (CO) formed from dichloromethane is more than twice as great as the half-life of CO itself, as measured in alveolar air of workers exposed for 8 hr by inhalation to either dichloromethane or to CO.[26,27] This is not because there is a real difference in CO half-life in the two cases, but rather because dichloromethane stored in body tissues continues to provide a source of CO subsequent to removal of the subject from the dichloromethane exposure atmosphere. In this way CO production, and hence its elimination, are prolonged.

Most of these considerations apply principally to single-dose studies. They are of lesser theoretical and practical concern when exposure is continuous or chronic. During chronic exposure the mean steady-state concentration of metabolite should be proportional to the rate of formation of metabolite ("DR" in Equation 14), as long as metabolite elimination remains first-order. Therefore, steady-state blood levels of metabolite may be constant and independent of exposure at high exposures where the rate of metabolite formation is saturated. If metabolite elimination is itself saturable at these high doses, Equation 16 could be used to predict metabolite steady-state concentration provided that the rate of formation of metabolite (the value of DR/V_D in Equation 16) does not exceed the rate of its elimination. Of course, metabolite, like its parent, may be eliminated by parallel first-order and saturable mechanisms. In this case metabolite concentration cannot increase indefinitely; there must be a steady-state metabolite concentration, albeit possibly a large one, at which formation rate is equal to elimination rate.

Experience has shown that approximating the amount of metabolite formed (or the steady-state concentration of metabolite) by estimating the rate of its formation over a limited time period can provide useful and toxicologically significant information. This was the approach adopted by Gehring et al.,[28] who estimated exposure to metabolites of vinyl chloride monomer

(VCM) by measuring the total amount of VCM metabolized during a 6-hr inhalation exposure of rats to VCM. Post-exposure metabolism was not taken into account. This ground-breaking study and the associated analysis in which VCM metabolism was successfully related to its tumor-producing action is discussed in greater detail in Section III.

This discussion has not dealt in any way with the possibility that both parent and metabolite may be active agents, perhaps with differing potencies. This is not at all an unusual situation, particularly with drugs whose metabolites are structurally similar to the parent drug and may bind reversibly to the same active site. It should be readily apparent that models become impracticably complex rather quickly in such situations. In cases of complex kinetics and dynamics, if concentrations in the blood can be measured it may be possible to relate them to a measured effect. This will, of course, be true only for relatively chemically stable or reversibly acting drugs and toxicants. A good example is the work of Hinderling and Garrett,[29] who were able to correlate the cardioactive effects of β-methyldigoxin with the total amounts of β-methyldigoxin and its active metabolite digoxin combined in specific compartments of a multicompartment kinetic model. While the model developed by Hinderling and Garrett was a linear one, the same approach could be adopted for reversibly acting drugs and toxicants that exhibit dose-dependent kinetics of elimination.

III. EXAMPLES OF THE APPLICATION OF THESE PRINCIPLES

In this section, several selected examples will be given in some detail. The paucity of examples of application of the principles discussed in the previous section to toxicological problems is striking. Indeed, the first three examples given below are taken from the pharmaceutical literature. Their inclusion illustrates the fact that although systematic investigations into toxicant and carcinogen kinetics are now being undertaken, the most detailed and complete kinetic studies in the literature to date remain studies of drugs. In addition, these examples of metabolic saturation even at pharmacologic dose levels should serve as a reminder of the generality of saturability of metabolic and other elimination processes and the strong possibility that at least one such pathway is likely to be saturated when exposures lie within a toxic range.

A limited number of investigations have been undertaken in which apparently anomalous dose-toxicity curves have been successfully resolved by relating toxicity to steady-state concentration or area under the concentration curve of the active moiety. Consideration of dose-dependent metabolism and its consequences has been the key. These analyses are also discussed in this section.

A. Chronic Exposure: Steady-State Concentration of Parent Compound: Three Drugs
Equation 14 states that steady-state concentration should be directly proportional to dose rate as long as all elimination mechanisms are first-order. This expectation has been amply verified for many compounds, at least at low dose rates. An interesting example is theophylline (1,3-dimethylxanthine), a bronchodilator used in treatment of asthma. The therapeutic plasma concentration range for theophylline is 10 to 20 μg/mℓ,[30] and within this range therapeutic effect correlates with plasma concentration.[31,32] However, theophylline has a low therapeutic index. Toxicity, which can be serious, is associated with plasma concentrations above about 20 μg/mℓ.[33,34] The magnitude of adverse effects is also correlated with plasma concentration.[35] Consequently, the nature of the relationship between dose regimen and plasma concentration at steady state is of considerable interest to the clinician.

Figure 2 is taken from a study of theophylline clearance.[36] It demonstrates that the relationship between theophylline infusion rate and steady-state plasma concentration is linear at least up to concentrations of 25 μg/mℓ in the six patients studied. On the basis of this and other evidence, theophylline elimination has been presumed to be first-order.

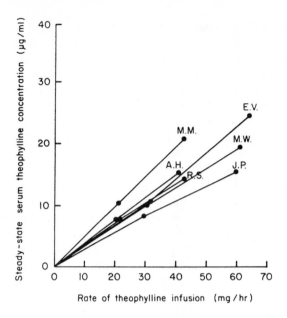

FIGURE 2. Serum theophylline concentrations resulting from constant intravenous infusions at two rates in each of six patients. (Adapted from Weinberger, M., Hudgel, D., Spector, S., and Chidsey, C., *J. Allergy Clin. Immunol.*, 59, 228, 1977. With permission.)

However, more careful examination of theophylline kinetics has shown that this premise is not justified, at least not at the higher doses associated with toxicity. Caldwell et al.[37] reported that while urinary elimination of theophylline itself and of two of its metabolites followed first-order kinetics in adult volunteers given a large single dose of theophylline, the major metabolite 3-methylxanthine, which accounts for as much as 35 to 40% of theophylline elimination, was excreted by Michaelis-Menten kinetics. Since 3-methylxanthine does not accumulate in body fluids, it is the biotransformation step itself that is saturable. Theophylline is eliminated by parallel first-order and saturable mechanisms. As might be expected when only one of multiple pathways for elimination is saturable, evidence for nonlinearity of overall theophylline elimination kinetics is equivocal. Systematic trends in deviation from the linearity of Figure 2 tend to be slight, and not statistically significant. Nonlinearity has been demonstrated most clearly in a group of children administered two separate infusions of theophylline.[38] The second infusion rate was chosen after the steady-state plasma theophylline concentration associated with the first infusion had been established, and was selected on the basis that it should produce a steady-state plasma concentration slightly less than 20 µg/mℓ, assuming a linear relationship between infusion rate and steady-state plasma concentration in each child. However, in 6 of 20 children the new steady-state plasma concentration exceeded 20 µg/mℓ, the highest being 31 µg/mℓ; and clearances at the lower infusion rates were slightly but statistically significantly higher than at the higher infusion rates. Figure 3 shows the relationship of steady-state concentration ratio to infusion rate ratio in these children. Plasma theophylline concentrations were followed for nearly 32 hr in another child who had suffered a seizure consequent to an inadvertent 50% increase in her daily dose of theophylline. This child's plasma theophylline concentration, which previously had not exceeded 18 µg/mℓ, reached 72 µg/mℓ after several days at the increased dose rate. Loss of theophylline from her plasma, once the medication error had been corrected, appeared to be a Michaelis-Menten process. This is a typical experience with theophylline: occasional patients exhibit unequivocal non-first-order kinetics,[38,39] while such

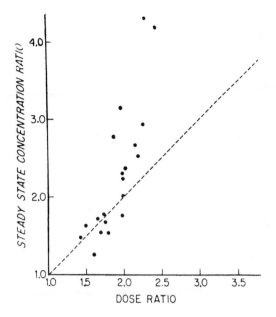

FIGURE 3. Relationship of the ratio of steady-state concentrations to the ratio of intravenous infusion rates of theophylline in 20 asthmatic children administered two separate
infusions of theophylline. The dotted line indicates the proportional changes that would be observed if elimination
kinetics were first-order. (Reproduced from Weinberger, M.
and Ginchansky, E., *J. Pediatr.*, 91, 820, 1977. With
permission.)

behavior may be difficult to detect when group means are compared, especially at low dose
rates.[40] Thus, the presence of a saturable pathway of theophylline metabolism may contribute
significantly to the wide variability in theophylline clearance among healthy individuals that
is a characteristic feature of theophylline kinetics.[33,41,42]

Other pharmacologically active agents are also metabolized by dose-dependent pathways.
Salicylic acid, produced by the rapid and nearly complete hydrolysis of its precursor ace-
tylsalicylic acid (aspirin), is a well-known example. Like theophylline, salicylic acid can
be toxic at concentrations only slightly in excess of its therapeutic range, so that metabolic
nonlinearity is a potential source of concern with regard to toxicity. Of the five routes by
which salicylic acid may be eliminated, two, both metabolic pathways, are saturable. Taken
together, these two pathways account for more than 90% of salicylic acid elimination at low
doses; however, the K_m's for both are well within the range of plasma concentrations expected
with common dosing patterns.[43] Consequently, it is to be expected that salicylic acid elimination should show much more clearcut dose dependence than theophylline elimination.
That this expectation is correct is shown in Figure 4, based on data from Aarons et al.,[44]
in which steady-state plasma concentration of free (not protein-bound) salicylic acid is given
as a function of the dose of aspirin taken every 8 hr by two human subjects. Both the
disproportionality and the intersubject differences are marked.

A final example from the pharmaceutical literature is phenytoin (diphenylhydantoin).
Although several metabolites of phenytoin have been identified, available data are compatible
with the premise that a single metabolic step is rate-limiting.[45] This step is saturable. Thus,
the rate of plasma concentration decline after a single dose of phenytoin should be describable
by Michaelis-Menten kinetics. A number of investigators have shown that the Michaelis-
Menten equation provides a good fit to phenytoin concentration data, and have estimated

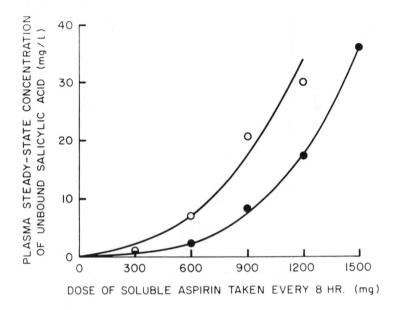

FIGURE 4.   Steady-state concentration of salicylic acid as a function of dose rate
in two healthy volunteers. Curves were drawn by inspection. (Data from Aarons,
L. J., Bochner, F., and Rowland, M., *Brit. J. Pharmacol.*, 61, 456, 1977. With
permission.)

K_m values in the range of 5 to 25 $\mu g/m\ell$.[45-48] Since the therapeutic concentration range is
10 to 20 $\mu g/m\ell$,[45] nonlinearity of phenytoin kinetics should be apparent even within the
therapeutic range. Further, the therapeutic index is small and central nervous system toxicity
may occur at plasma concentrations only slightly greater than 20 $\mu g/m\ell$. Thus, it is critically
important to control for dose-dependent kinetics of phenytoin if toxicity is to be avoided.
The relationship of steady-state plasma phenytoin concentration to phenytoin dose rate in 5
patients is shown in Figure 5.[49] The shaded area defines a therapeutic concentration range
of 10 to 25 $\mu g/m\ell$. The excellent Michaelis-Menten fit is apparent. The interindividual
variability is reduced if dose is expressed on the basis of body weight,[45] but even then
considerable interindividual variability remains.

All three of the drugs whose kinetics have been summarized illustrate the wide intersubject
variability in kinetic behavior that is a common property of substances eliminated largely
by metabolism. Since for each of these three drugs both therapeutic and toxic action have
been shown to be correlated with plasma concentration of parent (that is, the metabolites
are inactive or only slightly active), a dose-effect or dose-response curve could be developed
for each of them, relating toxicity to steady-state concentration of drug. However, the
published toxicity data are unfortunately not adequate for this purpose. Plasma drug concentrations are generally grouped into ranges, and insufficient individual data points are
available. The pharmacologist is, after all, concerned with avoidance rather than with quantitation of toxicity.

B. Continuous Exposure: Steady-State Concentrations of Parent and Metabolite: Dichloromethane

Human exposure to dichloromethane (DCM; also methylene chloride), a commercially
important solvent, is most commonly by inhalation. Elevated carboxyhemoglobin (COHb)
levels in humans exposed to DCM vapors were first noted and reported by Stewart et al.[50]
Within a short time it was established that the source of this excess COHb was DCM itself;
that is, that DCM is metabolized to carbon monoxide (CO).[51,52] CO is not the only metabolite,

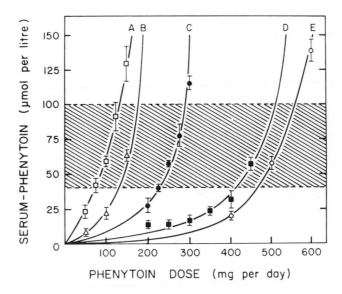

FIGURE 5. Relationship between daily dose of phenytoin and resulting serum concentration in five patients. Data points are the means of 3 to 8 values. The SEM is shown. The hatched area represents the therapeutic range of serum concentrations. The curves were fit by computer, using the Michaelis-Menten equation. (Reproduced from Richens, A. and Dunlop, A., *Lancet*, 2, 247, 1975. With permission.)

however. DCM is also biotransformed to CO_2[52,53] and to stable nonvolatile metabolites[54,55] and is exhaled unchanged.[52,55] The pathways leading to formation of CO and CO_2 are independent, the former being mediated by a microsomal cytochrome P-450-dependent mixed function oxidase system[56] and the latter by a cytosolic pathway involving glutathione.[57] It should be noted that this is an instance in which the putative intermediate glutathione conjugate, S-chloromethyl glutathione, may possess alkylating ability; it is a homolog of the mutagen S-chloroethyl glutathione,[58,59] and is also related to the halomethyl methyl ethers and bis-halomethyl ethers, established tumorigens in mice and rats.[60-64]

Both formation of CO and formation of CO_2 from DCM are saturable. The data of McKenna et al.[55] may be used to suggest the order of magnitude of the values of K_m and V_m for these two pathways in rats. In this study the rats were exposed for 6 hr by inhalation to chamber concentrations of 50, 500, or 1500 ppm [^{14}C]-DCM. Measurements of plasma DCM concentration and of percent carboxyhemoglobin (COHb) saturation made at 30-min intervals during the exposure period showed that DCM steady state was attained after about 2 hr while achievement of an apparent COHb steady state required 1 to 3 hr, depending on dose. Body burden of ^{14}C at the end of the 6-hr exposure was calculated as total radiolabel recovered during the first 48 hr after exposure. The amounts excreted as ^{14}CO and as ^{14}CO$_2$ and remaining in the carcass during the same 48 hr period are shown in Figure 6. ^{14}C present in the carcass, which was shown not to be DCM, may be in part nonvolatile metabolic intermediates in the pathways to CO or CO_2.

It appears that K_m is below the intermediate inhalation concentration of 500 ppm in both cases. Using the data of Rodkey and Collison,[65] Andersen[15] calculated that K_m for CO production from DCM should be less than 250 ppm.

As expected when two major pathways of metabolism are close to saturation, the percent of the ^{14}C body burden excreted as DCM during the first 48 hr after exposure increases with increasing chamber DCM concentration. This behavior is shown in Figure 7. Steady-state plasma DCM concentration also increases disproportionately with dose (Figure 8). It should

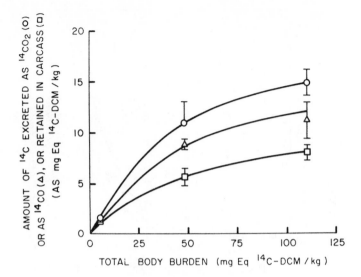

FIGURE 6.   The amount of ^{14}C excreted as $^{14}CO_2$ (○) or as ^{14}CO (△), or retained in the carcass (□), by 48 hr after termination of a 6-hr inhalation exposure of rats to ^{14}C-DCM. Calculation of initial body burden is described in the text. The SD is shown except where it lies within the symbol. Curves were drawn by inspection. (Data from McKenna, M. J., Zempel, J. A., and Braun, W. H., *Toxicol. Appl. Pharmacol.*, 65, 1, 1982. With permission.)

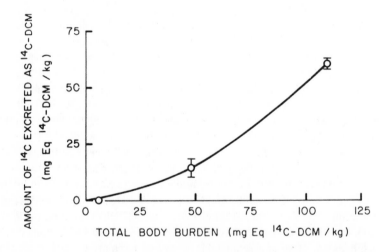

FIGURE 7.   The amount of ^{14}C excreted as ^{14}C-DCM by 48 hr after termination of a 6-hr inhalation exposure of rats to ^{14}C-DCM. Calculation of initial body burden is described in the text. The SD is shown except where it lies within the symbol. The curve was drawn by inspection. (Data from McKenna, M. J., Zempel, J. A., and Braun, W. H., *Toxicol. Appl. Pharmacol.*, 65, 1, 1982. With permission.)

be noted that body burden in this study is not equivalent to total dose, since considerable elimination of ^{14}C has occurred by the end of the 6 hr exposure. Further, since elimination is dose-dependent, ^{14}C body burden after 6 hr is not proportional to DCM concentration in the exposure atmosphere.

One important consequence of saturation of the metabolic pathway by which CO is produced is that percent COHb saturation does not exceed 10 to 13, as shown in Figure 9. No increase in steady-state COHb level was observed at the 1500 ppm chamber concentration

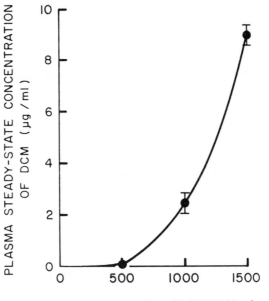

FIGURE 8. Steady-state plasma concentration of DCM in rats as a function of inhalation exposure concentration. Data points are the means of values from 3 rats. The SD is shown except where it lies within the symbol. The curve was drawn by inspection. (Data from McKenna, M. J., Zempel, J. A., and Braun, W. H., *Toxicol. Appl. Pharmacol.*, 65, 1, 1982. With permission.)

compared with the 500 ppm concentration. Whatever the overall relationship between DCM metabolism and toxicity, it is clear that the potentially toxic production of CO with formation of COHb is self-limiting as a result of saturation of the CO-producing mechanism.

It is not known whether CO production from DCM in humans approaches saturation within a comparable range of DCM inhalation exposures, although several observations suggest that this may be so. In controlled inhalation studies with human volunteers, DiVincenzo and Kaplan[66] showed that blood concentrations of DCM and percent COHb saturation in blood were both directly proportional to the magnitude of exposure up to 200 ppm. Stewart et al.[27] and Peterson[67] presented data very similar to those of DiVincenzo and Kaplan for blood concentrations of DCM in humans exposed by inhalation to up to 250 ppm DCM. However, at 500 ppm the blood concentration of DCM in both of these studies was slightly higher than would have been expected on the basis of linear kinetic behavior. Stewart et al.[27] stated that exhaled CO was directly proportional to the magnitude of DCM exposure. In contrast, the empirical equation developed by Peterson[67] to describe the elevation of percent COHb saturation above preexposure values reflects a nonlinear dependence of COHb on DCM exposure, consistent with approaching saturation of CO production, for exposures up to 500 ppm. At still higher exposures, up to 1000 ppm, Gamberale et al.[68] demonstrated that steady state concentrations of DCM in arterial blood increased disproportionately with the concentration of DCM in inspired air. These are concentrations at and above those that might be encountered in the workplace. Several studies have shown that within the range of workplace exposures, COHb rarely exceeds about 10% of saturation even in workers exposed daily.[66,67,69,70] This degree of saturation is below the level at which toxicity is anticipated except in persons with severe cardiovascular disease.[71]

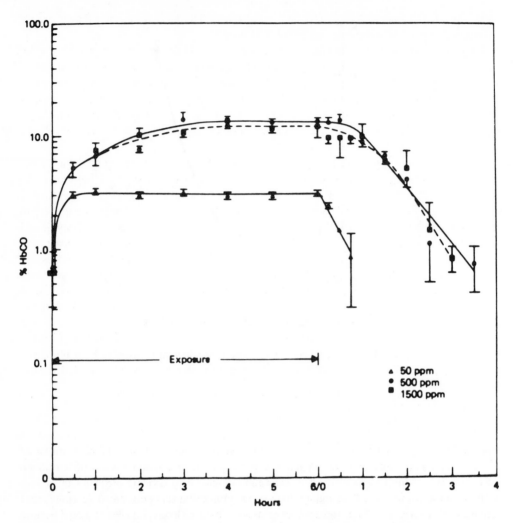

FIGURE 9.   Blood COHb levels (percent of saturation) in rats during and after a 6-hr DCM inhalation exposure. Data points are the means ± SEM of values from 2 to 4 rats. (Reproduced from McKenna, M. J., Zempel, J. A., and Braun, W. H., *Toxicol. Appl. Pharmacol.*, 65, 1, 1982. With permission.)

C. Chronic Exposure: Excretion of Stable Metabolites: Perchloroethylene and Tri-chloroethylene Hepatotoxicity.

It was pointed out in Section II above that the total amount of a reactive metabolite should be proportional to $AUC_{m\infty}$ as long as metabolite elimination mechanisms remain first-order, and that total stable end products may be used as an index of the amount of reactive metabolite produced provided that all end products originating from the reactive intermediate have been accounted for. A recently completed study from this author's laboratory[72] illustrates two of the ways in which total stable metabolite excretion can relate to dose of parent compound under these conditions.

Both trichloroethylene (TRI) and perchloroethylene (PER) are hepatotoxic in mice, although TRI is regarded as only slightly so.[73-75] Both compounds produced hepatocellular carcinomas when administered to mice in accordance with the carcinogenicity bioassay procedure of the National Cancer Institute.[76-78] In male mice, hepatocellular carcinoma prevalence was elevated to an extent independent of dose with both compounds, given orally at the maximum tolerated dose (1072 mg/kg/da for PER, 2339 mg/kg/da for TRI) and at half this dose rate. The results of other studies have been negative with respect to carcinogenicity of TRI and PER.[79,80] The NCI results with TRI have been questioned because mutagenic impurities were detected in the TRI used.[81]

It has been proposed that the carcinogenicity of both TRI and PER is due primarily to an epigenetic mechanism involving either recurrent cytotoxicity with regeneration resulting in increased likelihood of occurrence of a spontaneous transformation, or enhancement of oncogenic factors already established in the mouse strain.[82,83] Observations cited in support of this proposal include the relatively low level of binding of radiolabel derived from either compound to hepatic DNA, and the increase in rate of hepatic DNA synthesis that follows exposure of mice to either compound.

Both compounds have been thought to be metabolized through an epoxide to stable metabolites that are excreted in the urine.[84-86] Miller and Guengerich[87] have presented evidence supporting the proposition that the epoxide may not be an obligatory intermediate in metabolism of TRI. If end products of metabolism are to be used as indices of exposure to reactive intermediates, they must reflect total production of such intermediates. Thus, if end products do not all originate from a single hepatotoxic intermediate, they must at least vary in parallel with hepatotoxic metabolites. In mice, trichloroethanol (both free and as the glucuronide) and trichloroacetic acid are the metabolites of TRI found in the urine. Only trichloroacetic acid is found in the urine of PER-treated mice. Elevated levels of oxalic acid have been found in the urine of rats exposed by inhalation to PER.[88] ^{14}C-Oxalic acid has also been identified in the urine of mice exposed by inhalation to ^{14}C-PER,[89] but oxalic acid was not detected in greater than endogenous amounts in the urine of treated mice in the study reported here. Previous reports had indicated that metabolism of PER in humans[90] and in rats[88,90] is saturable, but evidence with respect to saturability of TRI metabolism has been mixed.[83,90,91]

In this study, TRI and PER were administered to male Swiss-Cox mice by daily gavage 5 days a week for 6 weeks, over the dose ranges 100 to 3200 mg/kg/da (TRI) and 20 to 2000 mg/kg/da (PER). Total metabolite formation from TRI or PER was estimated as cumulative urinary metabolite excretion during a 24-hr dosing interval. Although the study was based on a repeated-exposure experimental design, the results showed that 95% of each TRI dose and 85% of each PER dose had been eliminated by the end of the 24-hr dosing interval, so that the amount of metabolism occurring during this period can be considered a reasonable estimate of total metabolites generated by each dose. Figures 10 and 11 show the observed relationship of total metabolism to dose for each of these two compounds. For PER, the relationship appears to be Michaelis-Menten, as previously suggested by the work of Ikeda et al.,[90] so that the activity of the metabolizing enzyme system must be rate-limiting at all experimental concentrations. Fitting the Michaelis-Menten expression in the form

$$\text{Total daily metabolite excretion} = \frac{V_m D}{K_m + D}$$

to the data of Figure 11 gives V_m = 136 mg/kg in 24 hr and K_m = 660 mg/kg. It should be noted that the value of V_m is based on 24-hr urine collections. It represents the maximum amount of PER excreted as urinary metabolites at very high doses, as evaluated 24 hr after dosing. The maximum rate of metabolite excretion is probably much higher.

The relationship of TRI metabolism to TRI dose appears not to be Michaelis-Menten but, rather, to be composed of two linear segments with a short transition dose range (Figure 10). This behavior has been demonstrated for a number of low molecular weight volatile compounds most commonly administered by inhalation in experimental studies.[15,92-94] It is consistent with the idea that perfusion, not metabolism, is rate-limiting for these compounds at low doses. Only when the biotransforming enzyme system becomes saturated does metabolism become rate-limiting. Thus, there is an abrupt transition from perfusion-limited

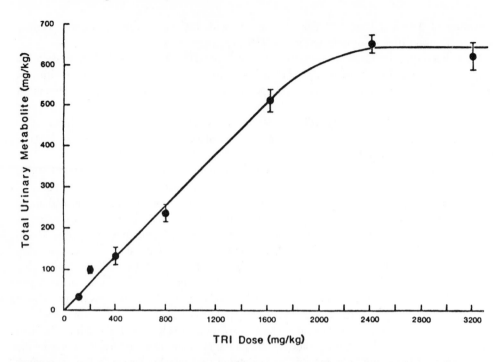

FIGURE 10.   Total urinary metabolites excreted within 24 hours of administration of an oral dose of TRI to mice. Data points are the means of values from 7 to 9 mice except at the lowest and highest dose where n = 4 and n = 3, respectively. The SEM is shown except where it lies within the symbol. The first 5 data points were fit by linear regression. (Unpublished data from Buben and O'Flaherty.)

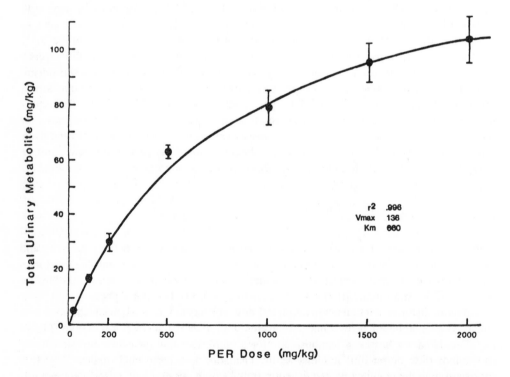

FIGURE 11.   Total urinary metabolites excreted within 24 hr of administration of an oral dose of PER to mice. Data points are the means of values from 9 to 11 mice except at the two highest doses where n = 4 (at 1500 mg/kg/day) and n = 5 (at 2000 mg/kg/day). The SEM is shown using the Michaelis-Menten equation. (Unpublished data from Buben and O'Flaherty.)

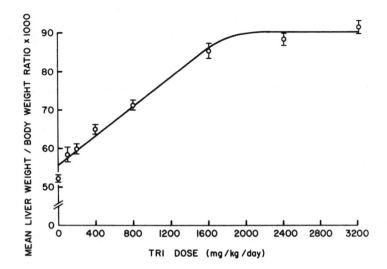

FIGURE 12. Liver weight to body weight ratio in mice after 6 weeks of daily oral administration of TRI, 5 day/week, as a function of the daily dose of TRI. Data points are the means of values from 12 mice except at the lowest and highest doses where n = 5 and n = 4, respectively. There were 24 mice in the control group. The SEM is shown except where it lies within the symbol. The first 5 data points were fit by liner regression. (Unpublished data from Buben and O'Flaherty.)

elimination at low doses to capacity-limited elimination at high doses. This behavior should be characteristic of compounds whose affinity for their biotransformation sites is high. Many of the halogenated ethylenes, as well as other low molecular weight halogenated compounds, appear to meet this criterion.[92]

Four hepatotoxic effects of graduated severity were evaluated: increase in liver weight to body weight ratio, increase in liver triglyceride concentration, inhibition of hepatic glucose-6-phosphatase activity, and increase in serum glutamate-pyruvate transaminase activity. PER exposure resulted in significant changes in all four measures. TRI exposure significantly affected only two. In Figures 12 and 13, the effects of TRI and PER on liver weight/body weight ratio are shown as functions of the daily dose of each compound. Comparison of Figures 12 and 13 with Figures 10 and 11, respectively, shows that the shape of each dose-effect curve is the same as the shape of the corresponding dose-metabolism curve. Consequently, when liver weight/body weight ratio is plotted as a function of metabolism, both relationships are linear. In all cases, the relationships between the metabolism of each compound and the magnitudes of the effects caused by it were linear while the relationships between dose and effect were not.

These findings demonstrate that the metabolism of both compounds is responsible for their toxicity. At the same time, they are consistent with the proposition that the mechanism of production of hepatocellular carcinoma by both TRI and PER is epigenetic, since both compounds cause hepatotoxicity whose severity is dose-related and since the metabolism, hepatotoxicity, and carcinogenic activity of both compounds all attain plateaus at high doses in male mice. Direct comparison between the carcinogenicity and metabolism/hepatotoxicity studies cannot be undertaken, however, because of marked species differences in the degree of TRI and PER metabolism. The B6C3F1 mouse strain used in the NCI bioassays transforms as much as 62% of the PER[82] or 75% of the TRI[83] taken up from 6-hr low-dose inhalation exposures into metabolites excreted in the urine within 50 to 72 hr after termination of exposure. The outbred Swiss-Cox mouse used in the metabolism/hepatotoxicity study metabolizes less than 30% of even low oral doses of either compound.

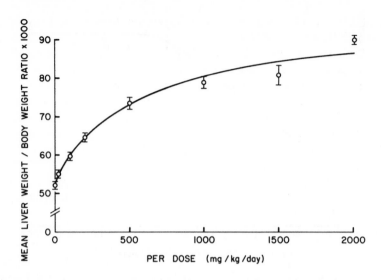

FIGURE 13. Liver weight to body weight ratio in mice after 6 weeks of daily oral administration of PER, 5 day/week, as a function of the daily dose of PER. Data points are the means of values from 13 to 19 mice except at the two highest doses where n = 6. There were 26 mice in the control group. The SEM is shown except where it lies within the symbol. The curve was fit using the Michaelis-Menten equation. (Unpublished data from Buben and O'Flaherty.)

D. Chronic Exposure: Rate of Transformation to an Active Metabolite: Vinyl Chloride Carcinogenesis.

Vinyl chloride has been studied with unusual thoroughness, perhaps because it has been shown to be carcinogenic in both animals and humans. In the early 1970s, it was observed that industrial exposure to vinyl chloride monomer in the manufacture of polyvinyl chloride was associated with development of a rare tumor, hepatic angiosarcoma.[95,96] In rats, vinyl chloride causes nephroblastoma and zymbal gland carcinoma as well as hepatic angiosarcoma.[97] While prevalence of zymbal gland carcinoma is approximately proportional to the dose of vinyl chloride, the prevalence of the other two tumor types reaches a constant maximum level at intermediate vinyl chloride doses; further increases in vinyl chloride dose do not result in further increases in tumor prevalence.

There is general agreement today that the active carcinogen is a metabolite of vinyl chloride, probably an epoxide.[98-100] If transformation of vinyl chloride to its carcinogenically active metabolite is saturable, then the observed constancy of the angiosarcoma response at high vinyl chloride doses could be understood as a reflection of constancy of active metabolite production as a consequence of saturation of the rate-limiting metabolizing enzyme.

Hefner et al.[101] and Watanabe et al.[21,102,103] investigated the metabolism of vinyl chloride. They established that its metabolism in rats is dose-dependent whether vinyl chloride is administered orally or by inhalation. Gehring et al.[28] fit the metabolism data for inhaled vinyl chloride (1.4 to 4600 ppm in exposure air) to the Michaelis-Menten equation. They showed that the rate of vinyl chloride metabolism in rats was related to exposure concentration as predicted by Michaelis-Menten kinetics with $K_m = 860 \pm 159$ (SD) µg vinyl chloride/ℓ of air and $V_m = 8558 \pm 1147$ (SD) µg vinyl chloride metabolized/6-hr exposure interval.

Maltoni and Lefemine[97] reported the prevalence of hepatic angiosarcoma in rats exposed to vinyl chloride by inhalation (6 doses ranging from 50 to 10,000 ppm in the exposure atmosphere) 4 hr/day, 5 days/week for 1 year. The progressive diminution of response increments that they observed at high vinyl chloride doses began at concentrations between 500 and 2500 ppm, or very roughly around the value of K_m for metabolism.

Gehring et al.[28] combined their data on metabolism with Maltoni and Lefemine's data on tumor prevalence, adjusting dose for the difference in duration of exposure period (6 hr/day in their study, 4 hr/day in Maltoni and Lefemine's). The difference in number of exposures in the two studies was not considered to be relevant, since Watanabe et al.[104] had shown that biotransformation rate was not induced by repeated exposure. Figure 14 shows the result of expressing prevalence as a function of the rate of biotransformation rather than as a function of vinyl chloride concentration in the inhalation atmosphere. The probit transform of the prevalence of hepatic angiosarcoma is linear with respect to the logarithm of the rate of vinyl chloride metabolism but not with respect to the logarithm of vinyl chloride dose. Thus, this analysis not only provides support for the concept that an active metabolite, whose production from vinyl chloride becomes saturated at high vinyl chloride doses, is responsible for angiosarcoma induction, but also permits all of the response date to contribute to establishing the slope of the dose-response line.

Reactive vinyl chloride metabolites are thought to be detoxified by conjugation with glutathione prior to excretion.[21] At inhalation doses at and above 100 ppm vinyl chloride for 6 hr, rat hepatic glutathione stores are significantly reduced. The magnitude of the reduction is dose-dependent; at 5000 ppm vinyl chloride, the hepatic glutathione pool of exposed rats is only 39% of the hepatic glutathione pool of control rats.[103] If reduction of glutathione stores represents a limitation on the rate of deactivation of reactive vinyl chloride metabolites, then vinyl chloride doses sufficiently high to result in biologically significant reductions in glutathione stores would be expected to be associated with disproportionate increases in angiosarcoma prevalence. These prevalence increments would result from proportional reductions in the ability of the rats to detoxify reactive metabolites. In the range of intermediate experimental exposures to vinyl chloride (up to about 1000 ppm for 6 hr), the reduction in hepatic glutathione pool is directly correlated with angiosarcoma incidence.[12] Thus, it is possible that depletion of hepatic glutathione in this dose range is a contributory factor in the induction of hepatic angiosarcoma, although the angiosarcoma prevalence data can be satisfactorily explained by considerations of metabolism alone. However, the constancy of angiosarcoma prevalence at concentrations above the K_m of 860 ppm suggests that availability of glutathione is not a critical factor determining the rate of detoxification of vinyl chloride metabolites at high dose rates; that is, that production of active metabolites has become rate-limiting.

E. Acute Exposure: Area Under the Curve of Parent Compound: Urethane Adenogenesis

Urethane, or ethyl carbamate, is a low molecular weight, water soluble compound whose ability to induce lung adenomas in the mouse has been known for many years.[105] When urethane is given as a single intraperitoneal injection, at doses ranging from about 0.5 g/kg up to 1.5 g/kg, the number of adenomas induced increases disproportionately with dose, as shown in Figure 15.[106] At urethane doses above 1.5 g/kg, the number of adenomas per mouse does not increase further with further increases in dose.[106,107] The reason for this plateau is not known.

Kaye[108] showed that a urethane dose of 0.75 g/kg i.p. was eliminated in mice by what appeared to be zero-order kinetics, suggesting that saturability of urethane metabolism should be considered in any analysis of the relationship between urethane dose and adenoma production. A series of experiments has been carried out in this author's laboratory, in which the kinetics of elimination of urethane from mouse blood have been more fully described. Urethane was given as a single intraperitoneal injection, at seven doses ranging from 0.4 to 1.8 g/kg, and the concentration in blood was monitored for up to 18 hr at the highest doses, using as an assay the determination of ethanol liberated from urethane by alkaline hydrolysis.[109] Urethane elimination was found to be not only saturable, but saturated at least down to the detection limit of urethane (about 0.1 mg/mℓ), with V_m = 0.087 ± 0.006 (SD) mg/mℓ/hr.

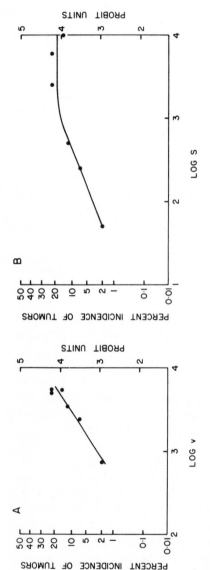

FIGURE 14.   (A) Metabolism of vinyl chloride expressed as log v (micrograms of VC metabolized/4 hr) versus percentage incidence of hepatic angiosarcoma (probability scale). (B) Exposure concentration expressed as log S (parts per million) versus the percentage incidence of hepatic angiosarcoma. The probit equivalents of the percentage incidence are shown on the right-hand ordinate. The solid line is the best fit for experimentally observed responses while the dashed line represents extrapolation below those doses producing an observable response assuming no threshold. (Reproduced from Gehring, P. J., Watanabe, P. G., and Park, C. N., *Toxicol. Appl. Pharmacol.*, 44, 581, 1978. With permission.)

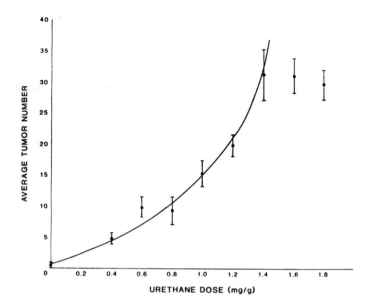

FIGURE 15. The number of lung adenomas induced in Swiss-Cox mice by single intraperitoneal injections of urethane. Data points are the means of values from 9 to 10 mice except for the two highest dose groups, each of which consisted of 17 mice. The SD is shown. The line was drawn by inspection. (Unpublished data from Sichak and O'Flaherty.)

At the lowest dose given, 0.4 g/kg, the initial concentration C_o was 0.50 mg/mℓ. Equation 8 and the accompanying discussion show that in this case, where C_o at even the lowest dose greatly exceeds K_m, AUC_{oo} is approximately $C_o^2/2V_m$. This curve is plotted in Figure 16 along with the observed values of AUC_{oo}. When the number of adenomas per mouse was expressed as a function of AUC_{oo} rather than as a function of administered dose, the relationship between dose and effect was linear (Figure 17).

A qualitative difference between this example and the vinyl chloride example should be noted. In the urethane study an effect, the number of adenomas per mouse, was measured while in the vinyl chloride study a response, the percent of rats with angiosarcoma, was measured. Thus, the ordinate in Figure 16 is properly expressed as a probit transform (other transforms could also have been used), while the ordinate in Figure 17 is linear.

The data transformation of Figure 17, like the other transformations discussed, enables use of a wide range of observations to define the slope of the dose-effect relationship. The active moiety in urethane adenogenesis is not known. It has been postulated that it is a reactive intermediate, but none has so far been unequivocally identified.[110] That use of the AUC_{oo} effectively linearizes the dose-effect curve does not necessarily suggest that urethane itself is the active tumorigen. All that can be said with assurance is that the active tumorigen occurs in the reaction sequence at some point prior to the action of the saturable enzyme, and varies directly with urethane concentration. Thus, this analysis does not rule out the possibility that a urethane metabolite may be responsible for urethane adenogenesis.

F. Continuous Exposure: Rate of Transformation to an Active Metabolite: 1,1-Dichloroethylene Toxicity

Like VC and TRI, 1-1-dichloroethylene (vinylidene chloride, VDC) is an unsymmetric chlorinated ethylene. All three of these unsymmetrically substituted molecules have been shown to be mutagenic in *E. coli K12* after metabolic activation with a liver microsomal preparation from phenobarbital treated mice.[111] The symmetrically chlorinated molecules *cis*

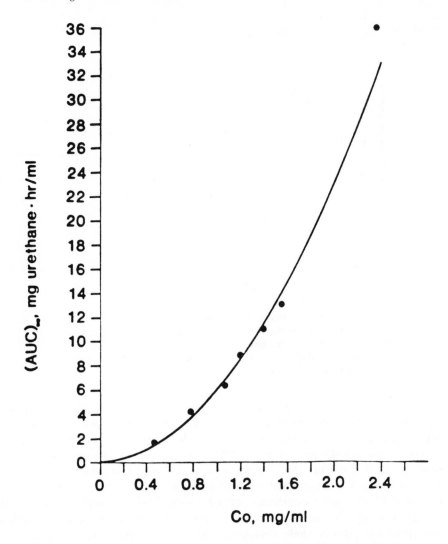

FIGURE 16.   Area under the blood urethane concentration, time curve as a function of initial urethane concentration. The curve represents the expected relationship, $AUC_x = C_o^2/2V_m$. Data points represent actual areas under the concentration, time curves for each of the seven urethane doses. Reproduced from O'Flaherty, E. J. and Sichak, S. P., *Toxicol. Appl. Pharmacol.*, in press 1983. With permission.)

and *trans* 1,2-dichloroethylene and perchloroethylene were not mutagenic in this test system. Attempts have been made to correlate the chemical instability of the unsymmetrically substituted ethylenes[112] and of their epoxides[83] with their reactivity and, thus, with their hepatotoxicity and potential mutagenicity or carcinogenicity. The epoxide of VDC is the least chemically stable of all the chloroethylene epoxides.[113] Its existence has been inferred from the nature of the end products of VDC metabolism.[85] Consistent with its greater reactivity, VDC appears to induce a pattern of hepatocellular injury different from that caused by the other chloroethylenes.[112]

It is generally agreed that VDC is activated by metabolism. Support for this premise comes from several sources: by analogy with other chloroethylenes, from the good correlation between the level of hepatic microsomal oxidizing activity possessed by rats of different ages and sexes and their susceptibility to acute VDC toxicity,[114] from the observed inhibition by VC of VDC hepatotoxicity suggestive of a competitive interference,[115] and from the

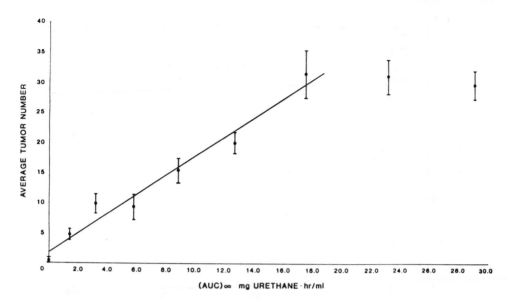

FIGURE 17. The number of lung adenomas induced in Swiss-Cox mice by single intraperitoneal injections of urethane, as a function of AUC_∞. Data points are the means of values from 9 to 10 mice except for the two highest dose groups, each of which consisted of 17 mice. The SD is shown. The line was fit by linear regression to the first 7 data points. (Unpublished data from Sichak and O'Flaherty.)

observation that microsomal enzyme inhibitors that block VDC metabolism also protect against acute VDC toxicity.[116,117]

Pretreatment of rats with the microsomal enzyme inhibitors pyrazole, aminotriazole, or carbon tetrachloride protects them from acute VDC lethality.[116] On the other hand, pretreatment with certain microsomal enzyme inducers, such as phenobarbital and Aroclor 1254, protects rats from VDC hepatotoxicity although it enhances VC hepatotoxicity.[112,118] Thus, it must be concluded that microsomal enzymes catalyze more than one step in the metabolism of VDC to stable end products. Glutathione is also central to VDC metabolism in rats, since VDC administration depletes glutathione[20,112] and since fasting or other treatments that deplete glutathione enhance VDC hepatotoxicity.[119]

Dose-mortality curves for VDC are not straightforward. Both oral[114] and inhalation[120] mortality curves for VDC exhibit maxima or extended plateaus within selected dose ranges. The mortality curve for a 4-hr inhalation exposure is shown in Figure 18. In the oral toxicity study,[114] hepatotoxicity as measured by increases in plasma transaminase activities in surviving rats paralleled mortality. Chieco et al.[121] observed similar plateaus in oral dose plasma transaminase activities in the same dose range. Together with the comparable plateau in the amount of intubated VDC retained and therefore, presumably, metabolized,[114] these data suggested that microsomal activation of VDC to (a) metabolite(s) responsible for hepatotoxicity and lethality might be saturable.

McKenna et al.[1,2] showed that the fraction of a VDC dose metabolized decreased with increase in dose in rats administered VDC either orally or by inhalation. Andersen et al.[117] studied the metabolism of VDC in groups of six rats exposed to VDC by inhalation in a closed chamber with maintenance of normal oxygen levels and removal of expired CO_2. In this system, once the exchange of VDC between the animal body and the chamber atmosphere has reached a dynamic steady state, the rate of loss of the test compound from the chamber air is taken to be its rate of metabolism.

Figure 19 illustrates the Michaelis-Menten dependence of this loss rate on concentration in chamber air, showing that loss of VDC approaches saturation in the exposure range

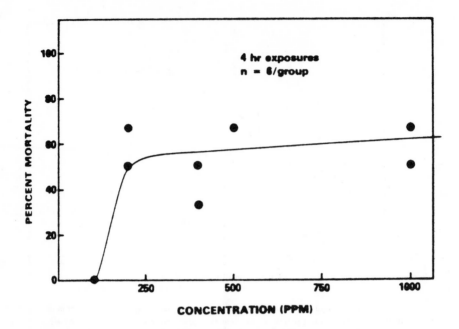

FIGURE 18. Concentration-mortality curve for exposure of mature male rats to VDC by inhalation for 4 hr. (Reproduced from Andersen, M. E., French, J. E., Gargas, M. L., Jones, R. A., and Jenkins, L. J., *Toxicol. Appl. Pharmacol.*, 47, 385, 1979b. (With permission.)

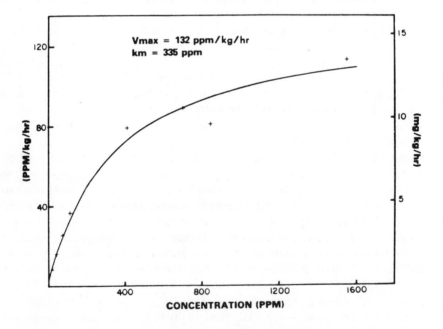

FIGURE 19. Dependence of rate of VDC metabolism on its concentration in the exposure atmosphere. The curve was fit using the Michaelis-Menten equation. (Reproduced from Andersen, M. E., Gargas, M. L., Jones, R. A., and Jenkins, L. J., *Toxicol. Appl. Pharmacol.*, 47, 395, 1979a. With permission.)

studied. If metabolites are indeed the toxic agents, then acute toxicity should be determined by the total "dose" of metabolites. This will be relatively independent of concentration at concentrations much above K_m but dependent on time, since the rate of production of

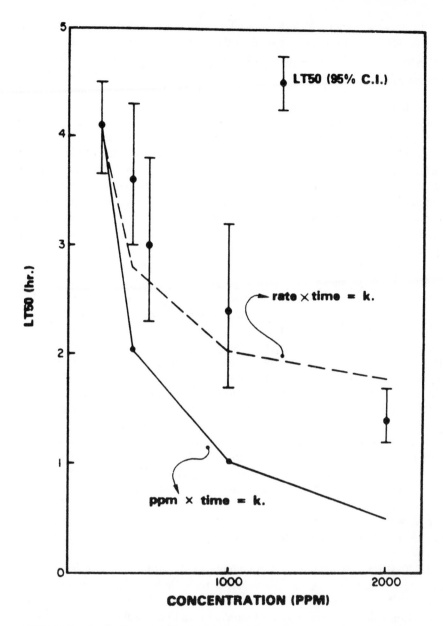

FIGURE 20. Comparison of observed LT50's for VDC at different exposure concentrations with predicted values calculated based either on the assumption that (—) toxicity is proportional to VDC concentration or on the assumption that (----) toxicity is proportional to the amount of metabolite formed during exposure. The data points are the observed LT50's together with their associated 95% confidence intervals. (Reproduced from Andersen, M. E., Jones, R. A., and Jenkins, L. J., *Toxicol. Appl. Pharmacol.*, 47, 395, 1979a. With permission.)

metabolites is constant throughout much of the exposure period. Since the dose-mortality curve (Figure 18) is relatively independent of chamber concentrations above 200 ppm for a 4-hr exposure, Andersen et al.[120] determined the LT50, or time required to kill half the exposed rats, at 6 different concentrations between 100 and 2000 ppm. At the lowest dose, 100 ppm, mortality was only 1/9 after 8 hr, but at the other doses LT50's were calculable. They are shown in Figure 20 as a function of chamber concentration, and are there compared with the expected dependence of LT50 on chamber concentration if mortality were proportional to the concentration of VDC as well as with the expected dependence calculated on the basis that mortality is proportional to the "dose" of metabolites. In this calculation, Andersen et al.[120] took into account the period of time during which rat body levels of VDC had not yet reached a dynamic steady-state relationship with chamber VDC, as well as the subsequent steady-state phase. It is clear that acute toxicity is much more closely correlated with metabolite production than with the concentration of VDC itself.

Resolution of the acute toxicity dose-response curve does not answer all the questions associated with VDC toxicity. At sufficiently high oral doses (800 to 2000 mg/kg), the VDC dose-mortality curve is conventional, with 100% mortality eventually achieved. The plateau or maximum in the mortality curve occurs at oral doses below about 800 mg/kg.[116] This behavior is consistent with the differential effects of various microsomal enzyme inducers and inhibitors on VDC toxicity, and suggests that total VDC metabolism probably correlates well with toxicity only within limited dose ranges and that toxicity reflects the balance between production of active intermediates and their elimination. Since certain microsomal enzyme inducers such as phenobarbital protect against VDC toxicity without altering its rate of loss from the chamber atmosphere (that is, its rate of metabolism),[117] it is reasonable to speculate that these agents may induce enzymes responsible for detoxification of active intermediates. Similarly, glutathione depletion enhances toxicity without significantly altering the V_m for VDC metabolism so that glutathione must be involved in a detoxification step not involving VDC itself. Indeed, two of the four major urinary metabolites of VDC in rats are derived from conjugation of metabolic intermediates with glutathione.[1,2] Andersen et al.[122] have investigated the relative importance of glutathione-dependent and glutathione-independent pathways of VDC metabolism.

Neither do these studies illuminate the questions surrounding the potential carcinogenicity of VDC. Although covalent binding of ^{14}C-VDC metabolites to liver protein is inversely proportional to hepatic glutathione content of rats,[20] this observation is relevant primarily to VDC hepatotoxicity. VDC-related tumors have been found in the kidneys of male mice,[123] but VDC has not been shown to be carcinogenic in rats.[123-125] Tumorigenic doses of VDC produced massive kidney tissue damage and an increase in kidney DNA replication in mice, but little liver or kidney DNA alkylation and only slight increases in kidney DNA repair.[126] VDC did not cause comparable tissue damage or comparable increases in DNA replication in the livers of exposed mice or in the kidneys or livers of exposed rats. Thus, it has been suggested that VDC is an epigenetic carcinogen in mice.[126]

G. The First-Pass Effect: Route Dependence of Bioavailability and Exposure

First-pass metabolism of the β-adrenergic receptor blocking agents propranolol,[127,128] alprenolol,[129-131] and metoprolol[132,133] has been studied with particular thoroughness. Two of these drugs, the structurally related alprenolol and metoprolol, present interesting similarities and contrasts.

Both alprenolol and metoprolol have high intrinsic clearances and are subject to significant first-pass effects. Systemic availability of both compounds is dose-dependent. Figure 21[133] illustrates the relationship between oral or intravenous dose of metoprolol and the area under the plasma concentration vs. time curve. While AUC_{oo} is directly proportional to the magnitude of an intravenous dose, the figure clearly indicates the nonlinear relationship between AUC_{oo} and oral dose in the dose range up to 20 mg. Bioavailability of the oral doses in this study was calculated to be 31, 41, and 46% for the three doses in order of increasing dose.[133]

The bioavailability of an oral 100-mg dose of alprenolol is only about 10%.[130] In the dose range 50 to 200 mg alprenolol, increases in dose are associated with disproportionately large increases in plasma concentration.[129] This dose dependency is coupled with a large interindividual variability in steady-state plasma concentration. For example, a 25-fold range of C_{ss} values has been reported in hypertensive patients treated with identical dose regimens

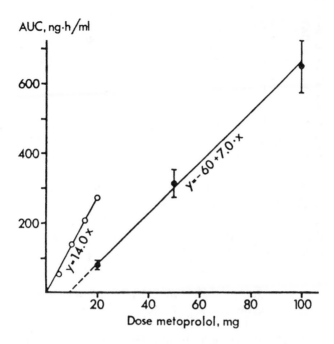

FIGURE 21. The relationship between the area under the plasma concentration curve (AUC) and the dose after (●) and intravenous (○) administration of metoprolol to five male subjects. Data points are the means ± SEM. (Reproduced from Johnsson, G., Regard, G., and Solvell, L., *Acta Pharmacol. Toxicol.*, 36, 31, 1975. With permission.)

of alprenolol.[134] Alván et al.[131] selected young adult volunteers on the basis that their steady-state plasma alprenolol concentrations after five doses of alprenolol, 200 mg every 12 hr, varied over a fourteenfold range. The purpose of this study was to establish whether first-pass metabolism was an important determinant of interindividual variation in steady-state concentration. The observed proportionality between steady-state concentration and systemic availability, calculated as the ratio of AUC's$_{oo}$ after oral and intravenous administration of equal doses, is shown in Figure 22. In contrast, half-life after an intravenous dose was unrelated to steady-state concentration during oral dosing. Thus, the variability in steady-state concentration is determined principally by interindividual variation in dose-dependent first-pass metabolism. Consistent with this observation, plasma concentrations of alprenolol in the slowest metabolizer greatly exceeded those of its metabolite 4-hydroxyalprenolol, while in the fastest metabolizer, plasma concentrations of the metabolite greatly exceeded those of alprenolol itself. Treatment with pentobarbital of the two subjects with the lowest capacities to metabolize alprenolol led to a marked decrease in the AUC$_{oo}$ of an oral dose, to 59% and 32% of pretreatment values in the two subjects. Nonetheless, alprenolol half-lives were not changed by pentobarbital pretreatment.

The relationship between reduction in exercise-induced tachycardia and plasma concentration of metoprolol was independent of whether the drug had been given orally or intravenously.[132,133] This observation indicates that metoprolol itself is responsible for this pharmacological effect and that none of its biotransformation products has clinically significant activity. For alprenolol, however, these relationships are different. Figure 23 shows that at any specific magnitude of reduction of exercise-induced tachycardia by alprenolol, plasma levels of alprenolol were lower after oral than after intravenous administration.[130] Thus, the β-blocking effect of alprenolol must be due partly to an active metabolite(s) as well as to alprenolol itself. A consequence of this observation is that when alprenolol is

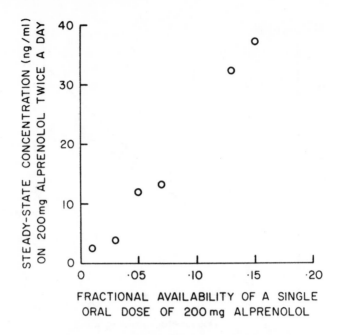

FIGURE 22.   The relationship between observed fractional availability
of an oral dose of alprenolol and alprenolol concentration at steady state
during repeated oral dosing (200 mg b.i.d.) in six subjects selected on the
basis of their wide range of steady-state plasma alprenolol concentrations.
(Data from Alván, G., Lind, M., Mellström, B., and von Bahr, C., *J.
Pharmacokinet. Biopharmaceut.*, 5, 193, 1977. With permission.)

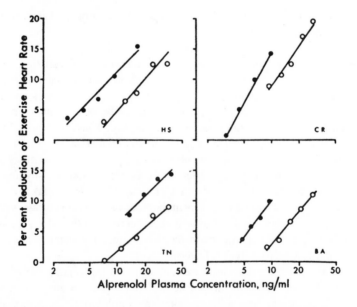

FIGURE 23.   The relationship between plasma concentration of alprenolol and effect
on exercise heart rate in four subjects given alprenolol either orally (●) or intravenously
(○). (Reproduced from Åblad, B., Borg, K. O., Johnsson, G., Regarth, G., and Solvell,
L., *Life Sci.*, 14, 693, 1974. With permission.)

given orally, plasma concentrations associated with a given magnitude of effect vary widely among individuals.[129]

Not only can the relationship of exposure to metabolite and exposure to parent be shifted by dose-dependent first-pass metabolism, but when several biotransformation pathways occur in parallel, patterns of metabolite formation can be sensitive to both dose and route of exposure. For example, the pattern of excretion of the four major metabolites of VDC is both route dependent and dose dependent.[1,2]

There is an additional important aspect of this route and dose dependence. If exposure to metabolites is associated with a spectrum of effects different from the effects of the parent compound, dose dependence of first-pass metabolism could be responsible for dose dependence of the nature as well as the magnitude of effect. Levy et al.[135] speculated that such a mechanism might be responsible for the poor correlation between serum carbamazepine concentrations and side effects of the drug in humans after oral administration of carbamazepine. Onset of side effects was rapid. Their maximum intensity occurred several hours before the maximum concentration of carbamazepine was reached, and their disappearance was complete while near-maximum concentrations of carbamazepine persisted. Even though first-pass metabolism of carbamazepine is not marked, first-pass production of a potent metabolite could have accounted for both the rapidity of onset and the transience of the observed side effects.

REFERENCES

1. **McKenna, M. J., Zempel, J. A., Madrid, E. O., Braun, W. H., and Gehring, P. J.**, Metabolism and pharmacokinetic profile of vinylidene chloride in rats following oral administration, *Toxicol. Appl. Pharmacol.*, 45, 821, 1978a.
2. **McKenna, M. J., Zempel, J. A., Madrid, E. O., and Gehring, P. J.**, The pharmacokinetics of [^{14}C] vinylidene chloride in rats following inhalation exposure, *Toxicol. Appl. Pharmacol.*, 45, 599, 1978b.
3. **Chiou, W. L.**, Quantitation of hepatic and pulmonary first-pass effect and its implications in pharmacokinetic study. I. Pharmacokinetics of chloroform in man, *J. Pharmacokinet. Biopharmaceut.*, 3, 419, 1975.
4. **Roth, R. A. and Wiersma, D. A.**, Role of the lung in total body clearance of circulating drugs, *Clin. Pharmacokinet.*, 4, 355, 1979.
5. **Jusko, W. J., Koup, J. R., and Alván, G.**, Nonlinear assessment of phenytoin availability, *J. Pharmacokinet. Biopharmaceut.*, 4, 327, 1976.
6. **Alván, G., Borgå, O., Lind, M., Plamér, L., and Siwers, B.**, First pass hydroxylation of nortriptyline: concentrations of parent drug and major metabolites in plasma, *Europ. J. Clin. Pharmacol.*, 11, 219, 1977.
7. **Raaflaub, J. and Dubach, U. C.**, On the pharmacokinetics of phenacetin in man, *Europ. J. Clin. Pharmacol.*, 8, 261, 1975.
8. **Talseth, T.**, Kinetics of hydralazine elimination, *Clin. Pharmacol. Therap.*, 21, 715, 1977.
9. **Quick, A. J.**, The conjugation of benzoic acid in man, *J. Biol. Chem.*, 92, 65, 1931.
10. **Jollow, D. J., Mitchell, J. R., Zampaglione, N., and Gillette, J. R.**, Bromobenzene induced liver necrosis, *Pharmacology*, 11, 151, 1974.
11. **Mitchell, J. R., Jollow, D. J., Potter, W. Z., Gillette, J. R., and Brodie, B. B.**, Acetaminophen-induced hepatic necrosis. IV. Protective role of glutathione, *J. Pharmacol. Exp. Therap.*, 187, 211, 1973.
12. **Watanabe, P. G., Young, J. D., and Gehring, P. J.**, The importance of nonlinear (dose-dependent) pharmacokinetics in hazard assessment, *J. Environ. Pathol. Toxicol.*, 1, 147, 1977.
13. **Rose, J. Q., Yurchak, A. M., and Jusko, W. J.**, Dose dependent pharmacokinetics of prednisone and prednisolone in man, *J. Pharmacokinet. Biopharmaceut.*, 9, 389, 1981.
14. **Gillette, J. R. and Pang, K. S.**, Theoretic aspects of pharmacokinetic drug interactions, *Clin. Pharmacol. Ther.*, 22, 623, 1977.
15. **Andersen, M. E.**, Saturable metabolism and its relationship to toxicity, *CRC Crit. Rev. Toxicol.*, 9, 105, 1981a.
16. **Wagner, J. G.**, Properties of the Michaelis-Menten equation and its integrated form which are useful in pharmacokinetics, *J. Pharmacokinet. Biopharmaceut.*, 1, 103, 1973.

17. **McNamara, B. P.,** Concepts in health evaluation of commercial and industrial chemicals, in *Advances in Modern Toxicology,* Vol. 1, Part 1: New Concepts in Safety Evaluation, Mehlman, M. A., Shapiro, R. E. and Blumenthal, H., Eds., Hemisphere Publishing Corp., Washington, D.C., 1976.

18. **Wagner, J. G., Northam, J. I., Alway, C. D., and Carpenter, O. S.,** Blood levels of drug at the equilibrium state after multiple dosing, *Nature,* 307, 1301, 1965.

19. **O'Flaherty, E. J.,** *Toxicants and Drugs: Kinetics and Dynamics,* John Wiley and Sons, Inc., New York, 1981, 229.

20. **McKenna, M. J., Watanabe, P. G., and Gehring, P. J.,** Pharmacokinetics of vinylidene chloride in the rat, *Environ. Health Perspectives,* 21, 99, 1977.

21. **Watanabe, P. G., McGowan, G. R., Madrid, E. O., and Gehring, P. J.,** Fate of [^{14}C] vinyl chloride following inhalation exposure in rats, *Toxicol. Appl. Pharmacol.,* 37, 49, 1976b.

22. **Bus, J. S., Deyo, D., and Cox, M.,** Dose-dependent disposition of n-hexane in F-344 rats after inhalation exposure, *Fund. Appl. Toxicol.,* 2, 226, 1982.

23. **Rollins, D. E. and Klaassen, C. D.,** Biliary excretion of drugs in man, *Clin. Pharmacokinet.,* 4, 368, 1979.

24. **Gillette, J. R.,** A perspective on the role of chemically reactive metabolites of foreign compounds in toxicity I. Correlation of changes in covalent binding of reactive metabolites with changes in the incidence and severity of toxicity, *Biochem. Pharmacol.,* 23, 2785, 1974a.

25. **Gillette, J. R.,** A perspective on the role of chemically reactive metabolites of foreign compounds in toxicity II. Alterations in the kinetics of covalent binding, *Biochem. Pharmacol.,* 23, 2927, 1974b.

26. **Ratney, R. S., Wegman, D. H., and Elkins, H. B.,** In vivo conversion of methylene chloride to carbon monoxide, *Arch. Environ. Health,* 28, 223, 1974.

27. **Stewart, R. D., Hake, C. L., and Wu, A.,** Use of breath analysis to monitor methylene chloride exposure, *Scand. J. Work Environ. Health,* 2, 57, 1976.

28. **Gehring, P. J., Watanabe, P. G., and Park, C. N.,** Resolution of dose-response toxicity data for chemicals requiring metabolic activation: example-vinyl chloride, *Toxicol. Appl. Pharmacol.,* 44, 581, 1978.

29. **Hinderling, P. H. and Garrett, E. R.,** Pharmacokinetics of -methyldigoxin in healthy humans. III. Pharmacodynamic correlations, *J. Pharm. Sci.,* 66, 326, 1977.

30. **Hendeles, W., Weinberger, M., and Johnson, G.,** Monitoring serum theophylline levels, *Clin. Pharmacokinet.,* 3, 294, 1978.

31. **Mitenko, P. A. and Ogilvie, R. I.,** Rational intravenous doses of theophylline, *N. Eng. J. Med.,* 289, 600, 1973.

32. **Pollock, J., Kiechel, F., Cooper, D., and Weinberger, M.,** Relationship of serum theophylline concentration to inhibition of exercise-induced bronchospasm and comparison with cromolyn, *Pediatrics,* 60, 840, 1977.

33. **Jacobs, M. H., Senior, R. M., and Kessler, G.,** Clinical experience with theophylline: relationships between dosage, serum concentration, and toxicity, *J. Am. Med. Assoc.,* 235, 1983, 1976.

34. **Zwillich, C. W., Sutton, F. D., Jr., Neff, T. A., Cohn, W. M., Matthay, R. A., and Weinberger, M. M.,** Theophylline-induced seizures in adults, *Ann. Intern. Med.,* 82, 784, 1975.

35. **Hendeles, L., Bighley, L., Richardson, R. H., Hepler, C. D., and Carmichael, J.,** Frequent toxicity from IV aminophylline infusions in critically ill patients, *Drug Intell. Clin. Pharm.,* 11, 12, 1977.

36. **Weinberger, M., Hudgel, D., Spector, S., and Chidsey, C.,** Inhibition of theophylline clearance by troleandomycin, *J. Allergy Clin. Immunol.,* 59, 228, 1977.

37. **Caldwell, J., Lancaster, R., Monks, T. J., and Smith, R. L.,** The influence of dietary methylxanthines on the metabolism and pharmacokinetics of intravenously administered theophylline, *Br. J. Clin. Pharmacol.,* 4, 637P, 1977.

38. **Weinberger, M., and Ginchansky, E.,** Dose-dependent kinetics of theophylline disposition in asthmatic children, *J. Pediatr.,* 91, 820, 1977.

39. **Jenne, J. W., Wyze, E., Rood, F. S., and MacDonald, F. M.,** Pharmacokinetics of theophylline. Application to adjustment of the clinical dose of aminophylline, *Clin. Pharmacol. Ther.,* 13, 349, 1972.

40. **Weinberger, M. M. and Bronsky, E. A.,** Evaluation of oral bronchodilator therapy in asthmatic children, *J. Pediatr.,* 84, 421, 1974.

41. **Piafsky, K. M., Sitar, D. S., Rangno, R. E., and Ogilvie, R. I.,** Theophylline kinetics in acute pulmonary edema, *Clin. Pharmacol. Therap.,* 21, 310, 1977.

42. **Ogilvie, R. I.,** Clinical pharmacokinetics of theophylline, *Clin. Pharmacokinet.,* 3, 267, 1978.

43. **Levy, G., Tsuchiya, T., and Amsel, L. P.,** Limited capacity for salicyl phenolic glucuronide formation and its effects on the kinetics of salicylate elimination in man, *Clin. Pharmacol. Therap.,* 13, 258, 1972.

44. **Aarons, L. J., Bochner, F., and Rowland, M.,** A chronic dose-ranging kinetic study of salicylate in man, *Brit. J. Pharmacol.,* 61, 456, 1977.

45. **Martin, E., Tozer, T. N., Sheiner, L. B., and Riegelman, S.,** The clinical pharmacokinetics of phenytoin, *J. Pharmacokinet. Biopharmaceut.,* 5, 579, 1977.

46. **Gerber, N. and Wagner, J. G.**, Explanation of dose-dependent decline of diphenylhydantoin plasma levels by fitting to the integrated form of the Michaelis-Menten equation, *Res. Commun. Chem. Pathol. Pharmacol.*, 3, 455, 1972.

47. **Mawer, G. E., Mullen, P. W., Rodgers, M., Robins, A. J., and Lucas, S. B.**, Phenytoin dose adjustment in epileptic patients, *Br. J. Clin. Pharmacol.*, 1, 163, 1974.

48. **Rambeck, B., Boenigk, H. E., Dunlop, A., Mullen, P. W., Wadsworth, J., and Richens, A.**, Predicting phenytoin dose — a revised nomogram, *Therap. Drug Monitoring*, 1, 325, 1979.

49. **Richens, A. and Dunlop, A.**, Serum-phenytoin levels in management of epilepsy, *Lancet*, 2, 247, 1975.

50. **Stewart, R. D., Fisher, T. N., Hosko, M. J., Peterson, J. E., Baretta, E. D., and Dodd, H. C.**, Carboxyhemoglobin elevation after exposure to dichloromethane, *Science*, 176, 295, 1972a.

51. **Kubic, V. L., Anders, M. W., Engel, R. R., Barlow, C. H., and Caughey, W. S.**, Metabolism of dihalomethanes to carbon monoxide. I. *In vivo* studies, *Drug Metab. Disp.*, 2, 53, 1974.

52. **DiVincenzo, G. D. and Hamilton, M. L.**, Fate and Disposition of [^{14}C] methylene chloride in the rat, *Toxicol. Appl. Pharmacol.*, 32, 385, 1975.

53. **Rodkey, F. L. and Collison, H. A.**, Biological oxidation of [^{14}C] methylene chloride to carbon monoxide and carbon dioxide by the rat, *Toxicol. Appl. Pharmacol.*, 40, 33, 1977a.

54. **Ahmed, A. E. and Anders, M. W.**, Metabolism of dihalomethanes to formaldehyde and inorganic halide. I. *In vitro* studies, *Drug Metab. Disp.*, 4, 357, 1976.

55. **McKenna, M. J., Zempel, J. A., and Braun, W. H.**, The pharmacokinetics of inhaled methylene chloride in rats, *Toxicol. Appl. Pharmacol.*, 65, 1, 1982.

56. **Kubic, V. L. and Anders, M. W.**, Metabolism of dihalomethanes to carbon monoxide. II. *In vitro* studies, *Drug Metab. Disp.*, 3, 104, 1975.

57. **Anders, M. W., Kubic, V. L., and Ahmed, A. E.**, Metabolism of halogenated methanes and macromolecular binding, *J. Environ. Pathol. Toxicol.*, 1, 117, 1977.

58. **Rannug, U. and Beije, B.**, The mutagenic effect of 1,2-dichloroethane on *Salmonella typhimurium*. II. Activation by the isolated perfused rat liver, *Chem. — Biol. Interact.*, 24, 265, 1979.

59. **Rannug, U., Sundvall, A., and Ramel, C.**, The mutagenic effect of 1,2-dichloroethane on *Salmonella typhimurium*. I. Activation through conjugation with glutathione *in vitro*, *Chem.-Biol. Interact.*, 20, 1, 1978.

60. **Van Duuren, B. L., Goldschmidt, B. M., Katz, C., Langseth, L., Mercado, G., and Sivak, A.**, Alpha-haloethers: a new type of alkylating carcinogen, *Arch. Environ. Health*, 16, 472, 1968.

61. **Van Duuren, B. L., Sivak, A., Goldschmidt, B. M., Katz, C., and Melchionne, S.**, Carcinogenicity of halo-ethers, *J. Natl. Cancer Inst.*, 43, 481, 1969.

62. **Leong, B. K. J., Macfarland, H. N., and Reese, W. H., Jr.**, Induction of lung adenomas by chronic inhalation of bis(chloromethyl) ether, *Arch. Environ. Health*, 22, 663, 1971.

63. **Kuschner, M., Laskin, S., Drew, R. T., Cappiello, V., and Nelson, N.**, Inhalation carcinogenicity of alpha halo ethers. III. Lifetime and limited period inhalation studies with bis(chloromethyl) ether at 0.1 ppm, *Arch. Environ. Health*, 30, 73, 1975.

64. **Laskin, S., Drew, R. T., Cappiello, V., Kuschner, M., and Nelson, N.**, Inhalation carcinogenicity of alpha halo ethers. II. Chronic inhalation studies with chloromethyl methyl ether, *Arch. Environ. Health*, 30, 70, 1975.

65. **Rodkey, F. L. and Collison, H. A.**, Effect of dihalogenated methanes on the *in vivo* production of carbon monoxide and methane by rats, *Toxicol. Appl. Pharmacol.*, 40, 39, 1977b.

66. **DiVincenzo, G. D. and Kaplan, C. J.**, Uptake, metabolism, and elimination of methylene chloride vapor by humans, *Toxicol. Appl. Pharmacol.*, 59, 130, 1981.

67. **Peterson, J. E.**, Modeling the uptake metabolism and excretion of dichloromethane by man, *Amer. Industr. Hygiene Assoc. J.*, 39, 41, 1978.

68. **Gamberale, F., Annwall, G., and Hultengren, M.**, Exposure to methylene chloride: II. Psychological functions, *Scand. J. Work Environ. Health*, 1, 95, 1975.

69. **Stewart, R. D., Fisher, T. N., Hosko, M. J., Peterson, J. E., Baretta, E. D., and Dodd, H. C.**, Experimental human exposure to methylene chloride, *Arch. Environ. Health*, 25, 342, 1972b.

70. **Åstrand, I., Övrum, P., and Carlsson, A.**, Exposure to methylene chloride: I. Its concentration in alveolar air and blood during rest and exercise and its metabolism, *Scand. J. Work Environ. Health*, 1, 78, 1975.

71. **Stewart, R. D.**, The effect of carbon monoxide on humans, *Annu. Rev. Pharmacol.*, 15, 409, 1975.

72. **Buben, J. A. and O'Flaherty, E. J.**, Delineation of the role of metabolism in the hepatotoxicity of trichloroethylene and perchloroethylene: A dose-effect study, *Toxicol. Appl. Pharmacol.*, in press.

73. **Kylin, B., Reichard, H., Sümegi, I., and Yllner, S.**, Hepatotoxicity of inhaled trichloroethylene, tetrachloroethylene and chloroform. Single exposure, *Acta Pharm. Tox.*, 20, 16, 1963.

74. **Kylin, B., Sümegi, I., and Yllner, S.**, Hepatotoxicity of inhaled trichlorethylene and tetrachloroethylene. Long-term exposure, *Acta Pharm. Tox.*, 22, 379, 1965.

75. **Klaassen, C. D. and Plaa, G. L.**, Relative effects of various chlorinated hydrocarbons on liver and kidney function in mice, *Toxicol. Appl. Pharmacol.*, 9, 139, 1966.

76. National Cancer Institute, Carcinogenesis Bioassay of Trichloroethylene, DHEW Publ. No. (NIH) 76, 1976.
77. National Cancer Institute, Bioassay of Tetrachloroethylene for Possible Carcinogenesis, DHEW Publ. No. (NIH) 77, 1977.
78. **Weisburger, E. K.,** Carcinogenicity studies on halogenated hydrocarbons, *Environ. Health Perspectives,* 21, 7, 1977.
79. **Van Duuren, B. L., Goldschmidt, B. M., Loewengart, G., Smith, A. C., Melchionne, S., Seldman, I., and Roth, D.,** Carcinogenicity of halogenated olefinic and aliphatic hydrocarbons in mice, *J. Natl. Cancer Inst.,* 63, 1433, 1979.
80. **Henschler, D., Romen, W., Elsässer, H. M., Reichert, D., Eder, E., and Radwan, Z.,** Carcinogenicity study of trichloroethylene by longterm inhalation in three animal species, *Arch. Toxicol.,* 43, 237, 1980.
81. **Henschler, D., Eder, E., Neudecker, T., and Metzler, M.,** Carcinogenicity of trichloroethylene: fact or artifact? *Arch. Toxicol.,* 37, 233, 1977.
82. **Schumann, A. M., Quast, J. F., and Watanabe, P. G.,** The pharmacokinetics and molecular interactions of perchloroethylene in mice and rats as related to oncogenicity, *Toxicol. Appl. Pharmacol.,* 55, 207, 1980.
83. **Stott, W. T., Quast, J. F., and Watanabe, P. G.,** The pharmacokinetics and macromolecular interactions of trichloroethylene in mice and rats, *Toxicol. Appl. Pharmacol.,* 62, 137, 1982.
84. **Daniel, J. W.,** The metabolism of ^{36}Cl-labelled trichloroethylene and tetrachloroethylene in the rat, *Biochem. Pharmacol.,* 12, 795, 1963.
85. **Henschler, D.,** Metabolism and mutagenicity of halogenated olefins — a comparison of structure and activity, *Environ. Health Perspectives,* 21, 61, 1977.
86. **Leibman, K. C. and Ortiz, E.,** Metabolism of halogenated ethylenes, *Environ. Health Perspect.,* 21, 91, 1977.
87. **Miller, R. E. and Guengerich, F. P.,** Oxidation of trichloroethylene by liver microsomal cytochrome P-450: Evidence for chlorine migration in a transition state not involving trichloroethylene oxide, *Biochemistry,* 21, 1090, 1982.
88. **Pegg, D. G., Zempel, J. A., Braun, W. H., and Watanabe, P. G.,** Disposition of tetrachloro (^{14}C) ethylene following oral and inhalation exposure in rats, *Toxicol. Appl. Pharmacol.,* 51, 465, 1979.
89. **Yllner, S.,** Urinary metabolites of ^{14}C-tetrachloroethylene in mice, *Nature,* 191, 820, 1961.
90. **Ikeda, M., Ohtsuji, H., Imamura, T., and Komoike, Y.,** Urinary excretion of total trichloro-compounds, trichloroethanol, and trichloroacetic acid as a measure of exposure to trichloroethylene and tetrachloroethylene, *Br. J. Indust. Med.,* 29, 328, 1972.
91. **Tanaka, S. and Ikeda, M.,** A method for determination of trichloroethanol and trichloroacetic acid in urine, *Br. J. Industr. Med.,* 25, 214, 1968.
92. **Filser, J. G. and Bolt, H. M.,** Pharmacokinetics of halogenated ethylenes in rats, *Arch. Toxicol.,* 42, 123, 1979.
93. **Andersen, M. E., Gargas, M. L., Jones, R. A., and Jenkins, L. J., Jr.,** Determination of the kinetic constants for metabolism of inhaled toxicants *in vivo* using gas uptake measurements, *Toxicol. Appl. Pharmacol.,* 54, 100, 1980.
94. **Andersen, M. E.,** A physiologically based toxicokinetic description of the metabolism of inhaled gases and vapors: analysis at steady state, *Toxicol. Appl. Pharmacol.,* 60, 509, 1981b.
95. **Creech, J. L., Jr. and Johnson, M. N.,** Angiosarcoma of liver in the manufacture of polyvinyl chloride, *J. Occup. Med.,* 16, 150, 1974.
96. **Heath, C. W., Jr., Falk, H., and Creech, J. L., Jr.,** Characteristics of cases of angiosarcoma of the liver among vinyl chloride workers in the United States, *Ann. N.Y. Acad. Sci.,* 246, 231, 1975.
97. **Maltoni, C. and Lefemine, G.,** Carcinogenicity bioassays of vinyl chloride: current results, *Ann. N.Y. Acad. Sci.,* 246, 195, 1975.
98. **Van Duuren, B. L.,** On the possible mechanism of carcinogenic action of vinyl chloride, *Ann. N.Y. Acad. Sci.,* 246, 258, 1975.
99. **Hathway, D. E.,** Comparative mammalian metabolism of vinyl chloride and vinylidene chloride in relation to oncogenic potential, *Environ. Health Perspect.,* 21, 55, 1977.
100. **Green, T. and Hathway, D. E.,** The chemistry and biogenesis of the S-containing metabolites of vinyl chloride in rats, *Chem. Biol. Interact.,* 17, 137, 1977.
101. **Hefner, R. E., Jr., Watanabe, P. G., and Gehring, P. J.,** Preliminary studies of the fate of inhaled vinyl chloride monomer (VCM) in rats, *Ann. N.Y. Acad. Sci.,* 246, 135, 1975.
102. **Watanabe, P. G., McGowan, G. R., and Gehring, P. J.,** Fate of [^{14}C] vinyl chloride after single oral administration in rats, *Toxicol. Appl. Pharmacol.,* 36, 339, 1976a.
103. **Watanabe, P. G., Zempel, J. A., Pegg, D. G., and Gehring, P. J.,** Hepatic macromolecular binding following exposure to vinyl chloride, *Toxicol. Appl. Pharmacol.,* 44, 571, 1978a.
104. **Watanabe, P. G., Zempel, J. A., and Gehring, P. J.,** Comparison of the fate of vinyl chloride following single and repeated exposure in rats, *Toxicol. Appl. Pharmacol.,* 44, 391, 1978b.
105. **Nettleship, A., Henshaw, P. S., and Meyer, H. L.,** Induction of pulmonary tumors in mice with ethyl carbamate (urethane), *J. Natl. Cancer Inst.,* 4, 309, 1943.

106. **Sichak, S. P. and O'Flaherty, E. J.,** Consideration of the mechanism of pulmonary adenogenesis in urethane-treated Swiss mice, *Toxicol. Appl. Pharmacol.,* in press.

107. **White, M.,** Studies of the mechanism of induction of pulmonary adenomas in mice, in Proceedings of the Sixth Berkeley Symposium, University of California Press, Berkeley, 1972, 287.

108. **Kaye, A. M.,** A study of the relationship between the rate of ethyl carbamate (urethan) catabolism and urethan carcinogenesis, *Cancer Res.,* 20, 237, 1960.

109. **O'Flaherty, E. J. and Sichak, S. P.,** The kinetics of urethane elimination in the mouse, *Toxicol. Appl. Pharmacol.,* in press 1983.

110. **Dahl, G. A., Miller, J. A., and Miller, E. C.,** Vinyl carbamate as a promutagen and a more carcinogenic analog of ethyl carbamate, *Cancer Res.,* 38, 3793, 1978.

111. **Greim, H., Bonse, G., Radwan, Z., Reichert, D., and Henschler, D.,** Mutagenicity *in vitro* and potential carcinogenicity of chlorinated ethylenes as a function of metabolic oxirane formation, *Biochem. Pharmacol.,* 24, 2013, 1975.

112. **Reynolds, E. S. and Moslen, M. T.,** Damage to hepatic cellular membranes by chlorinated olefins with emphasis on synergism and antagonism, *Environ. Health Perspectives,* 21, 137, 1977.

113. **Bonse, G., Urban, T., Reichert, D., and Henschler, D.,** Chemical reactivity, metabolic oxirane formation and biological reactivity of chlorinated ethylenes in the isolated perfused rat liver preparation, *Biochem. Pharmacol.,* 24, 1829, 1975.

114. **Andersen, M. E. and Jenkins, L. J., Jr.,** Oral toxicity of 1,1-dichloroethylene in the rat: effects of sex, age, and fasting, *Environ. Health Perspectives,* 21, 157, 1977.

115. **Jaeger, R. J., Conolly, R. B., and Murphy, S. D.,** Short-term inhalation toxicity of halogenated hydrocarbons: effects on fasting rats, *Arch. Environ. Health,* 30, 26, 1975.

116. **Andersen, M. E., Jones, R. A., and Jenkins, L. J., Jr.,** The acute toxicity of single, oral doses of 1,1-dichloroethylene in the fasted, male rat: effect of induction and inhibition of microsomal enzyme activities on mortality, *Toxicol. Appl. Pharmacol.,* 46, 227, 1978.

117. **Andersen, M. E., Gargas, M. L., Jones, R. A., and Jenkins, L. J., Jr.,** The use of inhalation techniques to assess the kinetic constants of 1,1-dichloroethylene metabolism, *Toxicol. Appl. Pharmacol.,* 47, 395, 1979a.

118. **Reynolds, E. S., Moslen, M. T., Szabo, S., Jaeger, R. J., and Murphy, S. D.,** Hepatotoxicity of vinyl chloride and 1,1-dichloroethylene, *Am. J. Pathol.,* 81, 219, 1975.

119. **Jaeger, R. J., Conolly, R. B., and Murphy, S. D.,** Effect of 18 hour fast and glutathione depletion on 1,1-dichloroethylene-induced hepatotoxicity and lethality in rats, *Exp. Molec. Pathol.,* 20, 187, 1974.

120. **Andersen, M. E., French, J. E., Gargas, M. L., Jones, R. A., and Jenkins, L. J., Jr.,** Saturable metabolism and the acute toxicity of 1,1-dichloroethylene, *Toxicol. Appl. Pharmacol.,* 47, 385, 1979b.

121. **Chieco, P., Moslen, M. T., and Reynolds, E. S.,** Effect of administrative vehicle on oral 1,1-dichloroethylene toxicity, *Toxicol. Appl. Pharmacol.,* 57, 146, 1981.

122. **Andersen, M. E., Thomas, O. E., Gargas, M. L., Jones, R. A., and Jenkins, L. J., Jr.,** The significance of multiple detoxification pathways for reactive metabolites in the toxicity of 1,1-dichloroethylene, *Toxicol. Appl. Pharmacol.,* 52, 422, 1980.

123. **Maltoni, C., Cotti, G., Morisi, L., and Chieco, P.,** Carcinogenicity bioassays of vinylidene chloride: research plan and early results, *Med. Lav.,* 68, 241, 1977.

124. **Viola, P. L. and Caputo, A.,** Carcinogenicity studies on vinylidene chloride, *Environ. Health Perspect.,* 21, 45, 1977.

125. **Quast, J. F., Humiston, C. G., Wade, C. E., Ballard, J., Beyer, J. E., Schwetz, R. W., and Norris, J. M.,** A chronic toxicity and oncogenicity study in rats and subchronic toxicity study in dogs on ingested vinylidene chloride, *Fund. Appl. Toxicol.,* 3, 55, 1983.

126. **Reitz, R. H., Watanabe, P. G., McKenna, M. J., Quast, J. F., and Gehring, P. G.,** Effects of vinylidene chloride on DNA synthesis and DNA repair in the rat and mouse: a comparative study with dimethylnitrosamine, *Toxicol. Appl. Pharmacol.,* 52, 357, 1980.

127. **Evans, G. H., and Shand, D. G.,** Disposition of propranolol. V. Drug accumulation and steady-state concentrations during chronic oral administration in man, *Clin. Pharmacol. Therapeut.,* 14, 487, 1973.

128. **Routledge, P. A. and Shand, D. G.,** Clinical pharmacokinetics of propranolol, *Clin. Pharmacokinet.,* 4, 73, 1979.

129. **Åblad, B., Ervik, M., Hallgren, J., Johnsson, G., and Sölvell, L.,** Pharmacological effects and serum levels of orally administered alprenolol in man, *Europ. J. Clin. Pharmacol.,* 5, 44, 1972.

130. **Åblad, B., Borg, K. O., Johnsson, G., Regårdh, C-G., and Sölvell, L.,** Combined pharmacokinetic and pharmacodynamic studies on alprenolol and 4-hydroxy-alprenolol in man, *Life Sci.,* 14, 693, 1974.

131. **Alván, G., Lind, M., Mellström, B., and von Bahr, C.,** Importance of "first-pass elimination" for interindividual differences in steady-state concentrations of the adrenergic — receptor antagonist alprenolol, *J. Pharmacokinet. Biopharmaceut.,* 5, 193, 1977.

132. **Borg, K. O., Carlsson, E., Ek, L., and Johansson, R.,** Combined pharmacokinetic and pharmacodynamic studies of metoprolol in the cat and the dog, *Acta Pharmacol. Toxicol.*, 36, 24, 1975.

133. **Johnsson, G., Regårdh, C-G., and Sölvell, L.,** Combined pharmacokinetic and pharmacodynamic studies in man of the adrenergic β-receptor antagonist metoprolol, *Acta Pharmacol. Toxicol.*, 36, Suppl. V., 31, 1975.

134. **Rawlins, M. D., Collste, P., Frisk-Holmberg, M., Lind, M., Östman, J., and Sjöqvist, F.,** Steady-state plasma concentrations of alprenolol in man, *Eur. J. Clin. Pharmacol.*, 7, 353, 1974.

135. **Levy, R. H., Pitlick, W. H., Troupin, A. S., Green, J. R., and Neal, J. M.,** Pharmacokinetics of carbamazepine in normal man, *Clin. Pharmacol. Therapeut.*, 17, 657, 1975.

Chapter 4

TOXICOLOGICAL EFFECTS ON CARCINOGENESIS

Ronald C. Shank and Louis R. Barrows

TABLE OF CONTENTS

I. INTRODUCTION

At the risk of stating the obvious, it is nevertheless important to keep in mind, in interpreting carcinogenicity data, that chemical carcinogens are also cytotoxic agents producing cell death in target organs after acute exposure. For many chemicals the carcinogenic response can be produced by exposure to doses below those which elicit widespread cell death in the target organ; such compounds appear to form highly reactive electrophiles in the target cell and covalently bind to nucleophilic sites in DNA. Other chemicals seem to cause cancer only after repeated exposure at maximally tolerated doses, levels which repeatedly cause cytotoxicity and restorative cellular regeneration; demonstration of covalent binding between DNA and these compounds has been difficult. Recently, however, some studies have suggested that the cytotoxic response to some chemical carcinogens may begin a series of biochemical events involving endogenous agents which damage DNA, and thus point to similarity in the mechanisms by which both classes of chemical carcinogens initiate cancer, by stimulating the formation of adducts with DNA.

II. CHEMICAL CARCINOGENESIS

A. Somatic Mutation Hypothesis

A number of hypotheses have been proposed to explain the mechanism by which chemicals can cause cancer; of these, the somatic mutation hypothesis has received considerable lasting support. Boveri[1] proposed in 1914 that cancer is a cellular process that parallels mutation but occurs in somatic cells rather than in germ cells. There have been many efforts to support or disprove the hypothesis, and early attempts to equate carcinogenicity with mutagenicity failed. At that time the most frequently used methods to detect mutagens relied on microbial systems which lacked the metabolic capabilities of mammalian cells, and it had not yet been recognized that many chemicals are inactive as carcinogens in the chemical state in which they exist outside the cell.

With the advent of mammalian and combined microbial-mammalian test systems in mutagenicity, such as the host-mediated assay[2] and the Ames assay,[3] it became even clearer that mammalian metabolism is necessary to activate chemically the carcinogens so that they would be both mutagenic and carcinogenic. Activation in most cases meant conversion of the procarcinogen to a highly reactive electrophile which served as the ultimate carcinogen by covalently binding to DNA in the target cell.[4] The Millers focussed the knowledge on chemical carcinogenesis, much of which they contributed, by pointing out that chemicals of such divergent structure as benzo(a)pyrene, dimethylnitrosamine, aflatoxin B_1, 2-acetylaminofluorene, etc. bind covalently to nucleophilic sites in target organ DNA.

Adduct formation in DNA has been shown to lead to genetic damage and mutagenic events,[5,6] yet such formation did not constitute obligatory transformation of the affected cell. In extensive comparative studies on aberrant methylation of target and non-target DNA by alkyl N-nitroso compounds, Magee and co-workers[7] have demonstrated that DNA alkylation itself does not always correlate with carcinogenicity. Goth and Rajewsky[8] were among the first to show a strong correlation between persistence of alkylation in DNA and the formation of cancer. Craddock[9] and others have offered considerable experimental evidence to stress the importance of DNA replication, after damage (alkylation) but before repair, in completing the process of initiating a cell in the many steps of carcinogenesis. The early sequence of events in chemical carcinogenesis appears to involve (1) conversion of a chemical agent to an electrophile which covalently binds to target organ DNA, constituting nonlethal damage to that macromolecule and (2) replication of that DNA before repair of the damage can be achieved, or induction of erroneous repair, such that of the resultant DNA leads to daughter cells which have an altered genetic structure compared to the parent (target) cell.

B. Indirect Mechanisms

The above "genetic mechanism," proposed to explain the mechanism of action of carcinogenic chemicals, applies well to a rapidly expanding list of compounds. All of these compounds (the polynuclear aromatic hydrocarbons, aflatoxins, N-nitroso compounds, aromatic amines, etc.) can be characterized by some or all of the following properties:

- they can induce cancer at exposures well below near lethal doses
- they can induce de novo cancers as well as increase the incidence of spontaneous tumors
- they can induce cancer in a short period of time relative to the life span of the test species
- they can form adducts with DNA in target organs

There is also a class of chemicals which induce cancer but have characteristics different from the above agents. Such compounds are chloroform, carbon tetrachloride, chlordane, hydrazine, etc. and share the following properties:

- they appear to induce cancer only at exposure levels which are near lethal doses (maximum tolerated dose which depresses growth rate 10 to 20%)
- many increase the incidence of spontaneous tumors but do not induce formation of tumors which are rarely seen in control populations of the test species
- cancers arise only after a long exposure relative to the life span of the test animal
- they do not form detectable levels of DNA adducts in in vivo tests

Such compounds have been given many classifications, and it has become popular to refer to their unknown mechanism(s) of action as "epigenetic", principally because no interaction between the carcinogen and the genetic template can be demonstrated. Although sufficient information is not yet available to scientifically place these two "types" of carcinogens into rigorously defined categories, one does develop intuitively a feeling for the distinction. A single low-level exposure to one of the latter agents would appear to be less likely to induce cancer than such an exposure to one of the former agents, merely because the animal work suggests greater difficulty in inducing cancer with an agent which appears to require repeated exposures to high doses.

One property of the latter group of carcinogens appears to be the association between cytotoxic damage and carcinogenicity. Rats,[10,11] mice,[12-14] and hamsters[15] develop liver tumors after receiving liver necrotizing doses of carbon tetrachloride repeatedly for several weeks but not when the exposure is to nonnecrotizing doses. Vinylidene chloride at renal necrotizing doses produces adenocarcinomas in mouse kidney but not in rat or hamster kidney when animals are given nonnecrotizing doses.[16,17] Rats exposed by inhalation to formaldehyde vapors at 15 ppm, 6 hours/day, 5 days/week for 18 months developed highly irritated nasal epithelial tissue including papillary hyperplasia and squamous atypia and then squamous cell carcinomas.[18] Rats exposed to 2 or 6 ppm formaldehyde developed less severe nasal irritation and no cancer; mice exposed to the same concentrations of formaldehyde failed to produce any nasal tumors. A similar experiment with hydrazine using rats, mice, and hamsters also produced carcinomas of the nasal turbinates only in rats at only that dose which was severely irritating to the nasal epithelium; exposure at lower doses, which were less irritating, failed to produce the tumors.[19]

The cancer bioassays on the above four compounds may be typical of a class of chemicals, those which require repeated cytotoxicity as part of the carcinogenic process. It is true that essentially all chemical carcinogens produce some toxicity during the carcinogenic regimen but the above class of compounds appears to require widespread necrosis as opposed to small foci of atypia and/or islands of necrosis.

If future studies are able to firmly establish a causal relationship between repeated wide-spread cytotoxicity and carcinogenesis, those experimental results will have significant impact on the interpretation of cancer bioassays that find carcinogenic effects of test compounds when exposure is at only the maximum tolerated dose and no increase in cancer incidence when exposures are below doses which cause such cytotoxicity. If such experimental results become available, the interpretative process necessary for extrapolations from high-dose bioassays to health risks for humans at low level environmental exposures may become increasingly complex. Attempts are currently being made to obtain experimental results which pertain to the causal role cytotoxicity may play in carcinogenesis. The weak carcinogen, hydrazine, has been used as the model.

III. HYDRAZINE AND INDIRECT DNA DAMAGE

It has recently been shown that administration of the inorganic hepatotoxin and carcinogen, hydrazine (H_2N-NH_2), results in the methylation of liver DNA guanine, with the methyl moiety arising from the 1-carbon pool.[20-22] The methylation profile in DNA after hydrazine administration is qualitatively the same as that seen after the administration of strong alkylating carcinogens such as dimethylnitrosamine, 1,2-dimethylhydrazine, or methylnitrosourea with the formation of 7-methylguanine and O^6-methylguanine. The mechanism of this indirect methylation of DNA and the universality with which it applies to other hepatotoxins and other tissues are not yet known.

A. Pharmacokinetic Studies on Methylguanines in Liver DNA in the Rat and Hamster

Becker and co-workers[23] studied the rate of formation and the persistence of 7-methylguanine and O^6-methylguanine in liver DNA of rats treated with 90 mg hydrazine/kg body weight, approximately the 7-day LD_{50}. Methylation of liver DNA guanine was detectable within 15 min after hydrazine administration; half-maximal alkylation levels were obtained in 30 to 45 min and maximum alkylation at about 6 hr (Table 1). The persistence of 7-methylguanine and O^6-methylguanine in the liver DNA of hydrazine-treated animals (Figure 1) was the same as that observed in rats treated with dimethylnitrosamine[24] or 1,2-dimethylhydrazine.[25] The study with hydrazine was repeated in the hamster;[26] longer persistence of O^6-methylguanine in hamster liver DNA compared to rat liver DNA is consistent with the results of Stumpf and co-workers,[27] who measured the persistence of this promutagenic base in liver DNA after treating hamsters with dimethylnitrosamine.

B. Role of S-Adenosylmethionine

If rats or mice are treated orally with a necrogenic dose of hydrazine and are given radiolabeled methionine intraperitoneally immediately thereafter and hourly for several hours to maintain label in the S-adenosylmethionine pool, the 7-methylguanine and O^6-methylguanine that form in the liver DNA are also radiolabeled. This suggests that S-adenosylmethionine is the source of the methyl group in the methylguanines.[20] Administration of ethionine, the antimetabolite of methionine, inhibits the formation of S-adenosylmethionine and concomitantly the methylation of DNA in hydrazine-treated rats; as the animals recover from the ethionine poisoning and S-adenosylmethionine begins to return to normal levels in the liver, the methylation of liver DNA in response to hydrazine administration also returns.[28]

C. Role of Monomethylhydrazine

The liver contains N-methylases which use S-adenosylmethionine in the methylation of primary amines, such as epinephrine[29] and histamine;[30] it would seem quite possible that these enzymes could methylate hydrazine to form monomethylhydrazine (CH_3NH-NH_2). Administration of monomethylhydrazine to mice has been shown to result in the formation

Table 1
LIVER DNA METHYLATION AFTER HYDRAZINE ADMINISTRATION TO RATS

Time after administration (hr)	μmol 7-MeG/mol G	μmol O⁶-MeG/mol G
0	ND[a]	ND[b]
	ND	ND
0.25	213	11
	409	19
	mean = 311	mean = 15
0.50	381	17
	912	33
	mean = 647	mean = 25
1	434	35
	758	53
	mean = 596	mean = 44
6	500	42
	1240	112
	mean = 870	mean = 77
12	902	91
	767	68
	mean = 835	mean = 80
24	838	52
	885	82
	mean = 862	mean = 67
48	600	14
	637	21
	mean = 619	mean = 18
72	355	trace
	558	trace
	mean = 447	
96	234	trace
	273	ND
	mean = 259	

Note: Young adult male Fischer 344 rats were fasted overnight and given by stomach tube 90 mg hydrazine/kg body wt. in 0.1 mℓ 0.1 *M* HCl and decapitated at various times therafter.

[a]   No 7-methylguanine detected (<50 μmol 7-MeG/mol G.
[b]   No O⁶-methylguanine detected (<2 μmol O⁶-MeG/mol G.

From R. A. Becker, L. R., Barrows, and R. C. Shank, *Carcinogenesis*, 2, 1181, 1981. With permission.

of 7-methylguanine in liver DNA,[31] and thus the formation of monomethylhydrazine as a result of hydrazine administration could explain the aberrant methylation of liver DNA in hydrazine-treated animals.[22,23]

Administration of equitoxic doses of hydrazine or monomethylhydrazine to rats results in more 7-methylguanine and O⁶-methylguanine in liver DNA in the hydrazine-treated animals; administration of equimolar doses of the two compounds to mice results in more methylation of liver DNA guanine in hydrazine-treated animals (Table 2).[28] Indeed, hydrazine administration to hamsters results in the expected levels of 7-methylguanine and O⁶-methylguanine, but administration of an equimolar dose, or even a lethal dose, of monomethylhydrazine

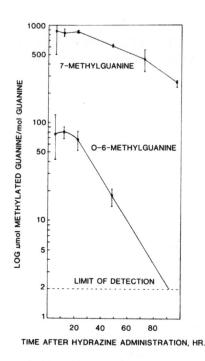

FIGURE 1.   Removal of 7-methylguanine and O^6-methylguanine from rat liver
DNA following a single oral administration of 90 mg hydrazine/kg body wt. Data
from Table 1 were plotted semilogarithmically to determine the removal rate of
these methylated purines. Trace amounts (2 to 5 μ mol/mol guanine) of O^6-
methylguanine were detected in liver DNA from rats killed 72 and 96 hr after
hydrazine treatment; extension of the curve from 48 to 96 hr using the same slope
as observed from 24 to 48 hr is consistent with detection of these trace levels of
O^6-methylguanine. (From Becker, R. A., Barrows, L. R., and Shank, R. C.,
Carcinogenesis, 2, 1181, 1981. With permission.)

yields no detectable methylguanines at all (Shank, unpublished data).[61] None of these results
is consistent with the proposal that monomethylhydrazine is an intermediate in the methylation of DNA in hydrazine-treated animals. If such were the case, then administration of
the more proximal methylating agent would be expected to be more efficient in methylating
DNA. All this is further complicated by the results of studies on hydrazine metabolism by
Dost and co-workers[32] who accounted for 75% of the administered toxicant as expired
nitrogen gas, and excreted hydrazine and monoacetylhydrazine, leaving only 25% or less
of the administered hydrazine available for possible methylation to monomethylhydrazine.
It is possible that hydrazine enters the liver cell more readily than does monomethylhydrazine,
so that administration of equimolar doses of the two results in a higher intracellular concentration of monomethylhydrazine as the methylation product of hydrazine. Route of administration has no effect on the acute toxicity (LD_{50}) of hydrazine or monomethylhydrazine,[33]
suggesting that the toxicants distribute with the body water. In in vitro studies rodent liver
slices metabolize monomethylhydrazine to carbon dioxide at a rate at least as fast as that
for glucose, indicating rapid adsorption of the toxicant into liver cells.[34] There is little
evidence available, then, to suggest that monomethylhydrazine enters the liver cells at a rate
appreciably slower than that for hydrazine.

Current methods of chemical analysis do not permit the quantitative measurement of both
hydrazine and monomethylhydrazine simultaneously in biological tissue, thus it is not feasible
at this time to determine the amount of monomethylhydrazine in liver tissue following the
administration of hydrazine.

Table 2
METHYLATION OF LIVER DNA GUANINE IN RATS AND MICE GIVEN HYDRAZINE OR MONOMETHYLHYDRAZINE

Agent[a]	Dose[b]	Toxicity	Kill Time, hr	DNA analyzed, mg	7-MeG[c]	O⁶-MeG[d]
			Rat			
HZ	60 (1.88)	≃ LD_{25}	13	13.3	193	22
MMH	15 (0.33)	≃ LD_{25}	13	19.6	ND[e]	ND
			Mouse			
HZ	10.4 (0.33)	≃$LD_{0.01}$	1	24.6	157	9
MMH	15.0 (0.33)	1/2 LD_{50}	1	23.9	52	2

Note: Young adult male Fischer 344 rats and Swiss Webster mice were given hydrazine or monomethyl-hydrazine by stomach tube; DNA alkylation levels were determined by fluorescence high performance liquid chromatography.

a HZ, hydrazine; MMH, monomethylhydrazine.
b mg/kg body wt. (mmol/kg body wt.).
c 7-MeG, 7-methylguanine (μ mol/mol guanine).
d O⁶-MeG, O⁶-methylguanine (μ mol/mol guanine).
e N.D., none detected.

D. Proposed Mechanisms of Action
1. Non-Enzymatic DNA Methylation by S-Adenosylmethionine
As stated above, S-adenosylmethionine is considered the most likely proximal methyl donor in hydrazine-induced DNA methylation. S-Adenosylmethionine is the major intracellular methyl donor in a wide variety of normal biochemical pathways in mammalian cells.[35] S-Adenosylmethionine contains an unstable sulfonium ion and decomposes at physiological pH to form methylthioadenosine with a half life of about 36 hr.[36] Paik and co-workers[37] showed that S-adenosylmethionine has the capacity to methylate nucleophiles nonenzymatically. They found the transfer of radioactivity from S-adenosylmethionine to acceptor proteins in vitro to yield proteins apparently containing esterified aspartyl and glutamyl residues. In unrelated studies, the kinetics of radioactive methionine uptake and incorporation in liver[38-40] were found to be consistent with the rapid appearance of radio-labeled 7-methylguanine in the DNA.[21] If the radiolabel had to pass through S-adenosylmethionine to a second methyl donor, such as tetrahydrofolic acid, a less extensive radiolabeling of the DNA would have been expected in the first 30 min after methionine administration. Nevertheless, it has been shown that mice treated with hydrazine and radioactive formate also contained radioactive 7-methylguanine in the liver DNA,[22] although the kinetics of this reaction have not been fully described. Further work comparing the relative contributions of formate and methionine to the toxicity-dependent DNA methylation could help identify the ultimate methyl source of the reaction. Methionine itself is not a likely candidate because it is a relatively stable compound, and there is no direct pathway for formate to generate the methylthioether moiety required.

It was, in part, because of the report by Paik and co-workers[37] that, in 1982, two laboratories independently published experimental results indicating that S-adenosylmethionine can methylate DNA nonenzymatically. Barrows and Magee[41] used physiological concentrations of S-adenosylmethionine to methylate calf thymus DNA in vitro. The putative 7-methylguanine co-migrated with authentic 7-methylguanine in two different high pressure liquid chromatography systems, and was found to have ultraviolet light absorption characteristics consistent with those of 7-methylguanine. It was also found that the DNA methylation increased linearly with increasing S-adenosylmethionine concentrations. At physiological concentrations of S-adenosylmethionine at 37°C and neutral pH, it was estimated that approximately 0.7 μ mole 7-methylguanine were formed per mole of guanine in the DNA per hour of incubation. The formation of minor DNA adducts was also suggested in this work, since low but significant amounts of radioactivity were consistently detected co-migrating with O^6-methylguanine and 3-methyladenine following chromatographic analysis of the DNA. The amount of O^6-methylguanine formed was estimated to be about 8% of the total 7-methylguanine formed. The analytical system used in these experiments has not been quantitated for the analysis of 3-methyladenine, nevertheless, radioactivity equaling about 1% of the total found in 7-methylguanine was always detected co-migrating with 3-methyladenine. The authors stress, however, that the slow rate of the methylation reaction made accurate quantitation of the minor products difficult.

The formation of 3-methyladenine was better quantitated in a study by Rydberg and Lindahl.[42] Their research into the mechanisms by which cells repair the specific methylated bases formed by simple methylating agents also suggested that S-adenosylmethionine was likely to methylate DNA nonenzymatically. The work provides strong evidence for the formation of 3-methyladenine as well as 7-methylguanine in these reactions; the investigators estimated the formation of 3-methyladenine to equal about 20% of the amount of 7-methylguanine formed. Rydberg and Lindahl also obtained evidence for the formation of O^6-methylguanine and estimated that the ratio of O^6-methylguanine to 7-methylguanine was less than 0.01; however it was also noted that the small amounts of radioactivity analyzed made accurate estimates difficult. Since the O^6-methylguanine/7-methylguanine and 3-methyladenine/7-methylguanine ratios are characteristic of the ultimate methylating species,[43] a more detailed description of these ratios in vivo and in vitro would provide a better understanding of the methylation mechanism in the animal.

In addition to the ability of S-adenosylmethionine to methylate DNA non-enzymatically in vitro, there are several in vivo observations that suggest that the toxicity-dependent DNA methylation might be a nonenzymatic reaction. There has been more than one methyl adduct identified in vivo so far. Both 7-methylguanine and O^6-methylguanine are produced. The presence of O^6-methylguanine suggests that other minor bases may be produced as well. This is similar to DNA methylation by methylating carcinogens such as methylnitrosourea and N-methyl-N'-nitro-N-nitrosoguanidine[43] and reflects the fact that DNA contains multiple reactive sites. The formation of more than one methyl adduct in vivo is inconsistent with the specificity normally attributed to enzymatic reactions. It would be particularly uncharacteristic of enzyme behavior in this case because O^6-methylguanine and 7-methylguanine are structurally dissimilar and because the O^6-position of guanine is involved in base pairing on the interior of α-helical DNA, while the 7-position of guanine is exposed on the outside of the helix.

Other in vivo evidence, obtained with the methionine antimetabolite, ethionine, is also consistent with a nonenzymatic methylation of DNA by S-adenosylmethionine. Immediately following ethionine administration to rats, liver S-adenosylmethionine concentrations fell to one third of normal levels (about 20 nmoles per gram liver), where they remained for at least 90 min.[40] When hydrazine was given to these animals, the 7-methylguanine and O^6-methylguanine formation was reduced in direct proportion to the reduced S-adenosylmethionine levels. Meanwhile, in the same samples, the known enzymatic synthesis of 5-methylcytosine was undiminished. Rat liver DNA methylase is thought to have a K_m around 2.5×10^{-6} (Reference 44) and would be expected to function normally at the reduced concentrations of S-adenosylmethionine. Thus the toxicity-dependent DNA methylation is distinct from 5-methylcytosine synthesis and is consistent with a nonenzymatic mechanism.

In view of the above discussion it appears possible that, during hydrazine toxicity, S-adenosylmethionine could methylate DNA directly. If this were the case, however, then a constant, although possibly lower level of DNA methylation would be expected in all living tissue; this has not been observed. 7-Methylguanine has never been detected in normal mammalian DNA despite several attempts.[21,45-47] If nonenzymatic methylation of DNA were normal to mammalian DNA, it would have to be below the limits of detection of current technology (0.1 μ mol methylguanine/mol guanine). The possibility of a constant low level methylation of cellular DNA was suggested in a recent report by Barrows and Magee.[48] Radioactivity was found to co-migrate with marker 7-methylguanine in DNA, analyzed by high pressure liquid chromatography, from mammalian cells cultured with radioactive methionine. If there is a constant nonenzymatic methylation of DNA in vivo, it is likely the resultant damage is kept to an acceptable level by the constitutive repair enzymes specific for these lesions (see Section III.D.3.). The rate of nonenzymatic methylation by S-adenosylmethionine in vitro, however, is too slow to account for the DNA methylation observed during the first half hour of hydrazine toxicity in vivo.[23] In order for nonenzymatic DNA methylation to be responsible for the in vivo observations, the concentration of S-adenosylmethionine in chromatin would have to be from 500 to 1000 times higher than the whole tissue levels of about 65 nmoles per gram liver. The concentration of S-adenosylmethionine in the cell nucleus during times of toxic stress is wholly unknown.

2. Aberrant Activity of DNA Methyltransferase

There is little available evidence to support other mechanisms of action for toxicity-dependent DNA methylation as proposed.[23] The enzymatic methylation of the 5-position of cytosine which follows DNA synthesis in mammalian cells has been well documented.[49] It is also well known that this methylation takes place primarily at specific sites in DNA involving palindromic sequences of 5'CG[50,51] and that the 5-position of cytosine is in close proximity to the 7-position of guanine, thus the normal methylation in DNA is stereochemically close to the site at which aberrant methylation may take place. It follows, then, that methylation in a cell poisoned by hydrazine may occur with a loss of specificity in the methylation site, due to either a loss of enzyme specificity or a stereochemical change in the nucleic acid, or both.

Little is known about the formation of 5-methylcytosine in DNA of animals treated with hydrazine, and the enzyme, DNA methyltransferase, has not been a focus in the hydrazine studies. It will be important to examine this proposed mechanism experimentally. The failure to explain the formation of O^6-methylguanine by a loss of specificity of DNA methyltransferase and the fact that methylation of RNA also results from hydrazine administration,[22] however, lessen the immediacy of these experiments.

3. Methylguanines as Normal Bases in Mammalian DNA

It has also been suggested[23] that detection of 7-methylguanine and O^6-methylguanine in liver DNA after hydrazine administration may represent not aberrant methylation of the macromolecule, but rather an inhibition of the removal of these methylguanines which are normally present in DNA. As indicated above, most efforts to demonstrate the presence of these bases in normal mammalian DNA have failed, although one report[48] suggests the possibility that methylguanines may exist at low levels in normal mammalian DNA. Also, considerable evidence is now available for the presence of endogenous enzymes for the removal of 7-methylguanine and O^6-methylguanine from DNA in normal mammalian cells.[52-55] The presence of such enzymes in normal cells implies a need for their activity and hence the presence of the methylguanines, the substrates for these enzymes. As methods of chemical detection of minor bases in DNA are improved, it may be possible to demonstrate clearly the presence of 7-methylguanine and O^6-methylguanine in normal mammalian DNA. Attempts will also have to be made to determine the effect of hydrazine toxicity on the activity of these "repair" enzymes.

IV. CYTOTOXICITY AND DNA DAMAGE

A. Hepatotoxins Other than Hydrazine

If hepatotoxicity, and not some intrinsic property of the hydrazine molecule, is the driving force that stimulates the S-adenosylmethionine-dependent methylation of liver DNA guanine, then other hepatotoxins, structurally unrelated to hydrazine, should also stimulate this aberrant methylation. Barrows and Shank[21] reported such methylation in response to carbon tetrachloride and ethanol toxicity. In addition, the formation of 7-methylguanine following administration of yellow phosphorus, thioacetamide, puromycin, and aflatoxin B_1 has been seen, but with poor reproducibility (Shank, unpublished data). In six trials with carbon tetrachloride, four trials with ethanol, and two with phosphorus, the methylation response was detected only half the time. In several experiments methylguanines have never been detected following administration of high doses of the hepatotoxins, diethylnitrosamine or ethionine. On the other hand, the methylation response is highly reproducible with N-nitrosopyrrolidine.[56] In this case administration of ring-labeled (^{14}C) N-nitrosopyrrolidine results in the formation of two fluorescent DNA adducts, one labeled with carbon-14 but as yet unidentified, and the second, unlabeled, and identified as 7-methylguanine. If rats are given unlabeled N-nitrosopyrrolidine and simultaneously (^{3}H-methyl)methionine, the former, unidentified, N-nitrosopyrrolidine-DNA adduct is unlabeled, but the 7-methylguanine in the DNA is labeled. Similar experiments have been done with dimethylnitrosamine which have shown reproducibly that, although dimethylnitrosamine is metabolized to a methylating agent itself, the carcinogen and hepatotoxin also stimulates S-adenosylmethionine-dependent methylation of DNA; approximately 0.4% of the total 7-methylguanine formed in liver DNA of dimethylnitrosamine-treated rats derives from methionine, rather than from the nitrosamine itself.[57]

Therefore, some evidence is available to suggest that S-adenosylmethionine-dependent DNA methylation may be a response to hepatotoxins in addition to hydrazine and thus may be a result of hepatotoxicity, but not hepatotoxicity alone; other contributing factors, not yet recognized, are likely to play an important role.

B. In Vitro Cell Culture Systems

While cytotoxicity is very difficult to define and quantitate in vivo, even with extensive histology, cytotoxicity in cultured cells can be described more rigorously. A number of biochemical end points can be followed easily in vitro. The inhibition of energy metabolism and the inhibition of protein, RNA, or DNA synthesis are examples of cytotoxicity which can be easily monitored in vitro. The most universal measure to cytotoxicity in vitro however, is the inhibition of cloning efficiency, that is, the inhibition of a cell's ability to divide and grow to form a colony. The inhibition of colony formation is considered a lethal event, and can be used to quantitate the effects of a wide variety of compounds on cultured cells.[58]

Preliminary experiments using this end point and looking for toxicity-dependent DNA methylation have been conducted in BHK 21/Cl 13 cells.[48] The cells were cultured with radioactive methionine and the DNA was analyzed by high pressure liquid chromatography. In these samples radioactivity was found to co-migrate with marker 7-methylguanine. The 7-methylguanine-associated radioactivity also increased in a dose-dependent fashion when toxic concentrations of either dimethylnitrosamine or hydrazine were added to the culture medium. This observation was similar to the observed DNA methylation in rat liver during hydrazine poisoning. Further experiments are now in progress to confirm the identity of the putative DNA methylation products in cultured cells. If this in vitro observation can be confirmed as toxicity-dependent DNA methylation, then several interesting determinations can be made. It may be possible to establish a quantitative dose-response relationship between cytotoxicity and the DNA methylation; in vitro systems have the capacity to test a number of toxicants relatively quickly. It may also be possible to test whether toxicity-dependent DNA methylation is mutagenic or oncogenic since mutation and transformation assays are already established in the BHK cell line.[40,59] In addition, a wide variety of mechanistic studies are possible in cell culture that might be impossible in the more complicated whole animal model. It is hoped that the in vitro and in vivo systems can be used in concert to determine the mechanism and biological significance of toxicity-dependent DNA methylation.

V. UNIFYING HYPOTHESIS

There is much evidence to support the hypothesis that most chemical carcinogens initiate the carcinogenic process through similar biochemical pathways that lead to the formation of electrophiles which covalently bind to target organ DNA; replication of the damaged DNA leads to transformation of the affected cells to cancer cells. If this hypothesis proves correct, it would be tempting to propose DNA binding studies as a screening test for predicting carcinogenic potential of chemical agents.

The studies with hydrazine, and a few other hepatotoxins, offer a note of caution, however, by indicating that DNA adducts may indeed form as a result of exposure to a carcinogen, but the adduct need not necessarily be a product of the nucleic acid and the carcinogen itself. Thus, failure to demonstrate covalent binding between a carcinogen and DNA does not necessarily mean that no DNA adduct has formed. The concept that chemical carcinogens form DNA adducts which lead to cell transformation remains intact however, whether the carcinogen itself binds to DNA or stimulates another chemical group to interact with the genetic material.

Roberts[60] has suggested that erroneous DNA repair and chromosomal aberrations during cellular regulation may explain induction of cancers by chemicals which do not appear to directly modify the genetic material. Non-alkylating toxicants produce cell killing which is followed by restorative hyperplasia; this hyperplasia takes place in an environment that may be abnormal and may be deficient in the normal regulatory feedback controls involved in homeostasis. Finding aberrant methylation in DNA following administration of a high dose of the inorganic toxicant, hydrazine, suggests that cytotoxicity may induce DNA methylation and therefore may be qualitatively equivalent to administration of a strong alkylating agent; this may add another consideration to Roberts' hypothesis, but ultimately the effect is the same: replication of damaged DNA presumably resulting in a somatic mutation. If this effect is a result of administration of a cytotoxic dose of the non-alkylating toxicant, rather than due to some intrinsic property of the toxicant itself, then it may be that such compounds induce somatic mutations following administration only at cytotoxic levels; lesser exposures which do not lead to DNA damage, cytotoxicity, and tissue regeneration would not be expected to lead to somatic mutation and cancer.

The observation that hydrazine toxicity results in aberrant methylation of liver DNA may be highly relevant to the argument that cytotoxicity can be causally associated with carcinogenesis. If this phenomenon is a general response to toxicity, understanding the mechanism by which the methylation occurs could assist in the interpretation of results from carcinogenicity bioassays in which increased cancer incidences are observed only at or near cytotoxic levels of the test compound.

REFERENCES

1. **Boveri, T.,** *Origin of Malignant Tumors,* (translated by M. Boveri), Williams and Wilkins, Baltimore, Md., 1929, 111.
2. **Gabridge, M. G. and Legator, M. S.,** A host-mediated microbial assay for the detection of mutagenic compounds, *Proc. Soc. Exptl. Biol. Med.,* 130, 831, 1969.
3. **Ames, B. N., McCann, J., and Yamasaki, E.,** Methods for detecting carcinogens and mutagens with the *Salmonella*/mammalian-microsome mutagenicity test, *Mutat. Res.,* 31, 347, 1975.
4. **Miller, J. A.,** Carcinogenesis by chemicals: an overview. G.H.A. Clowes Memorial Lecture, *Cancer Res.,* 30, 559, 1970.
5. **Loveless, A.,** Possible relevance of O^6-alkylation of deoxyguanosine to the mutagenicity and carcinogenicity of nitrosamines and nitrosamides, *Nature,* (London), 233, 206, 1969.
6. **Gerchman, L. L. and Ludlum, D. B.,** The properties of O^6-methylguanine in template for RNA polymerase, *Biochim. Biophys. Acta,* 308, 310, 1973.
7. **Swann, P. F. and Magee, P. N.,** Nitrosamine-induced carcinogenesis. The alkylation of nucleic acids of the rat by N-methyl-N-nitrosourea, dimethylnitrosamine, dimethylsulphate, and methyl methanesulphonate, *Biochem. J.,* 110, 39, 1968.
8. **Goth, R. and Rajewsky, M. F.,** Molecular and cellular mechanisms associated with pulse-carcinogenesis in the rat nervous system by ethylnitrosourea: ethylation of nucleic acids of different tissues, *Z. Krebsforsch.,* 82, 37, 1974.
9. **Craddock, V. M.,** Cell proliferation and experimental liver cancer, in *Liver Cell Cancer,* Cameron, H. M., Linsell, C. A., and Warwick, G. P., Eds., Elsevier/North Holland, Amsterdam, 1976, 153.
10. **Reuber, M. D. and Glover, E. L.,** Hyperplastic and early neoplastic lesions of the liver in Buffalo strain rats of various ages given subcutaneous carbon tetrachloride, *J. Natl. Cancer Inst.,* 38, 891, 1967.
11. **Reuber, M. D. and Glover, E. L.,** Cirrhosis and carcinoma of the liver in male rats given subcutaneous carbon tetrachloride, *J. Natl. Cancer Inst.,* 44, 419, 1970.
12. **Edwards, J. E.,** Hepatomas in mice induced with carbon tetrachloride, *J. Natl. Cancer Inst.,* 2, 197, 1941—42.
13. **Edwards, J. E. and Dalton, A. J.,** Induction of cirrhosis of the liver and hepatomas in mice with carbon tetrachloride, *J. Natl. Cancer Inst.,* 3, 297, 1942—43.
14. **Eschenbrenner, A. B. and Miller, E.,** Liver necrosis and the induction of carbon tetrachloride hepatomas in strain A mice, *J. Natl. Cancer Inst.,* 6, 325, 1945.
15. **Della Porta, G., Terracini, B., and Shubik, P.,** Induction with carbon tetrachloride of liver cell carcinomas in hamsters, *J. Natl. Cancer Inst.,* 26, 855, 1961.
16. **Maltoni, C.,** Recent findings on the carcinogenicity of chlorinated olefins, *Environ. Health Perspect.,* 21, 1, 1977.
17. **Maltoni, G., Gotti, G., Morisi, L., and Chieco, P.,** Carcinogenicity bioassays of vinylidene chloride. Research plan and early results, *Med. Lav.,* 68, 241, 1977.
18. **Swenberg, J. A., Kerns, W. D., Mitchell, R. I., Gralla, E. J., and Pavkov, K. L.,** Induction of squamous cell carcinomas of the rat nasal cavity by inhalation exposure to formaldehyde vapor, *Cancer Res.,* 40, 3398, 1980.
19. **MacEwen, J. D., Vernot, E. H., Haun, C. C., Kinkead, E. R., and Hall, A.,** Chronic Inhalation Toxicity of Hydrazine: Oncogenic Effects, *AFAMRL-TR-81-56,* Air Force Aerospace Medical Research Laboratories, Wright-Patterson Air Force Base, Ohio, 1981.
20. **Barrows, L. R. and Shank, R. C.,** Chemical modification of DNA in rats treated with hydrazine, *Toxicol. Appl. Pharmacol.,* 45, 324, 1978.
21. **Barrows, L. R. and Shank, R. C.,** Aberrant methylation of liver DNA in rats during hepatoxicity, *Toxicol. Appl. Pharmacol.,* 60, 334, 1981.
22. **Quinter-Ruiz, A., Paz-Neri, L. L., and Villa-Trevino, S.,** Indirect alkylation of CBA mouse liver DNA and RNA by hydrazine *in vivo.* A possible mechanism of action as a carcinogen, *J. Natl. Cancer Inst.,* 67, 613, 1981.
23. **Becker, R. A., Barrows, L. R., and Shank, R. C.,** Methylation of liver DNA guanine in hydrazine hepatotoxicity dose-response and kinetic characteristics of 7-methylguanine and O^6-methylguanine formation and persistence in rats, *Carcinogenesis,* 2, 1181, 1981.
24. **O'Connor, P. J., Capps, M. J., and Craig, A. W.,** Comparative studies of the hepatocarcinogen N,N-dimethylnitrosamine *in vivo*: reaction sites in rat liver DNA and the significance of their relative stabilities, *Br. J. Cancer,* 27, 153, 1973.
25. **Herron, D. C., and Shank, R. C.,** *In vivo* kinetics of O^6-methylguanine and 7-methylguanine formation and persistence in DNA of rats treated with symmetrical dimethylhydrazine, *Cancer Res.,* 41, 3967, 1981.
26. **Bosan, W. S. and Shank, R. C.,** Methylguanines in liver DNA after administration of hydrazine to hamsters, *Proc. Am. Assoc. Res. Cancer,* 23, 62, 1982.

27. **Stumpf, R., Margison, G. P., Montesano, R., and Pegg, A. E.,** Formation and loss of alkylated purines from DNA of hamster liver after administration of dimethylnitrosamine, *Cancer Res.,* 39, 50, 1979.

28. **Barrows, L. R.,** Methylation of DNA in Hydrazine-Treated Rats and Mice, Ph.D. Dissertation, Dept. Medical Pharmacol. Therap., University of Calif., Irvine, 1980.

29. **Kirshner, N. and Goodall, Mc. C.,** The formation of adrenaline from noradrenaline, *Biochim. Biophys. Acta,* 24, 658, 1957.

30. **Brown, D. D., Tomchick, R., and Axelrod, J.,** The distribution and properties of a histamine-methylating enzyme, *J. Biol. Chem.,* 234, 2948, 1959.

31. **Hawks, A. and Magee, P. N.,** The alkylation of nucleic acids of rat and mouse *in vivo* by the carcinogen 1,2-dimethylhydrazine, *Br. J. Cancer,* 30, 440, 1974.

32. **Dost, F. N., Springer, D. L., Krivak, B. M., and Reed, D. J.,** Metabolism of Hydrazine, *AMRL-TR-79-43,* Air Force Aerospace Medical Research Laboratories, Wright-Patterson Air Force Base, Ohio, 1979.

33. **Witkin, L. B.,** Acute toxicity of hydrazine and some of its methylated derivatives, *Arch. Ind. Health,* 13, 34, 1956.

34. **Shank, R. C.,** Comparative Metabolism of Propellant Hydrazine, *AMRL-TR-79-57,* Air Force Aerospace Medical Research Laboratories, Wright-Patterson Air Force Base, Ohio, 1979.

35. **Usdin, E., Borchardt, R. T., and Creveling, C. R., Eds.,** *Biochemistry of S-Adenosylmethionine and Related Compounds,* Macmillan Press, London, 1982.

36. **Parks, L. W. and Schlenk, F.,** The stability and hydrolysis of S-adenosylmethionine; isolation of S-ribosylmethionine, *J. Biol. Chem.,* 230, 295, 1958.

37. **Paik, W. K., Lee, H. W., and Kim, S.,** Non-enzymatic methylation of proteins with S-adenosyl-1-methionine, *F.E.B.S. Lett.,* 58, 39, 1975.

38. **Lombardini, J. B. and Talalay, P.,** Formation, functions and regulatory importance of S-adenosyl-1-methionine, *Adv. Enz. Reg.,* 9, 349, 1971.

39. **Craddock, V. M.,** The *in vivo* formation and turnover of S-adenosylmethionine from methionine in the liver of normal rats, of animals fed dimethylnitrosamine and of partially hepatectomised animals, *Biochem. Pharmacol.,* 23, 2452, 1974.

40. **Barrows, L. R., Shank, R. C., and Magee, P. N.,** Effect of ethionine on SAM metabolism and DNA methylation in hydrazine-treated rats, *Proc. Amer. Assoc. Cancer Res.,* 23, 53, 1982.

41. **Barrows, L. R. and Magee, P. N.,** Nonenzymatic methylation of DNA by S-adenosylmethionine *in vitro,* *Carcinogenesis,* 3, 349, 1982.

42. **Rydberg, B. and Lindahl, T.,** Nonenzymatic methylation of DNA by the intracellular methyl group donor S-adenosyl-1-methionine is a potentially mutagenic reaction, *EMBO J.,* 1, 211, 1982.

43. **Lawley, P. D.,** Carcinogenesis by alkylating agents, in *Chemical Carcinogens,* ACS Monogr. 173, Searle, C. E., Ed., American Chemical Society, Washington, D.C., 1976, 83.

44. **Simon, D., Grunert, F., Acken, U. V., Doring, H. P., and Kroger, H.,** DNA-methylase from regenerating rat liver: Purification and characterization, *Nucl. Acid Res.,* 5, 2152, 1978.

45. **Swann, P. F., Pegg, A. E., Hawks, A., Farber, E., and Magee, P. N.,** Evidence for ethylation of rat liver deoxyribonucleic acid after administration of ethionine, *Biochem. J.,* 123, 175, 1971.

46. **Craddock, V. M.,** Methylation of DNA in the intact animal and the effects of the carcinogens dimethylnitrosamine and ethionine, *Biochim. Biophys. Acta,* 240, 376, 1971.

47. **Shank, R. C. and Magee, P. N.,** Similarities between the biochemical actions of cycasin and dimethylnitrosamine, *Biochem. J.,* 105, 521, 1967.

48. **Barrows, L. R. and Magee, P. N.,** 7-Methylguanine formation in DNA of cultured cells, *Proc. 13th Int. Cancer Cong.,* 1982, 442.

49. **Ehrlich, M. and Wang, R. Y.-H.,** 5-Methylcytosine in eukaryotic DNA, *Science,* 212, 1350, 1981.

50. **Sinsheimer, R. L.,** The action of pancreatic deoxyribonuclease. II. Isomeric dinucleotides, *J. Biol. Chem.,* 215, 579, 1955.

51. **Doskocil, J. and Sorm, F.,** Distribution of 5-methylcytosine in pyrimidine sequences of deoxyribonucleic acid, *Biochim. Biophys. Acta,* 55, 953, 1962.

52. **Laval, J., Piere, J., and Laval, F.,** Release of 7-methylguanine residues from alkylated DNA by extracts of *Micrococcus leutes* and *Escherichia coli, Proc. Natl. Acad. Sci. USA,* 78, 852, 1981.

53. **Singer, B. and Brent, T. P.,** Human lymphoblasts contain DNA glycosylase activity excising N-3 and N-7 methyl and ethyl purines but not O^6-alkylguanines or 1-alkyladenines, *Proc. Natl. Acad. Sci. USA,* 78, 856, 1981.

54. **Margison, G. P. and Pegg, A. E.,** Enzymatic release of 7-methylguanine from methylated DNA by rodent liver extracts, *Proc. Natl. Acad. Sci. USA,* 78, 861, 1981.

55. **Craddock, V. M., Henderson, A. R., and Gash, S.,** Nature of the constitutive and induced mammalian O^6-methylguanine DNA repair enzyme, *Biochem. Biophys. Res. Comm.,* 107, 546, 1982.

56. **Hunt, E. J. and Shank, R. C.,** Evidence for DNA adducts in rat liver after administration of N-nitrosopyrrolidine, *Biochem. Biophys. Res. Comm.,* 104, 1343, 1982.

57. **Ruchirawat, M. M.,** Relationship Between Metabolism and Toxicity of Dimethylnitrosamine in the Rat, Ph.D. Dissertation, Dept. Nutrition and Food Sci., Mass. Inst. Tech., Cambridge, 1975.

58. **Bradley, M. D., Bhuyan, B., Francis, M. C., Lagenbach, R., Peterson, A., and Huberman, E.,** Mutagenesis by chemical agents in V7A Chinese hamster cells: a review and analysis of the literature, *Mutat. Res.,* 87, 81, 1981.

59. **Styles, J. A.,** A method for detecting carcinogenic organic chemicals using mammalian cells in culture, *Br. J. Cancer,* 36, 558, 1977.

60. **Roberts, J. J.,** Cellular responses to carcinogen-induced DNA damage and the role of DNA repair, *Brit. Med. Bull.,* 36, 25, 1980.

61. **Shank, R. C.,** unpublished data.

Chapter 5

PROBLEMS IN INTERSPECIES EXTRAPOLATION

David B. Clayson

TABLE OF CONTENTS

I. INTRODUCTION

The estimation of risk due to a chemical cannot easily be extrapolated from one experimental species to another or to man. Each species has its specific physiological, biochemical and anatomical characteristics that differentiate it from other species. These factors may play a major role in determining species response to toxic agents. Trans-species extrapolation becomes progressively more difficult the more complex the toxic process under consideration. The major obstacle to progress appears to be limited understanding of the fundamental mechanisms underlying complex toxic responses such as teratology, mutation and carcinogenesis. This presently makes prediction of species response highly empirical.

Another difficulty that assumes special significance in carcinogenesis and some similar areas in which an agent is generally regarded as having or not having an effect, is the adoption of a qualitative approach to risk assessment. This occurs despite Paracelcus (quoted by Sigerist[74]) clearly stating over four centuries ago, that it is the dose and not the agent that makes the poison. The reasons for this failure to think quantitatively are severalfold: first, there is little quantitative information about the levels of human exposure to any chemical that leads, for example, to cancer in man; second, the innate fear of the disease leads many people to regard any risk of carcinogen exposure to be unacceptable; and, third, the exquisitely complex mechanism of carcinogenesis has led pathologists and others to spurn a quantitative approach as unrealistic and possibly even dangerous in real-life situations. Nevertheless, the qualitative approach embodied, for example, in the Delaney Clause of the U.S. Food and Drug Act[88] is now becoming demonstrably unworkable.[85] It is becoming more apparent that not all carcinogenic agents may be eliminated from our environment. The need for a more quantitative approach is evident.

After considering examples of differences in general toxic response between various species, this chapter will concentrate on problems in carcinogenesis. A simple expression for carcinogenic potency will be developed that can be used to analyze data from even simple oncogenicity experiments in animals. Its utility in comparing species differences in response to carcinogens will be explored. Finally, in a speculative vein, the possibility that such a quantitative value may be generated for man will be discussed in the light of both existing and potential experimental techniques.

II. SPECIES DIFFERENCES

Simple toxic responses are dependent on the concentration of toxic agents present at the target receptor site and the time that this concentration persists. As the administered agent may need to be converted by the organism into its toxic form, activating and detoxifying metabolism, biodistribution and excretion of the administered chemical, as with pharmacologic agents, play an important role in determining the level of effect of the toxicant. Each of these features, but especially metabolism, may differ from species to species,[92] and between individual members of the same species.[65] Specific agents, such as enzyme inducers, may appreciably modify the metabolism of toxic agents.[27]

Other factors generally have a more specific effect. For example, DNA repair processes assume importance if the toxic agent interacts with DNA; receptor site antagonists will depend on the concentration and affinity of the specific receptor sites in the species and tissue for the antagonist. The anatomical structure of a tissue sometimes differs between species as with the number of membranes in the placenta which has been suspected to influence in utero toxicity. The balance between the distribution and metabolism of the toxic agent and its interaction with target tissues will be illustrated by a series of examples.

A. General Anesthetics

Anyone conducting animal research in or before the 1940s will realize that general anesthetics that are highly effective in one species may not be usable in a different species. The second species might demonstrate neurostimulation instead of anesthesia (which with larger animals can be dangerous), transient anesthesia, or fatal anesthesia. A useful drug in one species may be toxic in another. These differences in species response reflect the different distribution, metabolic detoxification and excretion of the anesthetic rather than differences in receptors in different species.[35] The use of an anesthetic is thus influenced by factors that affect its metabolism or excretion such as previous exposure to the anesthetic or to enzyme modifying agents (inducers and inhibitors), nutrition, body weight, age, sex, health status, pulmonary, renal, and cardiovascular function, etc.[35]

B. Teratogens

Few agents have been convincingly shown to induce birth defects in humans apart from radiation, rubella, thalidomide, folic acid antagonists, methylmercury and diethylstilbestrol.[31,51,52,75] In each of these examples there were adequate cases to create suspicion that a hazard existed and to permit epidemiological investigation. Many other agents have been shown experimentally to induce birth defects in animals but it is difficult to assess the relevance of these experimental findings to the human situation.

Teratogenesis is a complex process in which three major compartments have to be considered: the mother, the placenta and the embryo or fetus. Each of these compartments may differ in respect to the distribution of a toxic agent, its metabolic capabilities, and the clearance of the toxic agent and its metabolites. Furthermore, each of these parameters varies independently between different species as does the finer detail of the process of development from the blastocyst to the newborn.[6,42] The 9-month gestation period in humans means that the offspring develops certain of its extrauterine characteristics before parturition whereas these parameters do not develop similarly in the rat in its 21- to 22-day gestation period. For example, in rats some P-450 complex metabolic enzymes are not operational until about the time of parturition;[59] in humans, several fetal tissues demonstrate, albeit lower than usual, levels of such enzymes.[49] This means that in the rat, if a substance needs to be metabolized to be effective, the active metabolite will, if directly acting, have to be transferred from the maternal circulation through the placenta to the fetal circulation, before it can affect the fetal tissues. In contrast, the human fetus possibly can elaborate the active metabolite in situ. Therefore if the active metabolite is relatively unstable it will not survive to reach the rat fetus. Such considerations greatly help in understanding why in rodents some carcinogens such as ethylnitrosourea are very effective transplacentally while others such as certain nitrosamines, which need metabolic activation, are much less effective.[3,21,30]

Diethylstilbestrol is possibly an example of an agent that affects development. This agent was introduced in 1949 to prevent spontaneous abortion in women with a history of that condition.[77] By 1970, Herbst and Scully[40] reported six cases of a rare tumor, clear cell adenocarcinoma of the vagina, in young women whose mothers had received the medication. The observation was rapidly confirmed epidemiologically.[36] It now appears that perhaps as many as 1 to 2 million women were treated in this way but only about 300 cervical and vaginal cancers have been discovered. Non-malignant changes such as adenosis of the cervix and vagina appear to be much more common and suggest that the pre-natal use of diethylstilbesterol has led to a profound and prolonged disturbance of the hormonal balance in young women.[31] Animal studies suggest that these changes in hormonal status may affect the response to carcinogens and other toxic agents.[71]

The fact that in utero exposure to a drug such as diethylstilbestrol can alter the normal physiological behavior of the entire organism for, at least, a considerable part of the lifespan has some important implications. Such hormonal imprinting is well established. The response of the female hamster to renal tumorigenesis by diethylstilbestrol may be greatly enhanced by injecting testosterone during the first 48 hr of extra-uterine life.[53,54] The effect of hormonal preparations such as oral contraceptives that may inadvertently be taken during the first few weeks of human pregnancy needs to be investigated to ensure that they, too, do not lead to such imprinting.

More recently it has been demonstrated that the levels of, particularly, metabolic enzymes can be modified if the pregnant mother is exposed to certain agents.[57,58] For example, exposure of pregnant rats to 3 μg 2,3,7,8-tetrachlorodibenzodioxin 10 days after conception, leads even up to 25 days-partum to a fivefold increase in hepatic arylhydrocarbon hydroxylase.[57] Such experiments should stimulate the serious consideration of the total range of in utero toxic effects; that is, whether the more usually recorded teratologic effects, such as skeletal or histologic abnormalities, are really just the most extreme examples of a widespread "conditioning" of the developing animal to environmental agents. It is also relevant to ask whether part of the apparent species variability in response to teratogenic agents is due to a failure to look for less dramatic changes in the offspring of dams exposed to toxic agents.

C. Carcinogens

The fact that species differences occurred in response to carcinogens was realized at a very early stage in the development of the subject. The first fact to be established was that the mouse and rabbit responded to the painting of polycyclic hydrocarbon-containing oils and tars by developing cutaneous papillomas and carcinomas but the rat and guinea pig were resistant.[17,87,91]

Aromatic amines likewise show considerable variations in their effects on different species (Table 1). This fact, combined with the relatively large quantities of these agents required to induce tumors, thwarted earlier experimental attempts to reproduce human occupationally derived bladder cancer in animals.[12,56] Interspecies variability in response to aromatic amines involves not only the fact that some species are apparently unaffected by these carcinogens but also a considerable variation in the tissue or tissues affected.[24] Although the metabolic activation of the carcinogenic aromatic amines is fairly well comprehended,[62] the reasons for the different tissue susceptibility still need to be clarified.

In contrast to the examples quoted above, some carcinogens such as radiation[89] or diethylnitrosamine[72] appear to induce tumors in most species. Schmähl and his colleagues[72] describe cancer induction by diethylnitrosamine in all 23 species tested.

III. CARCINOGEN POTENCY

The realization that aflatoxin B$_1$ is a very effective carcinogen in rats but is less effective in mice, hamsters, and possibly man is scientifically interesting[14] but is of limited value for regulation that requires some form of quantitation. To overcome this lack of understanding of the effectiveness of carcinogens in different species, it has been customary to base regulations on the assumption that the human is at least as sensitive to a carcinogen as is the most sensitive experimental species. Such an assumption is necessary until a method for determining the relative effectiveness of specific carcinogens becomes available. It is not, however, a satisfactory approach as it requires the discarding of important parts of the data that can result from a carcinogen bioassay. Two sets of problems are involved in evaluating numerically the relative effectiveness of a carcinogen in different species: (1) there is a need for a method for the quantitation of animal bioassay data concerning tumor incidence and time to tumor, and (2) there is the much more difficult problem of how to determine the probable effectiveness of a carcinogen in the human species without doing an intentional or inadvertant chemical carcinogenicity bioassay in the human population.

Table 1
SPECIES RESPONSE TO CARCINOGENIC EFFECT OF OCCUPATIONAL BLADDER CARCINOGENS

Species	2-Naphthylamine	1-Naphthylamine	Benzidine	4-Aminobiphenyl
Man	Bladder	Bladder[a]	Bladder	Bladder
Dog	Bladder	None	Bladder	Bladder
Monkey	Bladder	— [b]	—	—
Hamster	Bladder	—	Liver	—
Rat	Bladder	—	Liver, earduct, intestines	Breast, intestine
Mouse	Liver	None	Liver	Liver
Rabbit	None	—	—	Bladder

[a] Contained 4 to 10% 2-naphthylamine.
[b] Not tested.

Adapted from Clayson, D. B., *Prevent. Med.*, 5, 228, 1976.

The term "carcinogen potency" as used in this chapter gives a measure of the effectiveness of a carcinogen in a particular situation. Carcinogen potency is not an absolute property of a carcinogen but depends on the conditions of exposure such as the nature and stage of development of the species tested, the route of exposure to the carcinogen, and certain environmental conditions such as adequacy of nutrition and environmental temperature.[81] The potency or strength of a carcinogen depends primarily on the yield of tumors obtained and the time to tumor with a certain dose rate of carcinogen.[22] Tumor multiplicity may be used as a criterion for determining carcinogen potency. It is omitted here because it is considered an extension at high dose levels of the innate ability of the carcinogen to increase tumor incidence. No correction is made for background (control) tumor incidences. Similarly, in determining carcinogen potency, the values obtained are dependent on the reliability of the bioassay data used. No numerical calculation can substitute for imperfect experimental data.

The three major factors to be used in determining potency are in each case self-limiting. Thus, the probability of obtaining a tumor in a tissue (or whole animal) cannot exceed one as the tissue either has or does not have a tumor. The time on test cannot exceed the lifespan of the test animal, and likewise, the dose of carcinogen cannot exceed the chronically toxic level or the animals will not survive to develop tumors.

This means that the probability of obtaining a tumor in an animal bioassay is a surface depending on the dose rate at which the carcinogen is applied and the time on test (Figure 1). There are very few sets of experimental data that enable such tumor surface diagrams to be plotted. Perhaps the most adequate data set may be derived from the U.S. National Center for Toxicological Research's ED_{01} experiment in which over 22,000 BALB/c mice were used to attempt to estimate the dose-rate of N,2-acetylaminofluorene required to induce a 1% incidence of liver or bladder tumors.[78,79] In this example, there appeared to be meaningful differences in the shape of the response surfaces between the induced liver and bladder lesions. Such an experiment that cost several million U.S. dollars to conduct is unlikely to be repeated.

Therefore it is necessary to look for a simpler data set on which to base values of carcinogen potency.[22] The simplest way to define potency is to use a fixed point on the dose rate, time to tumor surface (Figure 1). For example, the dose rate at which a 50% yield of a particular tumor is induced in a lifespan study is one parameter that could be used, although other points may be considered more appropriate. Using this particular point, carcinogenic potency (P) may be defined as:

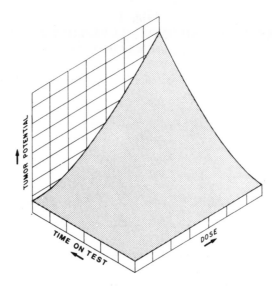

FIGURE 1.   The probability of obtaining a tumour in a tissue is a surface dependent on the dose rate and time to tumor. (From Clayson, D. B., Krewski, D., and Munro, I. C., *Reg. Toxicol. Pharmacol.*, 3, 329, 1983. With permission.)

$$P = 7 - \log_{10}ED_{50} \qquad (1)$$

where ED_{50} is the dose rate in μmoles/kg body weight/week required to induce a 50% tumor yield in a lifespan study and 7 is an arbitrary constant that ensures all values are positive. Unfortunately, few experiments give precisely 50% tumor yields in a lifespan study and therefore the experimental data need to be corrected. A series of approximate linear corrections is employed:

$$ED_{50} = d_o \times \frac{0.50}{P_o} \times \frac{S_o}{S_x} \qquad (2)$$

where d_o, P_o and S_o are the experimentally determined dose rate, tumor probability and overall survival time and S_x the lifespan of the species under consideration (Table 2). If experiments used for potency determination do not differ too greatly from lifespan studies and a 50% tumor yield, the error introduced on a log scale appears to be acceptable. Clearly, tumor yields in the ranges 0 to 10% or 90 to 100% are not suitable for potency determination since such values lie on the toes of the dose-response curve and thus lead to very inaccurate extrapolation. Potency derivations have been made by others, notably by Meselson and Russell[61] and Jones et al.[48]

This simple approach to the calculation of carcinogen potency does not consider two factors: (1) the background incidence of naturally occurring tumors against which the carcinogen acts and (2) the occurrence of deaths from competing causes during the study. In fact, neither of these factors need be critical in a well-conducted bioassay. If high incidences of naturally occurring tumors are present (over 10%) it is difficult to interpret the significance of the study as the inducing agent may be a carcinogen or a carcinogenesis enhancer.[20] Likewise, the number of animals dying from competing causes before the appearance of the earliest tumors is usually small in a well conducted bioassay.

Table 2
FACTORS USED FOR CALCULATING ED$_{50}$ IN ANIMALS

Factors	Mouse	Rat	Dog
Lifespan (years)	2.5	3.0	10
Food (g/day)	4—6	12—15	300—500
Drinking water (mℓ/day)	2.1	20.0	NK[a]
Gestation (days)	21.0	21.0	63
Weight (g)	25—40	100—500	10,000

[a] NK = not known.

Adapted from Peters, J. H., Miller, K. S., and Brown, P., *Pharmacol. Exp. Ther.*, 150, 298, 1965.

Table 3
THE POTENCY OF A RANGE OF CARCINOGENS TO RAT OR MOUSE LIVER FOLLOWING CONTINUOUS FEEDING

Chemical	Species	Potency
Aflatoxin B1	Rat	9.2
Michler's ketone	Rat	4.6
Dimethylnitrosamine	Rat	4.0
Carbon tetrachloride	Rat	3.0
2-Aminoanthraquinone	Rat	4.4
Trichloroethylene	Mouse	2.1

Adapted from National Academy of Sciences, National Research Council, Committee on Amines, Aromatic Amines: An Assessment of the Biological and Environmental Effects, National Academy Press, Washington, D.C., 1981.

Potency values for a range of carcinogens selected without reference to mechanisms of action are illustrated in Table 3. This shows that there is a seven order of magnitude or a ten million-fold range in potency between the most potent carcinogen, aflatoxin B$_1$, and the least potent, saccharin or trichlorethylene. In Table 4 values for N,2-acetylaminofluorene in rats and mice are compared. This example suggests that potency values determined in different experiments for tumors in different tissues in different strains of the same species are remarkably similar.

Tables 5 to 7 illustrate the differences in species response to specific carcinogens that have been adequately tested in three or more species. The approximately 1000-fold range of potency for diethylnitrosamine, the 150-fold range for 4-aminobiphenyl and 6-fold range for 2-naphthylamine contrast markedly with the lack of species differences in carcinogenic potency with N,2-acetylaminofluorene. They serve to indicate the limitations in our present efforts to assess the potency of individual carcinogens for man based on experimentally derived data.

IV. CARCINOGEN POTENCY DETERMINATION IN MAN: CAN KNOWLEDGE OF CARCINOGENESIS MECHANISMS BE HELPFUL?

Carcinogen potency values cannot be derived for man in the same way as for experimental animals because it is completely unethical to contemplate the relevant experimentation in

Table 4
THE CARCINOGENIC POTENCY OF N,2-FLUORENYLACETAMIDE IN DIFFERENT SPECIES AND STRAINS OF TEST ANIMALS[a]

Species	Route	Site of tumor	Potency
Dog	Diet	Liver, bladder	4.5
Rabbit	Gavage	Bladder, ureter	4.5
Hamster	Diet	Gall bladder	4.3
Rat			
Slonaker (M + F)[b]	Diet	Bladder	4.4
Wistar (M)	Diet	Liver	5.1
Wistar (F)	Diet	Breast	5.0
Piebald (M + F)	Diet	Intestine	4.9
Mouse			
BALB/c (F)	Diet	Liver	4.2
BALB/c (F)	Diet	Bladder	4.2

[a] Some evaluations based on early studies.
[b] M = male; F = female.

Adapted from National Academy of Sciences, National Research Council, Committee on Amines, Aromatic Amines: An Assessment of the Biological and Environmental Effects, National Academy Press, Washington, D.C., 1981.

Table 5
CARCINOGENIC POTENCY OF NDEA IN SEVERAL SPECIES AFTER CONTINUOUS ADMINISTRATION

Species	Stock	Route	Estimated lifespan months	Tissue of origin of tumors	Potency (log units)
Rat (*Rattus norvegicus*)	BD II	Oral	24	Liver	6.5
White-tailed rat (*Mystromys albicaudatus*)	—	Oral	72	Liver	6.3
Chicken (*Gallus domesticus*)	White leghorn	im[a]	100	Liver	5.3
Guinea pig (*Cavia procellus*)	Hybrid	Oral	84	Liver	4.2
Mouse (*Mus musculus*)	NMRI	Oral	18	Liver	4.0
	RF	Oral	18	Liver	3.9
Syrian golden hamster (*Mesocricetus auratus*)	—	Oral	18	Trachea	3.7

[a] Intramuscular injection.

Adapted from National Academy of Sciences, National Research Council, Committee on Nitrites and Alternative Curing Agents in Food, The Health Effects of Nitrate, Nitrite, and N-Nitroso Compounds, National Academy Press, Washington, D.C., 1981.

the human population. Where inadvertent exposure to carcinogens that are effective in man has occurred, there is usually a complete lack of accurate data on the extent of human exposure to the noxious agent(s).[44] A few drugs such as chlornaphazin,[82] cyclophosphamide[70] and phenacetin[7] provide very limited information. An indirect approach dependent on present knowledge of carcinogenesis mechanisms needs to be developed, if carcinogenic potency in man is to be estimated.

Table 6
POTENCY OF 4-AMINOBIPHENYL
FOLLOWING ADMINISTRATION TO
DIFFERENT SPECIES

Species	Route of administration	Tissue	Potency
Dog	Oral	Bladder	6.2
Mouse	Gavage	Liver	4.5
Rat	Subcutaneous	Intestine	4.4

Adapted from National Academy of Sciences, National Research Council, Committee on Amines, Aromatic Amines: An Assessment of the Biological and Environmental Effects, National Academy Press, Washington, D.C., 1981.

Table 7
POTENCY OF 2-NAPHTHYLAMINE IN DIFFERENT SPECIES FOLLOWING ORAL ADMINISTRATION

Species	Potency
Dog	4.3
Mouse	3.9
Rat	2.7
Hamster	2.1

Adapted from National Academy of Sciences, National Research Council, Committee on Amines, Aromatic Amines: An Assessment of the Biological and Environmental Effects, National Academy Press, Washington, D.C., 1981.

Carcinogenesis is a multistage process. The first evidence for this was adduced by Berenblum and Shubik[9-11] using mouse skin as the model system. They showed that there were two stages: a relatively rapid, irreversible stage in which normal cells were initiated to become 'latent tumor cells' and a promotional or developmental stage in which the latent tumor cell became expressed as a tumor. Different agents were effective for each stage. The two-stage concept has recently been shown applicable to, at least, eight other different tissues (Table 8).[69] Initiators are generally genotoxic, that is they induce genetic changes such as mutation, sister chromatid exchange, micronucleus, or related changes such as unscheduled DNA synthesis and cell transformation. This implies, but does not prove, that initiation may involve genetic change in the affected cell.[46]

Subsequent to Berenblum and Shubik's initial work a great deal has been learned about the events that probably contribute to initiation, but less about these that contribute to promotion.[20] Figure 2 gives a feeling for some major events in chemical carcinogenesis. The carcinogen is absorbed into the body from its site of administration, and depending on its physical properties will be retained near its site of administration and/or enter the circulation, reaching an equilibrium which may or may not be influenced by storage depots of, for example, lipophilic substances being established in fatty tissues.

Table 8

EXAMPLES OF THE TWO STAGE MECHANISM OF CARCINOGENESIS IN VARIOUS TISSUES

Species	Tissue	Initiating agent	Promoting agent	Ref.
Mouse	Skin	Benzo(a)pyrene, 7,12-dimethylbenz (a) anthracene	Croton oil	9—11
Rat	Bladder	FANFT[a]	Saccharin, tryptophan	26
Rat	Colon	MNNG[b]	Lithocholic acid	57
Rat	Bone marrow (leukemia)	2,7-Diacetylaminofluorene	Blood loss	80
Mouse	Forestomach	3-Methylcholanthrene Benzo(a)pyrene 7,12-Dimethylbenz (a) anthracene	Croton oil	8
Rat	Liver	2-AAF	Phenobarbital, DDT	67
Rat	Mammary gland	7,12-Dimethyl benz (a) anthracene	Phorbol, prolactin	5
Rat	Thyroid	AAF[c]	Methyl thiouracil	37

[a] = FANFT: N-(4-(5-nitro-2-furyl)-2-thiazolyl)formamide.
[b] = MNNG: N-methyl-N-nitro-N¹-nitrosoguanidine.
[c] = AAF: N,2-Fluorenylacetamide.

Abstracted from Pitot, H. C., and Sirica, A. E., *Acta Rev. Cancer*, 605, 191, 1980.

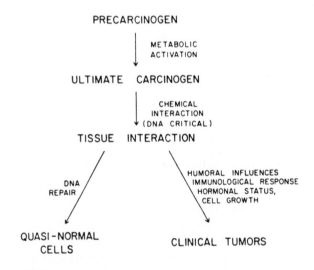

FIGURE 2. The mechanism of carcinogenesis is a multistage process consisting of the activation of the procarcinogen; interaction, probably with DNA; the fixation of the chemical lesion; and the development of the altered cell to frank neoplasia.

Metabolizing enzymes present in the liver or, usually to a lesser extent, in other tissues will either detoxify the carcinogen, converting it in multiple steps to a more easily excreted form, or will activate it to a highly reactive form which may be an electrophile[62] or a free radicle.[90] The reactive moiety will then interact with any available target in its vicinity including the cellular macromolecules protein, RNA and DNA. DNA is believed, but not proved, to be the critical receptor. However, DNA adducts of themselves are not now believed to be the ultimate genetic lesion. DNA-carcinogen adducts may be removed by some DNA repair mechanisms or may be converted to incorrect nucleotide sequences by

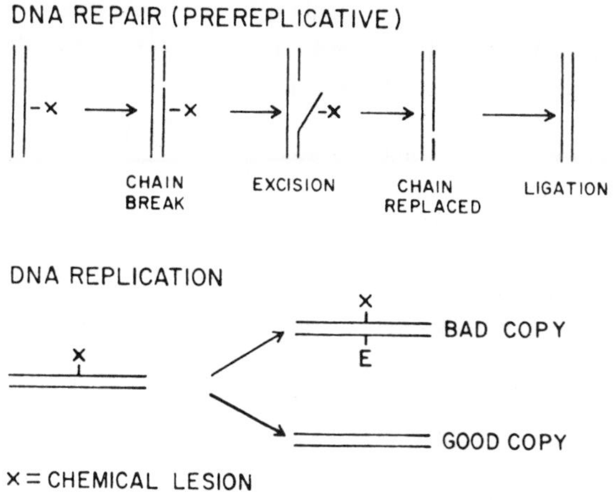

DNA REPAIR (PREREPLICATIVE)

CHAIN BREAK   EXCISION   CHAIN REPLACED   LIGATION

DNA REPLICATION

BAD COPY

GOOD COPY

X = CHEMICAL LESION

FIGURE 3. DNA excision-repair effectively removes a chemical lesion (×) from DNA; on the other hand DNA replication causes the chemical lesion (×) to be copied as an altered base (E) leading to a mutated cell.

other repair processes and by DNA replication (Figure 3). This fixation of chemical damage has been demonstrated by Gerschmann and Ludlum[34] for O-6-methylguanine but does not occur with N-7-methylguanine. Similar critical studies have not been performed with other DNA adducts. As DNA replication fixes the genetic damage as an altered base, whereas some DNA repair processes eliminate the adduct, the probability of obtaining a genetically modified cell depends on the level of adduct formation and the balance between DNA repair and DNA replication activity.

The suspicion that carcinogenesis involves a genetic process is essential to the suggestions to be put forward for estimating human risk from carcinogens. It is based on several observations. First, there is some degree of correlation between the results of whole animal bioassays and several of the recently introduced genotoxicity tests.[45,46] Second, skin cancer induction occurs much more frequently in Xeroderma pigmentosum patients, who lack the ability to remove ultraviolet light induced thymine dimers from their DNA.[25] DNA adduct formation also correlates in some, but not all, cases with the induction of chemical carcinogenesis. It is still only possible to speculate on the nature of the genetic lesion or lesions that lead to a cell to develop malignant potential.[16]

Promotion or carcinogenesis enhancement is much less adequately understood.[20] One reason for this appears to be that the enhancement of tumor development may follow many different pathways. Thus, any agent or process that enhances one or more of the critical events in tumor initiation, such as increasing the amount of active metabolite formed, increasing target cell replication, or decreasing the capacity of cells faithfully to repair their DNA, will be reflected in increased tumor yields and may be mistaken for a carcinogen rather than an enhancer of a promotional nature.[20]

The developmental stage of cancer may be visualized as first a survival competition between the initiated latent tumor cells and the normal cells in a tissue and secondly, in some cases, as a series of changes in tumor cells that increase their malignancy (i.e., progression as defined by Foulds[32]). Attention has recently focussed on the inhibition of cell to cell cooperation as the primary lesion underlying tumor promotion. Interaction of, for example, phorbol esters with receptors on cell membranes may be visualized as increasing the ability of all cells (including latent tumor cells) in the tissue to proliferate. Such a process is in fact analogous to the release of "contact inhibited" cells in culture and their subsequent release from proliferation inhibition.[76,86]

The question remains to be answered whether differences in promotional activity between species represent differences in receptor activity towards different promoting agents or reflect different anatomical structures or other factors that affect the access of the initiating or promoting agent to their receptors. For example, to what extent is the inutility of the rat and guinea pig in skin initiation-promotion studies[73] a reflection of the different receptor activities of the cells compared to physical factors such as thickness of the keratin layer of the skin? It is clear that this area needs study.

If it were possible, using in vitro techniques with both animal and human tissues to measure the effects of a series of animal carcinogens on each stage in the carcinogenic process and if it were possible to weight such data for the contribution they might make to the total development of tumors, it would be practicable to determine, indirectly, carcinogenic potency for man. Such an ideal situation is still a long way off and depends on a vastly increased knowledge of the mechanisms of cancer induction and the development of new quantitative techniques for the many factors that may influence tumorigenesis. Any approach at this point in time will have to be based on many approximations and assumptions. The following speculation is offered as a possible way to begin to investigate the problem.

As has been described, the "initiation phase" of carcinogenesis consists of metabolic activation of the procarcinogen, DNA interaction, DNA repair and replication. While each parameter can doubtless be determined independently, genotoxicity tests may offer some simplification in the approach. What is needed is first a rapid genotoxicity test that will give a quantitative expression of relative carcinogen initiating potency of a chemical. The Ames *Salmonella typhimurium* test[2-4] does not appear to do this because in the preparation of the metabolizing enzyme S-9 fraction, the activating and detoxifying enzymes and the levels of their essential co-factors may be seriously perturbed.[19,92] On the other hand, mammalian cell mediated mammalian cell mutagenesis, according to presently available results, appears much more promising. Langenbach et al.[55] put several pancreatic carcinogens based on N-nitrosobis(2-oxopropyl)amine into the order of their ability to induce pancreatic cancer in hamsters by using V79 cells as the mutatable organism and intact hamster hepatocytes as the metabolizing system. Use of the Ames test and S-9 fraction put these agents in almost inverse order of carcinogenic activity. Jones et al.[18] also using V79 cells with rat hepatocytes obtained a good correlation between carcinogenic and mutagenic potency with 26 nitrosamines ($r = 0.93$). Langenbach and his colleagues showed that this system is capable of measuring mutational activity with other tissue cells: such as fibroblasts, transitional cells from the urothelium, lung, and kidney cells.[43,60] This system therefore seems ideally suited for attempts to measure species or tissue differences in response to, at least, the initiating phase of carcinogenesis. This should include the use of human cells.

Since species vary in their capacity to repair DNA,[33,39] the second factor that may need to be examined in a quantitative fashion is the level of DNA repair capacity in the different species and tissues used for carcinogenicity determination. A variety of techniques is available for this purpose. Similarly we may anticipate the need to know something about the rate of cell replication in a tissue exposed to high or, more realistically, low doses of carcinogen. Putting the quantitative mutagenicity data together with the DNA repair and replication data will, it is speculated, give a reasonable approximation to the initiating ability of a carcinogen in different species, including man.

If reports that DNA repair activity in different species is related to the longevity or lifespan of the species[29,33,38,50] are established, the possibility exists that a correction for DNA repair capacity may not be necessary. Longer lived species have more time in which to develop tumors and may therefore possibly be responsive to lesser levels of DNA adduct formation and fixation. The higher activity of DNA repair systems would lead longer lived species more effectively to reduce their burden of DNA adducts than a shorter lived species possibly producing a balance between these two factors.

Quantitation by in vitro methods of the promotional or developmental phase of carcinogenesis appears to be a difficult problem insofar as there are multiple factors that may be involved. Such factors may include enhanced cell proliferation, hormonal stimulation, or reduced host-mediated immunocompetence, among others. Recent developments have suggested that a possible factor of major concern in tumor promotion may be a membrane-related loss in cell to cell cooperation and methods have been elaborated to study this process.[76,86] If promotion can be shown to depend on a single biological process such as loss of cell to cell cooperation it may be possible to quantitate the promotional aspects of carcinogenesis. The in vitro quantitation of human response to this aspect of chemical toxicity could then be contemplated.

It must be emphasized, however, that the preceding discussion is speculative in that it does not describe a practical method by which carcinogen potency may now be established in humans. It merely points to certain possible ways in which components of the value of carcinogen potency could be determined. However, if we are to take the better assessment of human risk from carcinogens as a real and serious problem, some approach to the actual potency of these agents in man must be established.

V. INDIVIDUAL VARIABILITY

Laboratory animals used in toxicological research are usually either inbred (pure line), F_1 hybrids (cross between two inbred strains), or random bred. Although the degree of genetic heterozygosity clearly increases the more outbred the animal, it is likely that random bred experimental animals will be a great deal more uniform than the general human population. This is due to the fact that the most outbred stocks of animals are maintained as closed colonies and therefore lack the opportunity for completely random breeding. Furthermore, experimental animals are maintained in controlled environments and will not differ markedly in environmentally mediated variations, such as imprinting during the developmental phase, enzyme induction, or hormonally mediated effects. If potency calculations are to help in determining differences between species in response to toxic agents, such as carcinogens, it is clearly necessary to determine whether the range of human variability does or does not surpass species differences in response.

There are many examples of differences in human susceptibility to carcinogens but little evidence to explain why this should be so. Even the large lung cancer burden experienced by heavy cigarette smokers involves only about 1 in 12 of that population and coronary heart disease perhaps another 2 of the 12.[28,29] On the other hand, massive occupational exposures to carcinogens may sometimes lead to nearly 100% cancer incidences. Williams,[81] for example, reported that 95% of men who pulverized or flaked freshly distilled 2-naphthylamine developed bladder cancer. At this stage, we know very little about the magnitude of human variability in response to toxic agents or whether this variability depends on chance or on observable characteristics.

Booth et al.[14] measured aflatoxin B_1-DNA adduct formation in liver slices derived from rats, mice, hamsters, and human biopsy specimens. They wished to determine whether this factor correlated with the observed experimental carcinogenicity of aflatoxin B_1 in rodents and would therefore give an indication of the likely magnitude of the carcinogenic response in man. The 6 human samples had a range of aflatoxin B_1-DNA binding levels from 0.7 to 8.5 ng AFB_1/mg DNA. The levels in rats, hamsters and mice were 31.7 ± 9.0, 11.3 ± 3.4, and 1.3 ± 0.4 ng/AFB_1/mg DNA, respectively, suggesting that, based on this metabolic experiment, the human should have an intermediate carcinogenic responsiveness between that of the hamster and mouse.

There is paucity of similar information for other carcinogens. Certain genetic factors clearly play a determining role in the induction of human cancer as, for example, the lack of DNA repair enzyme capacity in Xeroderma pigmentosum leading to early and frequent cutaneous cancer, or the development of colon cancer among those whose genetic constitution leads them to develop familial polyposis. Such out and out genetic disturbances are relatively uncommon and possibly should be considered only as outliers to the general human sensitivity to carcinogens. On the other hand, differences in the ability to metabolize drugs, such as in the acetylation of isoniazid,[15,68] may produce much more subtle changes in the response of an animal to a carcinogen. Differences in the levels of circulating hormones and their tissue receptors, different degrees of immunocompetence and many other such considerations may each modify the response of man to specific carcinogens. There is a need to organize studies of such factors if we are able to understand and eventually use such differences in the determination of human susceptibility to carcinogens.

VI. CARCINOGEN POTENCY, TRANS-SPECIES INTERACTION AND THE CONTROL OF CARCINOGENS

The two major problems in carcinogen regulation are perceived to be high to low dose extrapolation and trans-species extrapolation. Man is generally exposed to much lower doses of carcinogens than are experimental animals because, for reasons of economy, it is not possible to use a sufficient number of animals to demonstrate a statistically significant tumor response below the 5 to 10% tumor incidence level. The purport of this chapter is to suggest that it may be possible to establish methodology for the trans-species extrapolation of the results of carcinogenicity tests. The eventual goal of such a program would be to predict quantitatively the effects that a specific carcinogen might have in man.

Such an endeavor requires a form of quantitation of the results of animal-based carcinogenicity bioassays. Experience now indicates that it is highly unlikely that complete carcinogens, that combine initiating and promoting action, will demonstrate qualitative differences in different species. Where experimental results have indicated that such differences exist, they are always open to the challenge that a greater level of carcinogen, or a more effective mode of administration, might have led to cancer. Bonser et al.[13] among others, reported that rats were unresponsive to 2-naphthylamine. Hicks and Chowaniec,[41] however, demonstrated that infrequent but very high levels of exposure to this chemical induced bladder carcinoma.

It is desirable to eliminate as many chemical carcinogens from the environment as possible. Unfortunately, the complete elimination of cancer-causing chemicals is not possible because, first, some essential substances, such as selenium[47,66] exhibit carcinogenicity at high doses and, second, certain chemicals that are essential to our current civilization and that have no apparent alternative are carcinogenic. For these essential chemicals, protection of the human population from cancer must involve regulation. The present assumption, that man is as sensitive to a carcinogen as the most sensitive species, can only be regarded scientifically as an article of faith. It is a prudent assumption although it has certain major drawbacks. First, most chemical carcinogens are tested in only one or two species, normally mice and/ or rats.[83,84] There is no certainty that these species will be the most sensitive and a low estimate of the carcinogenic risk in man will be accepted. Secondly, if indeed man is less sensitive to a carcinogenic agent than the most sensitive species, this may result in wasted effort in protecting, for example, the factory worker to a higher degree than is needed. Although it may be argued that exposure to the lowest possible level of a carcinogen is the only ethical solution to the problem of carcinogen containment, it must be remembered that the overall volume of human resources is limited and that overexpenditure in an unnecessary direction will curtail possibly more meaningful protective effort in another area.

Therefore, there is a need for methodology to determine by indirect means the potency of individual chemical carcinogens to man. The fact that individuals vary from each other suggests that initial potency determinations of carcinogens for man need not be accurate to more than one order of magnitude. Work on individual sensitivity may eventually enable the most sensitive section of the population to be screened from contact with carcinogens, for example, in the workplace. Such an approach combining both carcinogenic potency calculations and individual susceptibility estimation would greatly help to reduce chemically induced human cancer.

The need is therefore to develop and validate methods for determining the potency of a carcinogen in experimental species, using techniques that may eventually lead to the capability of determining carcinogenic potency in man. The analysis put forward in this chapter suggests that such an approach may be a real possibility for the future although the methodology still needs to be elaborated, tested, and validated.

REFERENCES

1. **Althoff, J. and Grandjean, C.,** *In vivo* studies in Syrian golden hamsters; a transplacental bioassay of ten nitrosamines, *Natl. Cancer Inst. Monogr.,* 51, 251, 1979.
2. **Ames, B. N.,** Environmental Chemicals Causing Cancer and Genetic Birth Defects: Developing a Strategy for Minimizing Human Exposure, Calif. Policy Seminar, Calif. 1977, 1.
3. **Ames, B. N., Durston, W. E., Yamasaki, E., and Lee, F. D.,** Carcinogens are mutagens — a simple test system combining liver homogenates for activation and bacteria for detection, *Proc. Natl. Acad. Sci.,* 70, 2281, 1973.
4. **Ames, B. N., Lee, F. D., and Durston, W. E.,** An improved bacterial test system for the detection and classification of mutagens and carcinogens, *Proc. Natl. Acad. Sci.,* 70, 782, 1973.
5. **Armuth, V. M. and Berenblum, I.,** Promotion of mammary carcinogenesis and leukemogenic action by phorbol in virgin female Wistar rats, *Cancer Res.,* 34, 2704, 1974.
6. **Beck, F.,** Comparative placental morphology and function, in *Developmental Toxicology,* Kimmel, C. A. and Buelke, J., Eds., Raven, New York, 1981.
7. **Bengtsson, U., Angervall, L., Ekman, H., and Lehmann, L.,** Transitional cell tumours of the renal pelvis in analgesic abusers, *Scand. J. Urol. Nephrol.,* 2, 145, 1968.
8. **Berenblum, I. and Haran, N.,** Influence of croton oil and of Polyethylene Glycol-400 on carcinogenesis in forestomach of mouse, *Cancer Res.,* 15, 510, 1955.
9. **Berenblum, I. and Shubik, P.,** The role of croton oil applications, associated with a single painting of a carcinogen, in tumour induction of the mouse's skin, *Brit. J. Cancer,* 1, 379, 1947.
10. **Berenblum, I. and Shubik, P.,** A new, quantitative approach to the study of the stages of chemical carcinogenesis in the mouse's skin, *Brit. J. Cancer,* 1, 383, 1947.
11. **Berenblum, I. and Shubik, P.,** The persistence of latent tumour cells induced in the mouse's skin by a single application of 9, 10-dimethyl-1, 2-benzanthracene, *Brit. J. Cancer,* 3, 384, 1949.
12. **Bonser, G. M.,** Experimental cancer of the bladder, *Brit. Med. Bull.,* 4, 379, 1947.
13. **Bonser, G. M., Clayson, D. B., Jull, J. W., and Pyrah, L. N.,** The carcinogenic properties of 2-amino-1-naphthol hydrochloride and its parent amine, 2-naphthylamine, *Brit. J. Cancer,* 6, 412, 1952.
14. **Booth, S. C., Bosenberg, H., Garner, R. C., Hertzog, P. J., and Norpoth, K.,** The activation of aflatoxin B_1 in liver slices and in bacterial mutagenicity assays using livers from different species including man, *Carcinogenesis,* 2, 1063, 1981.
15. **Bouraoui, K.,** Penotype d'acetylation de l'isoniazide, *Rev. Med.,* 3, 135, 1981.
16. **Cairns, J.,** The origin of human cancers, *Nature,* 289, 353, 1981.
17. **Clayson, D. B.,** *Chemical Carcinogenesis,* J and A Churchill, London, 1962.
18. **Clayson, D. B.,** Occupational bladder cancer, *Prevent. Med.,* 5, 228, 1976.
19. **Clayson, D. B.,** ICPEMC Working paper 2/1: comparison between in vitro and in vivo tests for carcinogenicity: an overview, *Mutat. Res.,* 75, 205, 1980.
20. **Clayson, D. B.,** ICPEMC Working paper 2/3: carcinogens and carcinogenesis enhancers, *Mutat. Res.,* 86, 217, 1981.
21. **Clayson, D. B.,** Carcinogenesis in the developing organism: could protocols be improved? *Biol. Res. Preg.,* 2, 150, 1982.

22. **Clayson, D. B.,** Trans-species and trans-tissue extrapolation in carcinogenesis, in Proceedings of a Conference held in Raleigh, N.C., March 2—4, 1981.

23. **Clayson, D. B.,** Limitations of the Carcinogenesis Bioassay, Toxicology Forum Winter Meeting, Arlington, 1982.

24. **Clayson, D. B. and Garner, R. C.,** Carcinogenic aromatic amines and related compounds, in *Chemical Carcinogens — ACS Monograph No. 173* Searle, C. E., Ed., American Chemical Society, Washington, D.C., 1976.

25. **Cleaver, J. E. and Bootsma, D.,** Xeroderma pigmentosum: biochemical and genetic characteristics, *Ann. Rev. Genet.*, 9, 19, 1975.

26. **Cohen, S. M., Arai, M., Jacobs, J. B., and Friedell, G. H.,** Promoting effect of saccharin and DL-tryptophan in urinary bladder carcinogenesis, *Cancer Res.*, 39, 1207, 1979.

27. **Conney, A. H., Miller, E. C., and Miller, J. A.,** The metabolism of methylated aminoazodyes, V. Evidence of induction of enzyme synthesis in the rat by 3-methylcholanlthrene, *Cancer Res.*, 16, 450, 1956.

28. **Doll, R. and Peto, R.,** Mortality in relation to smoking: 20 years observations on male British doctors, *Br. Med. J.*, 2, 1525, 1976.

29. **Doll, R. and Peto, R.,** The Causes of Cancer: Quantitative Estimates of Avoidable Risks of Cancer in the United States Today, Oxford University Press, Oxford, 1981.

30. **Druckrey, H., Ivankovic, S., and Preussmann, R.,** Teratogenic and carcinogenic effects in the offspring after single injection of ethylnitrosourea to pregnant rats, *Nature*, 200, 1378, 1966.

31. **Forsberg, J. G.,** Permanent changes induced by DES at critical stages in female development: 10 years experience from human and model systems, *Biol. Res. Pregnancy.* 2, 168, 1981.

32. **Foulds, L.,** *Neoplastic Development*, Academic Press, London and New York, 1969.

33. **Francis, A. A., Lee. W. H., and Regan, J. D.,** The relationship of DNA excision repair of ultraviolet-induced lesions to the maximum life span of mammals, *Mech. Ageing Dev.*, 16, 181, 1981.

34. **Gerchman, L. L. and Ludlum, D. B.,** The properties of O^6-methylguanine in templates for RNA polymerase, *Biochem. Biophys. Acta*, 306, 310, 1973.

35. **Green, C. J.,** Animal Anesthesia: Laboratory Animal Handbooks 8, Laboratory Animals Ltd., London, 1979.

36. **Greenwald, P., Barlow, J. J., and Nasca, P. C.,** Vaginal cancer after maternal treatment with synthetic estrogens, *N. Engl. J. Med.*, 285, 390, 1971.

37. **Hall, W. H. and Bielschowsky, F.,** The development of malignancy in experimentally induced adenomata of the thyroid, *Brit. J. Cancer*, 3, 534, 1949.

38. **Hart, R. W., Sacher, G. A., and Hoskkins, T. L.,** DNA repair in a short and a long-lived rodent species, *J. Gerontol.*, 34, 808, 1979.

39. **Hart, R. W. and Setlow, R. B.,** Correlation between deoxyribonucleic acid excision-repair and life-span in a number of mammalian species, *Proc. Nat. Acad. Sci.*, 71, 2169, 1974.

40. **Herbst, A. L. and Scully, R. E.,** Adenocarcinoma of the vagina in adolescence: a report of 7 cases including 6 clear cell carcinomas (so called mesonephromas), *Cancer*, 25, 745, 1970.

41. **Hicks, R. M. and Chowaniec, J.,** The importance of synergy between weak carcinogens in the induction of bladder cancer in experimental animals and humans, *Cancer Res.*, 37, 2943, 1977.

42. **Hoar, R. M. and Monie, I. W.,** Comparative development of specific organ systems, in *Developmental Toxicology*, Kimmel, C. A. and Buelke-Sam, J., Eds., Raven, New York, 1981.

43. **Huberman, E. and Sachs, L.,** Mutability of different genetic loci in mammalian cells by metabolically activated carcinogenic polycyclic hydrocarbons, *Proc. Nat. Acad. Sci. U.S.A.*, 173, 188, 1976.

44. **Hueper, W. C.,** *Occupational Tumors and Allied Diseases*, Charles C Thomas, Springfield, Illinois, 1942.

45. **ICPEMC Committee 1,** Recommendations for development of a genetic screening program, *Mutat. Res.*, 114, 117, 1983.

46. **ICPEMC Committee 2,** Mutagenesis testing as an approach to carcinogenesis, *Mutat. Res.*, 99, 73, 1982.

47. **Jacobs, M. M., Janssen, B., and Griffin, A. C.,** Inhibitory effects of selenium on 1,2-dimethylhydrazine and methylazoxymethanol acetate induction of colon tumors, *Cancer Lett.*, 2, 133, 1977.

48. **Jones, C. A., Marlino, P. J., Lijinsky, W., and Huberman, E.,** The relationship between the carcinogenicity and mutagenicity of nitrosamines in a hepatocyte-mediated mutagenicity assay, *Carcinogenesis*, 2, 1075, 1981.

49. **Juchau, M. R., Nankung, M. J., Berry, D. L., and Zachariah, P. K.,** Oxidative biotransformation of 2-acetylaminofluorene in fetal and placental tissues of humans and monkeys: correlations with aryl hydrocarbon hydroxylase activities, *Drug. Metab. Dispos.*, 3, 494, 1975.

50. **Kato, H., Harada, J., Tsuchiya, K., and Moriwaki, K.,** Absence of correlation between DNA repair in ultraviolet irradiated mammalian cells and life span of the donor species, *Jap. J. Genet.*, 55, 99, 1980.

51. **Khera, K. S.,** Adverse effects in humans and animals of prenatal exposure to selected therapeutic drugs and estimation of embryo-fetal sensitivity of animals for human risk assessment: a review. In *Issues and Reviews in Teratology*, Vol. 2, Kalter, H., Ed., Plenum Press, N.Y., 1984, 399.

52. **Khera, K. S.,** in *Issues and Reviews in Teratology*, Plenum Press, New York, (in press).

53. **Kirkman, H.,** Estrogen-induced tumors of the kidney. IV. Incidence in female Syrian hamsters, *Natl. Cancer Inst. Monogr.*, 1, 59, 1959.

54. **Kirkman, H. and Bacon, R. L.,** Estrogen-induced tumors of the kidney. I. Incidence of renal tumors in intact and gonadectomized male golden hamsters treated with diethylstilbestrol, *J. Natl. Cancer Inst.*, 13, 754, 1952.

55. **Langenbach, R., Gingell, R., Kuszynski, C., Walker, B., Nagel, D., and Pour, P.,** Mutagenic activities of oxidised derivatives of *N*-nitrososodipropylamine in the liver cell mediated and *Salmonella typhimurium* assays, *Cancer Res.*, 40, 3463, 1980.

56. **Leitch, A.,** Annual Reports of the British Empire Cancer Campaign, 1929.

57. **Lipkin, M.,** Proliferative changes in the colon, *Am. J. Digest. Dis.*, 19, 1029, 1974.

58. **Lucier, G. W., Somawane, B. R., McDaniel, O. S., and Hook, G. E. R.,** Postnatal stimulation of hepatic microsomal enzymes following administration of TCDD to pregnant rats, *Chem. Biol. Interact.*, 11, 15, 1975.

59. **Lucier, G. W., Lui, E. M., and Lamartiniere, C. A.,** Metabolic activation/deactivation reactions during prenatal development, *Environ. Health. Perspect.*, 29, 7, 1979.

60. **Malick, L. E. and Langenbach, R.,** In vitro metabolic activation of chemical carcinogens to mutagens by urinary bladder epithelial cells, *In Vitro*, 16, 206, 1980.

61. **Meselson, M. and Russel, K.,** Comparisons of carcinogenic and mutagenic potency, in *Orgins of Human Cancer*, Proceedings of the Cold Spring Harbor Conference, Hiatt, H., Watson, J. D., and Winstein, J. A., Eds., Cold Spring Harbor Laboratory, N.Y., 1977, 1473.

62. **Miller, E. C. and Miller, J. A.,** The metabolism of chemical carcinogens to reactive electrophiles and their possible mechanisms of action in carcinogenesis, in *Chemical Carcinogens*, Searle, C. E., Ed., American Chemical Society, Washington, D.C., 1976, 737.

63. National Academy of Sciences, National Research Council, Committee on Amines, Aromatic Amines: An Assessment of the Biological and Environmental Effects, National Academy Press, Washington, D.C., 1981.

64. National Academy of Sciences, National Research Council, Committee on Nitrites and Alternative Curing Agents in Food, The Health Effects of Nitrate, Nitrite, and N-Nitroso Compounds, National Academy Press, Washington, D.C., 1981.

65. **Nebert, D. W. and Jensen, N. M.,** The Ah Locus: genetic regulation of the metabolism of carcinogens, drugs, and other environmental chemicals by cytochrome P-450-mediated monooxygenases, *Crit. Rev. Biochem.*, 6, 401, 1979.

66. **Nelson, A. A., Fitzhugh, O. G., and Calvery, H. O.,** Liver tumors following cirrhosis caused by selenium in rats, *Cancer Res.*, 3, 230, 1943.

67. **Peraino, C., Fry, R. J. M., Staffeldt, E., and Kisieleski, W. E.,** Effects of varying the exposure to phenobarbital on its enhancement of 2-acetylaminofluorene-induced hepatic tumorigenesis in the rat, *Cancer Res.*, 33, 2701, 1973.

68. **Peters, J. H., Miller, K. S., and Brown, P.,** Studies on the metabolic basis for the genetically determined capacities for isoniazid inactivation in man, *Pharmacol. Exper. Therap.*, 150, 298, 1965.

69. **Pitot, H. C. and Sirica, A. E.,** The stages of initiation and promotion in hepatocarcinogenesis, *Biochem. Biophys. Acta Rev. Cancer*, 605, 191, 1980.

70. **Puri, H. C. and Campbell, R. A.,** Cyclophosphamide and malignancy, *Lancet*, 1, 1306, 1977.

71. **Rustia, M. and Shubik, P.,** Effects of transplacental exposure to diethylstilbestrol on carcinogenic susceptibility during postnatal life in hamster progency, *Cancer Res.*, 39, 4636, 1979.

72. **Schmähl, E., Habs, M., and Ivankovic, S.,** Carcinogenesis on N-nitrosodiethylamine (DENA) in chickens and domestic cats, *Int. J. Cancer*, 22, 552, 1978.

73. **Shubik, P.,** Studies on the promoting phase in the stages of carcinogenesis in mice, rats, and rabbits, and guinea pigs, *Cancer Res.*, 10, 13, 1950.

74. **Sigerist, J. L.,** *The Great Doctors: A Biographical List of Medicine*, Paul, E. and Paul, C., Eds., Doubleday, New York, 1958.

75. **Sikov, M. R.,** Carcinogenesis following prenatal exposure to radiation, *Biol. Res. Pregnancy*, 2, 159, 1981.

76. **Sivak, A.,** ICPEMC Working paper 2/8 an evaluation of assay procedures for detection of tumor promoters, *Mutat. Res.*, 98, 375, 1982.

77. **Smith, O. W. and Smith, G. V. S.,** Use of diethylstilbestrol to prevent fetal loss from complications of late pregnancy, *N. Engl. J. Med.*, 241, 562, 1949.

78. Society of Toxicology, ED_{01} Task Force, Reexamination of the ED_{01} study, *Fundamental and Applied Toxicology*, 1, 26, 1981.

79. **Staffa, J. A. and Mehlman, M. A.,** Innovations in Cancer Risk Assessment (ED_{01} Study), in *Proceedings of a Symposium Sponsored by the National Center for Toxicology Research, U.S. Food and Drug Administration, and the American College of Toxicology*, Pathotox Publishers, Park Forest South, Illinois, 1979.

80. **Takayama, S. and Fujiwara, M.,** Effect of repeated bloodletting on the incidence of 2.7-FAA-induced rat leukemia, *Acta Path. Jap.,* 26, 435, 1976.

81. **Tannanbaum, A. and Silverstone, H.,** Nutrition and genesis of tumors, in *Cancer,* Raven, R. W., Ed., Butterworth, London, 1957, 1, 301.

82. **Thiede, T. and Christensen, B. C.,** Blaeretumoret inducerede af klornafazinbehandling, *Ugeskrift for Laeger,* 137, 661, 1975.

83. **Tomatis, L.,** The value of long-term testing for implementation of primary prevention, in *Origins of Human Cancer,* Hiatt, H. H., Watson, J. D., and Winsten, J. A., Eds., Cold Spring Harbor Laboratory, New York, 1977.

84. **Tomatis, L., Agthe, C., Bartsch, H., Huff, J., Montesano, R., Saracci, R., Walker, E., and Wilbourn, J.,** Evaluation of the carcinogenicity of chemicals: a review of the monograph program of the International Agency for Research in Cancer, *Cancer Res.,* 38, 877, 1981.

85. Toxicology Forum, Transcript Winter Meeting, Stouffers Hotel, Arlington, Va., 1982.

86. **Trosko, J. E., Dawson, B., Yotti, L. P., and Chang, C. C.,** Saccharin may act as a tumor promoter by inhibiting metabolic cooperation between cells, *Nature,* 285, 109, 1980.

87. **Tsustui, H.,** Über das künstlich erzeagte Cancroid bei der Maüse, *Ganñ,* 12, 17, 1918.

88. U.S. Food and Drug Act, Public Law, 85th Congress H. R. 13254, 85, 1958.

89. **Upton, A. C.,** Radiation effects, in *Origins of Human Cancer,* Hiatt, H. H., Watson, J. D., and Winsten, J. A., Eds., Cold Spring Harbor Conference on Cell Proliferation, Cold Spring Harbor Laboratory, New York, 1977, 477.

90. **Vasdev, S., Tsuruta, Y., and O'Brien, P. J.,** A free radical mechanism for arylamine induced carcinogenesis involving peroxides, *Biochem. Pharmac.,* 31, 607, 1982.

91. **Williams, M. H. C.,** Environmental and industrial bladder cancer. Preventative measures, *Acta Unio. Int. Cancrum,* 18, 676, 1962.

92. **Williams, R. T.,** *Detoxication Mechanisms, the Metabolism and Detoxication of Drugs, Toxic Substances and Other Organic Compounds,* Chapman and Hall, London, 1959.

93. **Wright, A. S.,** ICPEMC Working Paper 2/2: the role of metabolism in chemical mutagenesis and chemical carcinogenesis, *Mutat. Res.,* 75, 215, 1980.

94. **Yamagiwa, K. and Ichikawa, K.,** Experimental study of the pathogenesis of carcinoma, *J. Cancer Res.,* 3, 1, 1918.

Section B—Statistical Criteria

Chapter 6

STATISTICAL DESIGN AND ANALYSIS OF THE LONG-TERM CARCINOGENICITY BIOASSAY

Mikelis Bickis and Daniel Krewski

TABLE OF CONTENTS

I. INTRODUCTION

Carcinogenic risk assessment is a complex process which may draw on a variety of toxicological and epidemiological data in order to determine the magnitude of the risk involved.[1,2] Because human exposure necessarily precedes epidemiological investigations, however, current estimates of risk are based largely on toxicological experiments. Until in vitro prescreening procedures become sufficiently well developed, moreover, bioassays which use animal models for man will remain one of the toxicologist's key tools for risk assessment.

There are generally three reasons for conducting a carcinogenicity bioassay. First, the experiment may be part of a screening program for the detection of potential carcinogens. Second, the experiment may enable estimation of risks at low levels of exposure. Finally, the experiment may allow verification of scientific hypotheses about the mechanisms of carcinogenesis. The specific purpose of the experiment has to be kept firmly in mind when considering questions of statistical design and analysis. Since a particular experiment may have more than one objective, moreover, the actual procedures used may represent a compromise that is not best for any one purpose, but is reasonably good for all.

Some recent guidelines on experimental design for carcinogenicity bioassays are summarized in Table 1. Three or more dose levels are often recommended, with at least 50 animals of each sex assigned to each dose. The high dose is generally taken to be the maximum tolerated dose (MTD), which is defined as the dose that is sufficiently great to elicit minimal signs of toxicity, yet not high enough to reduce survival from causes other than tumor occurrence. Statistical procedures for the analysis of carcinogenicity studies have also been the subject of much recent discussion,[3] with extensive recommendations having been made by the International Agency for Research on Cancer.[4]

While the recently published guidelines are fairly specific about the experimental design, their rationale is generally vague. In this article, however, we discuss some statistical principles (Section II) which form the basis for our guidelines for experimental design presented in Section III. Suitable methods of statistical analysis are discussed in Section IV. These ideas will then be synthesized into a number of general principles for the statistical design and analysis of carcinogenicity studies (Section V).

II. STATISTICAL PRELIMINARIES

Experiments with biological organisms generally involve sufficient variability to impart some degree of uncertainty to any conclusions drawn from the observed results. Proper evaluation of such experiments thus requires the application of sound statistical methods. Judicious use of these methods will allow one not only to quantify this uncertainty but also to reduce it. Statistical considerations have to be included in both the design and analysis of an experiment, since the two are interdependent. The appropriate analysis will depend on the design and, conversely, the choice of design will be influenced by the analysis required. Both the design and analysis will of course be determined by the purpose of the experiment.

A. Significance Tests

The purpose of a screening study is simply to decide whether the test compound does or does not display carcinogenic potential. Since one of two decisions is made, the operating characteristics of any procedure can be expressed in terms of the probabilities of making the wrong decision. The probability of declaring a noncarcinogen to be carcinogenic is called the false positive rate and the probability of declaring a carcinogen to be noncarcinogenic is called the false negative rate. This latter probability will depend on the potency of the carcinogen, since more potent carcinogens will be easier to detect.

Table 1
SUMMARY OF SELECTED RECENT GUIDELINES ON EXPERIMENTAL DESIGN FOR CARCINOGENICITY BIOASSAYS

Ref.	No. of dose levels	No. of animals	High dose	Low dose	Intermediate dose
5	3+	50+	Induces slight toxicity but no substantial reduction in longevity due to effects other than tumors	Less than 1/2 of intermediate dose but not less than 1/10 of high dose	1/4 to 1/2 of high dose
6	1+	Number of animals required to provide adequate assurance of safety if the test failed to detect carcinogenicity	Can be administered for the lifetime of the test animal and not produce (1) clinical signs of toxicity or pathological lesions other than those related to a neoplastic response (2) alteration of the normal longevity of the animals from toxic effects other than carcinogenesis and (3) appreciably inhibit normal weight gain		
7	2	50+	Elicits some toxicity when administered for the duration of the test period, but does not induce, (1) overt toxicity (2) toxic manifestations which are predicted materially to reduce the life span of the animals except as the result of neoplastic development, or (3) 10% greater retardation of body weight gain as compared with control animals. Should not be significantly detrimental to conception rate, fetal or neonatal survival or postnatal development		
8	3	Each group including the concurrent control should contain at least 50 animals of each sex	Elicit signs of toxicity without substantially altering the normal lifespan due to effects other than tumours. Signs of toxicity are those that may be indicated by alterations in serum enzyme levels or slight depression of body weight gain (less than 10%). For diet mixtures, the ingested concentration should not exceed 5%	Should not interfere with normal growth, development and longevity of the animal or result in any indication of toxicity. In general, not less than 10% of high dose	Mid-range between high and low doses, depending upon the toxicokinetics of the chemical

Although more general decision procedures are possible, screening studies are commonly evaluated using significance tests. The data from the experiment are tested for statistical significance to determine whether there is sufficient evidence of carcinogenicity. (It should be emphasized that statements of statistical significance are statements about the experiment and not about the test compound. In other words, such statements pertain to the strength of the experimental evidence rather than to the potency of the compound itself.)

The logical basis of significance tests is as follows. The results of any experiment can be considered to be the output of some random process. In the absence of any intrinsic differences between the treatment groups, any observed differences will be due solely to chance. If the observed outcome is improbable under this assumption, then one could say that the experiment provides evidence against the ''null hypothesis'' of no differences between treatments.

Unfortunately, this simple description is not quite adequate because in a large experiment, any particular outcome is very unlikely. For example, suppose two groups of fifty animals each were exposed to treatments that both induce an expected tumour incidence rate of 10%. While the probability of observing exactly five tumours in each group would be .034 in this case, one would scarcely say that this small probability provides evidence against the hypothesis that the two treatments are identical. What is needed is an ordering of all possible outcomes according to the amount of evidence they provide against the null hypothesis. The result is then deemed significant if the combined probability of all outcomes at least as extreme as the observed one is sufficiently small. (One outcome will be called more extreme than another if it provides more evidence against the null hypothesis.)

Although the idea is conceptually simple, there remain several logical gaps in the above description. First, there is the question as to what constitutes a small probability. Traditionally, ''small'' has meant less than 5%, although there is no substantive reason why this bound has been chosen. The important point is that the procedure guarantees that the false positive rate will also be small. Thus, if we accept the traditional bound, then the false positive rate will be no greater than the nominal 5% level (and can be considerably less in certain situations). It is important to note that the procedure makes no guarantees about the false negative rate.

The second logical gap is the indefinite meaning of one outcome providing more evidence against the null hypothesis than another. The dilemma is usually resolved by calculating a statistic or numerical score for each outcome and then ranking the outcomes according to the values of their score. However, this solution just transforms the problem to one of defining a suitable statistic. Rival scoring procedures can however be evaluated in terms of their false negative rates calculated with reference to a particular alternative to the null hypothesis. The one giving the lowest false negative rate is the best one, and is termed the most powerful procedure for that alternative. It is important to note that a procedure is generally best only for a particular alternative. Only in the simplest situations do there exist procedures that are uniformly most powerful against all alternatives. Thus, the choice of procedure is dictated largely by the alternatives of most concern.

The third logical gap is the assumption that the probabilities of the various outcomes are known. In the simpler cases these can be explicitly calculated. In many situations, however, one has to be satisfied with approximations derived from certain idealized assumptions, and some deep theorems in probability theory.

B. Estimation

In addition to a qualitative classification, the experimenter may require a quantitative measure of carcinogenic potential, such as the risk associated with low levels of exposure. The estimation of such a quantity generally involves a mathematical model relating the probabilities of the observed outcomes to other quantities called parameters of the model. The true value of the quantity of interest can be expressed in terms of the unknown model parameters, whereas the estimate is expressed in terms of the observed data.

Since different experiments on the same compound will give different estimates, the estimate is a random variable, subject to experimental error. The uncertainty can be quantified by a confidence interval. That is, instead of giving a single number as the estimate, one gives a range of numbers that includes the true value with high probability. This probability is called the confidence coefficient of the interval. For a given confidence coefficient, one would like to make the interval as short as possible.

If the statistic used to estimate the quantity of interest has a normal distribution, then the length of the confidence interval depends only on the variance of the statistic. And since most reasonable statistics have approximately normal distributions for large samples, short confidence intervals correspond to small variances. It should be kept in mind that the meaning of the term "large sample" depends on the quantity being estimated. In some cases, a sample of thirty may be considered large, whereas a sample of several thousand might still be too small for the normal distribution to be a good approximation in other cases.[9]

C. Validity and Efficiency

The terms "validity" and "efficiency" are often used in discussing statistical procedures. These terms have technical meanings which are similar to but not identical with their popular meanings. A procedure is called valid if the probability statements made therein are true. In particular, a valid test is one for which the actual probability of a false positive is no greater than the nominal probability. Similarly, a valid confidence interval is one whose actual probability of including the true value is at least as great as the stated confidence coefficient. It should be noted that a valid procedure is not necessarily a good procedure. For example, the procedure of considering all compounds to be noncarcinogenic regardless of the experimental results is valid since the false positive rate is zero.

A procedure is called efficient if it makes the best use of all the information available. Thus, an efficient test has as low a false negative rate as possible. Similarly, an efficient confidence interval is, on the average, as short as possible. The efficiency of a statistical analysis is limited by the amount of information available in the experiment, which, in turn, is limited by cost considerations. Since the most important cost consideration is usually the number of animals used, it is often useful to evaluate procedures according to the amount of information they provide per animal.

Since fully efficient procedures are often not attainable, it is important to be able to compare the efficiencies of suboptimal competitors. Such comparisons are often expressed in terms of relative efficiency. To define this term we require a concept of quantity of information. Although more comprehensive definitions are possible, it will be adequate for our purposes to express the quantity of information in terms of false negative rates for qualitative procedures and shortness of confidence intervals for quantitative procedures. Thus two screening procedures can be said to be equally informative if for a given false positive rate they have equal false negative rates, and two estimation procedures can be said to be equally informative if they produce confidence intervals of equal length. Suppose now that we have applied an optimal procedure to an experiment with a given number of animals. We can achieve the same quantity of information with a suboptimal procedure simply by having a larger experiment. The relative efficiency of the second procedure is defined as the ratio of the number of animals in the first experiment to the number of animals in the second experiment.

III. EXPERIMENTAL DESIGN

A sound experimental design is essential for the results of any bioassay to be useful. No amount of toxicological, pathological, or statistical expertise can recover much information from a poorly designed study. A well designed experiment, on the other hand, has many

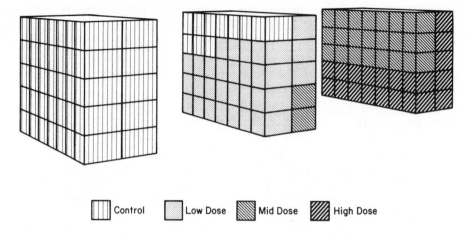

Control | Low Dose | Mid Dose | High Dose

FIGURE 1.   A systematic block design (not recommended).

advantages. Not only does it facilitate the application of valid and efficient statistical procedures, but the results are often easier to analyze, easier to interpret, and more comparable with those in other studies.

The concept of an experimental unit is central to a proper understanding of experimental designs. The experimental unit is that entity actually receiving the treatment, and encompasses all attributes of that entity. In a feeding study with two or more animals per cage, for example, the entire cage is the experimental unit since the treatment is given in the feed ration placed in the cage.[10] In a two generation study, the entire litter of the second generation is the experimental unit, since this is the entity that receives the treatment in utero.[11] It must be remembered that all attributes of the experimental unit must be considered. Thus, if a block of cages on the same treatment is placed in a particular location in the laboratory, then the entire block rather than the individual cage becomes the experimental unit.

A. Randomization

A crucial part of any good design is randomization. Although the need for randomization is widely recognized, there is often confusion as to what constitutes a valid randomization scheme. The purpose of randomization is twofold. First, it tends to eliminate biasing effects of unsuspected factors on the experimental results. Second, it provides a basis for statistical inference. These objectives can be achieved by designs satisfying the following two principles of randomization.

P1.   Nothing distinguishes the treatment groups other than the treatments themselves.
P2.   The experimental units are assigned to the treatment groups at random.

The first principle in particular requires that the treatment given to a cage should be unrelated to its position.

Consider the particular design shown in Figure 1. Here, the animals have been randomly assigned to treatment groups. However, the control animals are all in the first block of cages, the animals in the low dose group are all in the next block, and so on, with the high dose animals appearing entirely in the last block of cages.

Although such a design is logistically convenient, it violates both principles of randomization. In the first place, the treatment groups are clearly identifiable by their location. This identifiability effectively diminishes the number of experimental units: instead of the treatments being independentl given to 200 animals, we really only have treatments given to four blocks of cages. Secondly, the treatments are not randomly assigned to the experimental

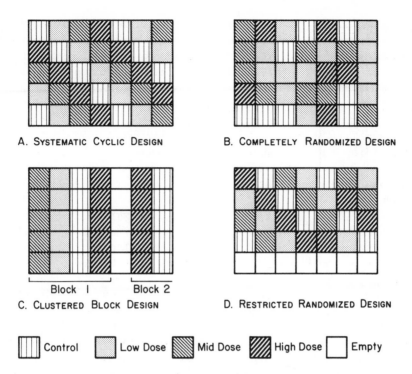

FIGURE 2. Cage face arrangements for four experimental designs.

units. (Even if the animals had been randomly assigned to the cages, P2 would not be satisfied because the experimental units are defined by the cage blocks.)

To examine the consequences of the flaws in this design, suppose there is an environmental gradient in the room resulting in a greater incidence of tumours on one side of the room than the other. If the gradient goes from left to right, then it may induce a difference between the dose groups which would appear to be due to the treatments. If, on the other hand, the gradient goes from right to left, then it could mask a real treatment effect.

Although concerns such as these have long been addressed in agricultural field trials where the existence of fertility gradients is well known, it seems to be generally assumed that such gradients do not exist in the carefully controlled laboratory environment. However, such a belief does not appear to have any empirical support. In one recent study, for example, substantial differences in reticulo-endothelial tumor rates were found between animals in different cage positions in the same treatment group.[12]

A tempting solution to the problem of positional effects is the rotation of cage positions during the course of the experiment. Although such a practice will ensure a more uniform environment for the different dose groups, it will not provide a basis for statistical inference if such rotation maintains the original contiguity of the cages.

A somewhat better design is shown in Figure 2a. Here the dose groups were assigned to consecutive cages in a systematic manner. This design does not violate the first principle of randomization, since the dose groups are dispersed throughout the experimental environment. However, because the allocation of treatment groups is not random, the second principle is not satisfied.

A design satisfying both principles is given in Figure 2b. In this example, the treatments assigned to the individual cages were determined using a table of random numbers. The patterns displayed by the dose groups would be different for the different cage racks, and it is extremely unlikely that two studies would have the same pattern. Thus, artifacts due to positional effects would not be reproducible, and will hence be recognized as such.

One objection that has been voiced against the use of this design is that the random dispersement of treatments within the cage banks will increase the chance of errors in administering the different treatments. It is undeniable that the proper conduct of a randomized experiment demands careful record keeping and well trained personnel. Although these requirements may increase the overall cost of the bioassay, such costs must be accepted as the price of ensuring scientific validity. Experience with trained personnel in our own laboratories indicates that mix up of treatments is not a serious problem.[10] (A practical way of implementing the treatment allocations is discussed below.) A more serious drawback of randomized designs is the potential for cross-contamination with volatile agents or through spillage of feed. In such cases, a clustered block design such as that illustrated in Figure 2c may be considered, although the experimental unit now becomes the column rather than the individual cage.

One must not overlook the fact that all aspects of the experiment should satisfy the two principles enunciated above. The first requirement, in particular, dictates that nothing in the experimental environment such as color coded cage labels identifies the animal's treatment group. The knowledge of an animal's treatment may affect the way it is handled by the animal care personnel, and such a bias should be avoided. Instead, the treatments should be prepared in advance in single dose containers by a person not otherwise involved in the experiment. The containers should then be labelled with the numbers of the cages that are to receive the respective treatments. (The labelling can be facilitated by having a computer produce a supply of preprinted stickers.) The containers should then be arranged in the cage number sequence and forwarded to the animal care personnel. The latter should verify that the number on the container agrees with the number on the cage. The list specifying the treatments for each cage should be kept confidential until all the data have been collected.

Similarly, the pathology should be done blindly.[13] Strictly speaking, the pathology report is part of the experimental unit, and hence the sequence in which necropsies are performed and the slides are read should be randomized among the treatment groups. If the experimental environment has been properly randomized, then presenting the animals in the caging sequence is a good approach. The practice of doing pathology on the high dose or control animals first should be firmly avoided. (If the pathologist requires material to practice upon, then a few extra animals, which will not be used in the final evaluation, could be added to the experiment for this purpose.)

B. Design Parameters

Given that validity has been ensured by proper randomization, the experimenter can manipulate a number of design parameters to improve efficiency. These include the number of animals, selection of blocking factors, number of dose groups, magnitude of dose levels, distribution of animals among dose groups, and duration of exposure.

The number of animals used is usually constrained by cost considerations. However, it is important to evaluate how informative an affordable experiment may be. If resources are limited, even the most efficient experiment may provide so little information that it is not worth doing at all.

Blocking refers to the deliberate attempt to reduce variation by partitioning the experimental units into homogeneous blocks, and then allocating treatments at random within these blocks. In this way, treatment differences will be less obscured by the variation among animals, and efficiency will be enhanced. Factors used in defining blocks could be attributes of the animals or of the environment. Examples of the former include sibling relationships and body weight; examples of the latter are cage position and initiation or autopsy date.

Complex schemes for blocking on several factors are possible such as in the balanced block design (Figure 2d). Note that the dose groups are balanced in the sense that they occur the same number of times in each column. Also, each dose group is missing in precisely one row, and the other dose groups in that row appear exactly twice. The cages are randomly assigned dose groups within these restrictions. The balance within columns protects against horizontal positional effects. The more complicated balance within rows does not directly prevent positional artifacts, but does allow one to make a simple adjustment for them. In addition, the magnitude of the positional effects themselves can be estimated.

Even more complex schemes involving latin squares for balancing positional effects have been proposed.[12] Although such designs are commonly used in agricultural research, their utility for toxicological studies is questionable. They can appreciably reduce experimental error in the presence of large environmental gradients, but can be somewhat less efficient than the completely randomized design if the gradient is slight. Furthermore, much of the advantage of these designs is a consequence of their symmetry. In chronic studies, intercurrent mortality could greatly disturb the symmetry, thereby reducing any such advantage. Another practical consideration is that these designs require certain relationships among the numbers used, relationships which may not be true of the dimensions of cage racks. (In the previous example, note that the bottom row of cages is not used.)

The efficiency of an experiment can depend greatly on the number of dose groups used, and the magnitude of the doses. A good choice will depend on the purpose of the experiment, with different guidelines being appropriate for screening, low dose extrapolation, and mechanistic experiments.

Once the number of animals and the number of dose groups have been determined, there remains the question of animal allocation. Traditionally, all dose groups have been assigned equal weight, with a somewhat larger number of animals being allocated to the control group on occasion. Such balanced or near-balanced allocations are not always the best strategy, as will be discussed later.

Another parameter that can be manipulated is the duration of exposure. Typically, the animals are exposed for a substantial portion of their lifetime, at which time any survivors are killed. Maximal exposure, however, does not always give the best design. There are experiments where one is interested in mechanisms such as reversibility or initiation/promotion, in which case intermittent exposures are needed. However, even screening studies may sometimes benefit from shorter exposure times. If a chemical manifests its carcinogenicity quickly then sufficient evidence is available before the full exposure time, and the experiment could be terminated early.[14,15] The resources so saved could be better used in screening other compounds, or in running larger studies.

Shorter exposure times will also result from planned interim sacrifices. Such sacrifices may be required to study the progressive pathogenesis of the lesion of interest or to estimate the distribution of times to tumor. Unless tumor appearance is directly observable in the living animals, the time to tumor distribution cannot be readily estimated without information on the cause of death.[16] Cause of death may be difficult to establish for nonsacrificed animals.

C. Designs for Screening Studies

Increased efficiency in a screening study is achieved by a decreased false negative rate. Since the false negative rate will be minimized by maximizing the expected response, it would appear that the optimal design will contain a dose as high as possible. If only lifetime tumor incidence is considered, the optimal design will have two dose groups: the MTD and control. The optimal allocation between test and control depends on the actual tumor incidence rates. However, equal allocation is frequently used, and is generally reasonably efficient in comparison with optimal allocation.[17]

Table 2 gives the false negative rates for an experiment with a control and single test group, each with 50 animals. It is evident that a bioassay of this size will not be very successful at detecting carcinogens unless the excess tumor incidence rate at the MTD is 20% or greater. Although the use of optimal allocation will reduce these false negative rates

Table 2
FALSE NEGATIVE RATES FOR A
SIMPLE CARCINOGENICITY
SCREEN[a]

Excess over spontaneous rate[b] (%)	Spontaneous rate (%)			
	0	1	5	20
5	90	88	87	90
10	43	49	61	77
15	11	18	34	58
20	2	5	15	36
25	1	1	5	19

[a]   Based on Fisher's exact test with 50 animals in each of a control and test group and assuming that all animals respond independently.

[b]   Difference between the response rates in the test and control groups respectively.

somewhat, the reduction will be slight except when the spontaneous response rate is extremely low.

The use of more than two dose groups will also decrease efficiency. For example a design with four equally spaced dose groups will have only about 60% of the efficiency of a design with two dose groups covering the same range. A middle dose group is frequently included in case the high dose exceeds the MTD. Although such a strategy is prudent, it must be remembered that this extra dose group has little effect on the false negative rate.

If the design is such that the experimental unit is an entire litter or cage then efficiency may be reduced. The reduction in efficiency will depend on the correlation of tumor incidence between animals in the same litter or cage.[18] This problem can sometimes be easily avoided through the use of designs in which the individual animal represents the experimental unit. The selection of one pup/sex/litter to continue on test on the second generation of a two generation study and the use of single caging may be advantageous in this regard.

D. Designs for Low Dose Extrapolation

While a screening study using relatively high dose levels is a useful tool for qualitatively assessing the carcinogenic potential of chemicals, it is also important to determine the magnitude of risk at lower doses typical of human exposure levels. Since direct estimates of risk at low levels of exposure would require prohibitively many animals, such estimates must be based on the downward extrapolation of the high dose results using some mathematical model relating the probability of tumor occurrence to the administered dose.

Six dose-response models that have been used for this purpose are the probit, logit, Weibull, one hit, gamma multi-hit, and multi-stage (Table 3). The biological basis and statistical properties of these models have been recently reviewed by Munro and Krewski[19] and Krewski and Van Ryzin.[20] Although all of these models imply no response at zero dose, background response can be accommodated by postulating either that this response is independent of chemically induced responses (independent background) or that the background response is due to an effective background dose (additive background). It is also possible to include both types of background in the model.[21]

Optimal designs for low dose extrapolation when only lifetime incidence rates are used have been studied by Krewski et al.[22] for the probit, logit, Weibull, and gamma multi-hit models as well as certain special cases of the two-stage model. Portier and Hoel[23] have also considered special cases of the multi-stage model. The former results are based on exact

Table 3
DOSE RESPONSE MODELS FOR QUANTAL
RESPONSE TOXICITY DATA

Model	Probability of occurrence at dose	
Probit	$(2\pi)^{-1/2} \int_{-\infty}^{\alpha+\beta \log d} \exp(-t^2/2)dt$	$(\beta > 0)$
Logit	$[1 + \exp(-\alpha - \beta \log d)]^{-1}$	$(\beta > 0)$
Weibull	$1 - \exp(-\lambda d^m)$	$(\lambda, m > 0)$
One-hit	$1 - \exp(-\lambda d)$	$(\lambda > 0)$
Gamma multi-hit	$\int_0^{\lambda d} e^{-t} t^{k-1}/\Gamma(k)dt$	$(\lambda, k > 0)$
Multi-stage	$1 - \exp\left(-\sum_{i=1}^{k} \beta_i d^i\right)$	$(\beta_i > 0)$

derivations for large samples, and the question of how large the experiment has to be for the results to apply is still under investigation. Portier and Hoel's results are based on exact derivations for large samples, and Monte Carlo simulations for moderate samples. These latter results suggest that the large sample theory for the multi-stage model may not be adequate.

Krewski et al.[22] found that for the models considered, optimal designs for low dose extrapolation will generally have three dose groups including one group at the MTD and one control. The dose given to the intermediate dose group depends on the curvature of the dose response curve, with greater curvature requiring a larger fraction of the MTD. The allocation of animals among the dose groups depends on a number of parameters, including the acceptable risk and background response rate. However, a 1:2:1 allocation with half of the animals on the middle dose and the other half divided evenly between the control and high dose appears to result in a reasonably efficient design. An interesting property of these designs is that they are practically independent of the particular model assumed.

A serious drawback of such optimal designs is that one has to know something of the shape of the dose response curve in order to determine the optimal design. For this reason, both Krewski et al. and Portier and Hoel have considered the efficiencies of suboptimal designs in an attempt to find one that is reasonably efficient for most situations. In spite of the different approaches and models, both of these investigations have yielded similar conclusions. The former investigators have proposed a design with a control and three equally spaced dose groups with a 1:2:2:1 allocation. Among other designs, Portier[24] has recommended a design with the same dose levels and a 2:3:3:2 allocation.

Instead of deriving optimal designs under an assumed mathematical model, Crump and Langley[25] consider the case where one extrapolates linearly from an upper confidence limit in the observed response in a single dose group. In the case of zero background, their results indicate that a near-optimal dose for extrapolation would be about half of that dose producing a 10% response. (Note that this does not generally correspond to that dose inducing 5% response.)

One question of great concern in low dose extrapolation is the matter of what mathematical model to use. Both Chambers and Cox[26] and Crump[27] have presented designs for discriminating between particular dose response models. Unfortunately, their results are not particularly encouraging. Even with optimal designs, several thousand animals are required to ensure adequate discrimination between plausible models.

E. Designs for Examining Mechanisms of Carcinogenesis

When the purpose of the experiment is to discriminate between rival hypotheses of carcinogenic mechanisms, no general guidelines can be given, since the best design will depend heavily on the particular hypothesis being tested. Specific aspects of the carcinogenic process

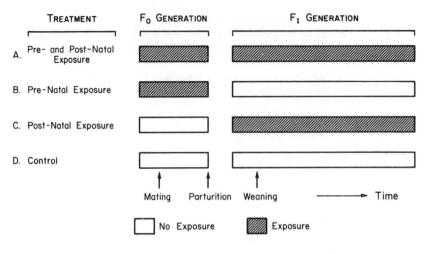

FIGURE 3.   Treatment regimens for two generation studies.

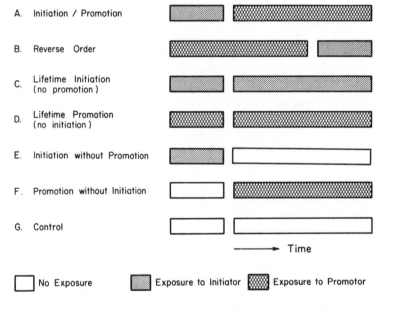

FIGURE 4.   Treatment regimens for initiation/promotion studies.

that could be studied include in utero vs. post weaning exposure,[11] initiation/promotion phenomena,[28] reversibility of lesions,[29] and the effects of mixed exposures.[30] All of these situations require special experimental protocols. Two generation studies, for example, may be employed in cases where the carcinogen is suspected of exerting its effects as a result of in utero exposure. In order to fully distinguish between prenatal and postnatal effects, several dosing regimens encompassing these two stages of development are required (Figure 3.)

A complete study of initiation/promotion would require at least the seven dosing regimens presented in Figure 4. A smaller set of treatments would suffice to test a more specific hypothesis. For example, if compound A was known to be a promoter, then the hypothesis that B is an initiator could be tested with only two dose groups, the first receiving control followed by A, the second receiving B followed by A. (Note that no pure control is necessary in this case.)

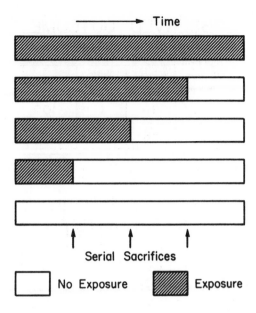

FIGURE 5. Treatment regimens for reversibility studies.

Dosing regimens involving initial exposure to the test agent followed by a return to control conditions would be required to study the possible reversibility of induced effects (Figure 5). Although rarely applied in the past, simultaneous exposure to two or more agents is required in order to assess interactive effects.

IV. STATISTICAL ANALYSIS

Just as a proper experimental design is needed to provide an informative experiment, so also is an appropriate statistical analysis essential to extract that information. Generally, the correct analysis will depend on the design used, which will again depend on the purpose of the experiment. We now discuss, in turn, the analysis of screening studies and of studies intended for low dose extrapolation. Although ideally the analysis should be performed on times to tumor, such data is not always available, and some information can be gleaned from the crude lifetime tumor incidence.

A. Screening Studies
1. Tests Based on Lifetime Tumor Incidence
Let us examine a significance test for the very simplest case, a completely randomized design with a control and a single test group, where the only information available for analysis is the lifetime incidence of tumors. The data can be summarized by a 2×2 table giving the number of animals in each dose group with or without tumors (Figure 6). In this example, 1/100 controls and 4/50 treated animals had tumors.

Because the design was randomized, we can carry out a significance test without making any further assumptions, since the probability of each possible outcome can be calculated exactly from the randomization alone. Under the null hypothesis of no difference between the two groups, the fact that 4 out of the 5 tumors appear in the test group is solely due to the random manner in which the animals were assigned to the groups. The other possible outcomes, along with their probabilities of occurrence under the null hypothesis, are also given in Figure 6. In this case there is no dispute about how the outcome should be ordered:

OBSERVED OUTCOME

Treatment Group	NUMBER OF ANIMALS		
	Without Tumor	With Tumor	Total
Control	99	1	100
Test	46	4	50

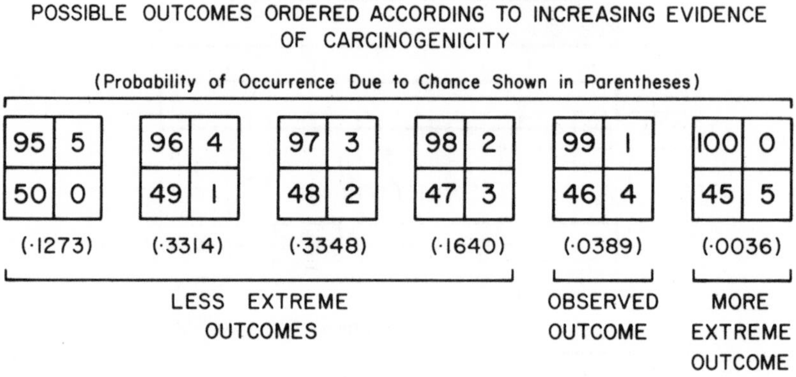

POSSIBLE OUTCOMES ORDERED ACCORDING TO INCREASING EVIDENCE
OF CARCINOGENICITY

(Probability of Occurrence Due to Chance Shown in Parentheses)

95	5		96	4		97	3		98	2		99	1		100	0
50	0		49	1		48	2		47	3		46	4		45	5
(·1273)			(·3314)			(·3348)			(·1640)			(·0389)			(·0036)	

LESS EXTREME OUTCOMES	OBSERVED OUTCOME	MORE EXTREME OUTCOME

FIGURE 6.   An example of Fisher's exact test.

the more tumors in the test group, the more evidence of carcinogenicity. Since the probability of outcomes at least as extreme as that observed is .043 which is less than the nominal .05 level, the result is significant. This procedure is commonly called "Fisher's exact test".

A more complicated example is given in Figure 7. Here we have four treatment groups: a control with 120 animals and three groups of 40 animals each on increasing doses. We observe three animals with tumors in the middle dose group and no tumors elsewhere. Is this result significant? The 20 possible outcomes are enumerated in Figure 7, along with their probabilities of occurrence under the null hypothesis. The difficulty in this case is deciding upon the ordering. Although the outcome with all three tumors in the top dose is clearly more extreme, what can one say about two tumors in the top dose, and one in the control?

One way out of this dilemma is to calculate a trend statistic

$$T_1 = \Sigma \, d_i \, x_i$$

where d_i is the ith dose level and x_i is the number of animals with tumor in the ith group. This statistic gives the ordering presented in Figure 7a. Under this ordering, the result is significant. This test will be most powerful against alternatives of a linear dose response curve. If we suppose a priori that the dose response curve is quadratic, then a statistic calculated as

$$T_2 = \Sigma \, d_i^2 \, x_i$$

may be appropriate. With this statistic, the ordering is different, and the result in the example is no longer significant (Figure 7b). This disagreement between the tests can be interpreted as follows: If one believes that any dose response curve must be quadratic, then the experiment does not provide significant evidence for a dose response. If however, linearity is possible,

OBSERVED OUTCOME

DOSE	NUMBER OF ANIMALS		
(Fraction of MTD)	Without Tumor	With Tumor	Total
0	120	0	120
1/8	40	0	40
3/4	37	3	40
1	40	0	40

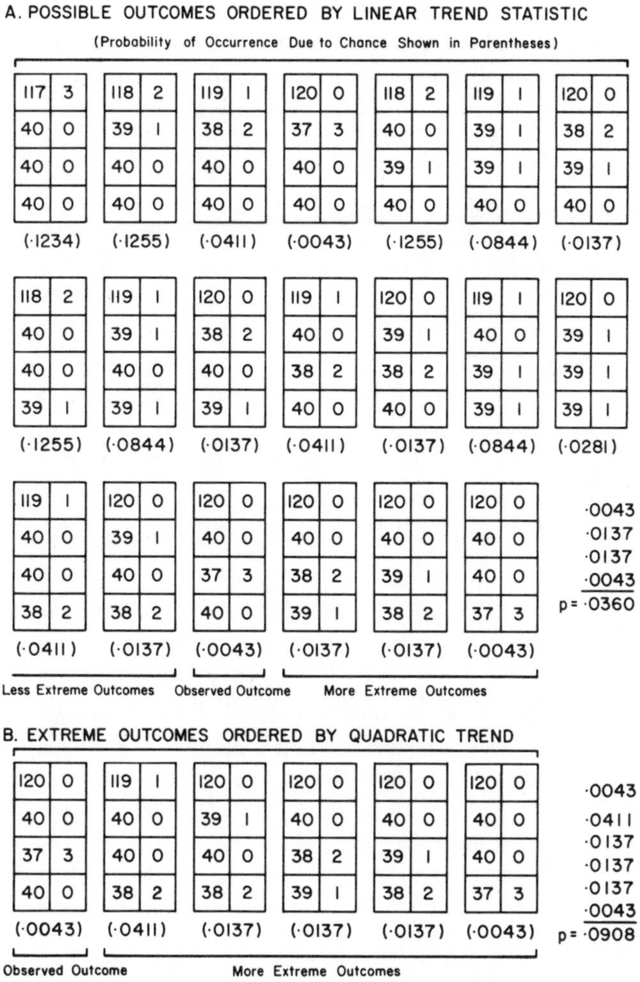

A. POSSIBLE OUTCOMES ORDERED BY LINEAR TREND STATISTIC

(Probability of Occurrence Due to Chance Shown in Parentheses)

Row 1:

117	3		118	2		119	1		120	0		118	2		119	1		120	0
40	0		39	1		38	2		37	3		40	0		39	1		38	2
40	0		40	0		40	0		40	0		39	1		39	1		39	1
40	0		40	0		40	0		40	0		40	0		40	0		40	0
(·1234)			(·1255)			(·0411)			(·0043)			(·1255)			(·0844)			(·0137)		

Row 2:

118	2		119	1		120	0		119	1		120	0		119	1		120	0
40	0		39	1		38	2		40	0		39	1		40	0		39	1
40	0		40	0		40	0		38	2		38	2		39	1		39	1
39	1		39	1		39	1		40	0		40	0		39	1		39	1
(·1255)			(·0844)			(·0137)			(·0411)			(·0137)			(·0844)			(·0281)		

Row 3:

119	1		120	0		120	0		120	0		120	0		120	0
40	0		39	1		40	0		40	0		40	0		40	0
40	0		40	0		37	3		38	2		39	1		40	0
38	2		38	2		40	0		39	1		38	2		37	3
(·0411)			(·0137)			(·0043)			(·0137)			(·0137)			(·0043)		

·0043
·0137
·0137
·0043
p = ·0360

Less Extreme Outcomes   Observed Outcome   More Extreme Outcomes

B. EXTREME OUTCOMES ORDERED BY QUADRATIC TREND

120	0		119	1		120	0		120	0		120	0		120	0
40	0		40	0		39	1		40	0		40	0		40	0
37	3		40	0		40	0		38	2		39	1		40	0
40	0		38	2		38	2		39	1		38	2		37	3
(·0043)			(·0411)			(·0137)			(·0137)			(·0137)			(·0043)		

·0043
·0411
·0137
·0137
·0137
·0043
p = ·0908

Observed Outcome   More Extreme Outcomes

FIGURE 7.   An example of permutation tests for trend.

then there is significance. A point to remember is that the ordering must be chosen *a priori*. If one first looks at the data, and then decides on the statistic, then the false positive rate is no longer maintained.

Unless the tumors are few in number, calculation of exact probabilities can be very time-consuming, even using a high-speed computer. Therefore, one frequently uses approximate methods. The approximation of Fisher's exact test is the familiar one-tailed χ^2 test with the continuity correction.[31] Armitage's trend test with a continuity correction[32] is the approximation to the procedure presented in Figure 7a.

Other significance tests are also possible. Schaafsma's test[33] is similar in structure, but weights the treatment groups on a worst case basis. That is, this test is designed to be most powerful for dose response curves that yield the lowest power. Bartholomew's test[31,33] is based on a similar philosophy, but on a different mathematical procedure. This latter test assumes nothing about the dose response curve save that it is increasing. Before calculating the test statistic, any apparent reversals in the observed dose response curve are first eliminated by averaging adjacent dose groups that imply a decreasing effect. By virtue of their construction, these two procedures will be more efficient than the trend test in some situations. Whether these tests should be used in practice depends on whether these special situations are likely to occur. One drawback of both procedures is that the dose levels used are not taken into account in the analysis of the data.

While more research is needed to examine the trade offs between the alternative procedures, the selection of a particular significance test is generally not crucial, for the region where they disagree is often small. Any of these tests will usually be more efficient than the common practice of comparing each test group with the control, and considerably more efficient than the practice of comparing the control with all of the dose groups combined.

A complication of significance testing in the carcinogenicity bioassay is that the particular tumor site of concern is generally not known until after the data have been analyzed. Thus, instead of a single significance test, many such tests may be performed, one for each site. Although the rate of false positives per site remains below the significance level, the chance of at least one false positive over all the sites could become unacceptably high. It is sometimes proposed that the false positive rate be controlled by restricting the significance level by the so-called Bonferroni bound, achieved by dividing the desired false positive rate by the number of tests made. Such an adjustment will ensure the validity of the bioassay as a whole, but the false negative rate will rise to possibly unacceptable levels. This problem is addressed by Gart, Chu, and Tarone,[3] who point out that because the true false positive rate in most such cases is much smaller than the significance level, a Bonferroni correction is unnecessary.

It has been proposed that incidence rates in control groups of the same strain in other experiments can help in evaluating the significance of the result.[34,35] If the historical control rates are fairly stable and similar to the concurrent controls, the additional information on the spontaneous response rate could strengthen a marginally significant result. If either of these criteria is not met, however, the historical data will be of little value.

It is sometimes argued[35] that a historical control range that encompasses the high dose incidence nullifies any significance obtained using the concurrent control. This argument is based on the presumption that the concurrent control incidence is, by chance, atypically low. However, in a properly randomized experiment the usual significance test already takes into account any such chance variation. Furthermore, any factor that might depress the concurrent control incidence should, in the absence of treatment effects, depress incidence in the treated groups as well.

Tarone[34] and Dempster et al.[36] have proposed similar procedures for quantitatively incorporating historical control information into the Armitage test for linear trend. These procedures effectively increase the number of control animals in accordance with the stability of the historical data. If the control incidence is highly variable, then the adjustment is slight as suggested above.

2. Tests Based on Time to Tumor Data

Although an assessment of lifetime tumor incidence is often the first step in the analysis of a carcinogenicity study, such an analysis can be misleading.[3,37] Ignorance of the time at which the tumors appeared can affect both the validity and efficiency of the statistical procedure. If the test chemical both reduces life expectancy and causes tumors, then the

Table 4

**A HYPOTHETICAL BIOASSAY OUTCOME WITH AN AGENT
CAUSING BOTH INCREASED TUMOR INCIDENCE AND
INTERCURRENT MORTALITY**

Number of animals observed	Time on test (months)					
	0—12		12—24		0—24	
	Control	Treated	Control	Treated	Control	Treated
With tumors	1	18	24	7	25	25
Dying or sacrificed	20	90	80	10	100	100
% With tumors	5	20	30	70	25	25

shortened lifespan will reduce the length of time the test animals will be at risk, and could mask a carcinogenic effect. As an example, consider a carcinogenic agent that increases the age specific tumor incidence at all ages and yet results in greater intercurrent mortality because of toxic effects unrelated to tumor induction. Under these conditions, a typical experiment could produce the hypothetical outcome shown in Table 4. Note that the proportion of animals with tumors is greater in the exposed group than in controls in both the early and later stages of the experiment, yet the lifetime tumor incidence rates are the same in both groups.

This problem can be readily solved if the neoplasm is observable in the living animal, such as would be the case with skin or mammary tumors. Statistical procedures for dealing with this situation, involving right-censored life table analysis, have been developed by numerous authors.[38,39,40]

If, however, the neoplasm is only detected at necropsy then another possible bias occurs. If the test compound decreases life expectancy but does not cause tumors, then the mere fact that the test animals are necropsied earlier could give the illusion of an earlier onset of tumors. The resolution of this problem requires that tumors be classified as being either fatal or incidental. For fatal tumors, one can use a life table analysis to determine whether the death rate from tumors is increasing with dose. For incidental tumors, a prevalence analysis may be used to determine whether the prevalence of tumors among autopsied animals increases with dose. Note that the response is defined differently in the two cases. In the first it is death from tumor, whereas in the second it is presence of tumor at death.

Either analysis involves setting up a series of tables at a number of points in time. The tables all have the following structure.

Dose group	0	1	...	k	Total
Number at risk	n_o	n_1	...	n_k	n
Number responding (O)	y_o	y_1	...	y_k	y
Expected responses (E)	$n_o\, y/n$	$n_1\, y/n$	...	$n_k\, y/n$	y
Deviation (O-E)	$y_o - n_o\, y/n$	$y_1 - n_1\, y/n$	...	$y_k - n_k\, y/n$	0

One of these tables is set up for each time at which an animal dies from the tumor in question. The number at risk in each column is the number of animals in the corresponding dose group that are still alive immediately prior to the time point. The number responding is the number of animals that died from the tumor at this time.

One such table is also set up for non-tumor deaths at intervals throughout the study. In this case, the number at risk is the number of animals autopsied during the interval that did not die from the tumor in question. The number responding is the number of animals that were observed to have the tumor in an incidental context.

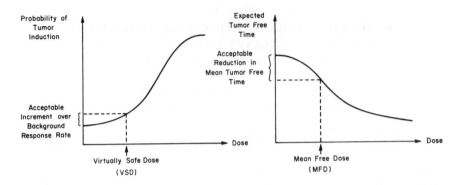

FIGURE 8.   Characterizations of low dose risk.

Once these tables have been defined, the deviations (O-E) can be combined across time points, and across the two kinds of tumor. Peto et al.[4] suggest simple addition, although giving different weights to the different time points would still give a valid test. It is again a question of maintaining efficiency against alternatives of particular concern. Simple addition results in a test that is powerful against the alternative that the age-specific death-from-tumor rate is magnified by a factor that is constant across time (the so called proportional hazards case). If there is concern that the chemical may have a more pronounced effect on younger animals, then the earlier time points should be given more weight.

Once the tables have been combined, one can do a test for trend by calculating the sum of (doses × combined (O-E)) and dividing by a denominator that is a complicated function of the entries in the separate tables. Exact formulas are given in Peto et al.[4]

Tests of this type are not very efficient in cases of tumor acceleration, such as was suspected in the case of the food color additive FD and C red 40.[12] To illustrate, suppose that there is a susceptible subpopulation in which the test chemical diminishes the tumor's latent period but does not otherwise affect its incidence. In such a case, the age-specific tumor incidence rate will be increased in the test group early on in the experiment, but will be decreased later in the experiment because the susceptible animals will have been removed from those at risk. Hence, combination of the (O-E) terms across time will tend to cancel out these two effects. A more powerful test against such an alternative has been proposed by Fleming et al.[41]

B. Low Dose Extrapolation

The purpose of low dose extrapolation is to estimate the carcinogenic risk of a chemical at the low doses typical of chronic human exposure. In the absence of a threshold level, any dose, no matter how small, will result in some degree of risk. While absolute safety may then be guaranteed only at zero dose, virtual safety may still be defined in terms of some small acceptable increase in risk.

The low dose risk may be expressed in several ways[16] (Figure 8). The most commonly used is the virtually safe dose (VSD) defined as the dose for which the incremental lifetime probability of tumor occurrence is equal to the acceptable risk. A rational choice of this acceptable risk would involve any number of sociopolitical considerations, but at present it is set arbitrarily at a small round number in the range 10^{-5} to 10^{-7}.[42] The unambiguous definition of the VSD requires specification of the time at which the accumulated tumors are counted, usually termination of the experiment. An alternative measure which can be used if time to tumor information is available is the mean free dose (MFD) of Sielken.[43] This is defined as the dose that reduces the expected time to tumor by a suitably small fraction.

Table 5
DOSE RESPONSE MODELS FOR TIME TO RESPONSE
TOXICITY DATA

Model	Probability of occurrence by time t at dose d	
Log-normal	$(2\pi)^{1/2} \int_{-\infty}^{\alpha + \beta \, \log \, d + \gamma \, \log \, t} \exp(-u^2/2)du$	$(\beta, \gamma > 0)$
Log-logistic	$(1 + \exp(-\alpha - \beta \log d - \gamma \log t))^{-1}$	$(\beta, \gamma > 0)$
Weibull	$(1 - \exp(-\lambda \, d^m t^k)$	$(\lambda, m > 0)$
Gamma	$\int_0^{\lambda dt} e^{-u} u^{k-1}/\Gamma(k)du$	$(\lambda > 0)$
General Product	$1 - \exp(-\sum_{i=1}^{m} d_i d^i \sum_{j=1}^{k} \beta_j t^j)$	$(\alpha_i, \beta_j > 0)$

No matter how the low dose risk is expressed, its estimation will necessarily involve extrapolation from results obtained at accelerated doses that produce measurably high response rates.[44] Extrapolation requires a mathematical model relating the probability of tumor occurrence to the dose. Models for lifetime incidence rates are given in Table 2, and models including time to tumor are given in Table 5. These models are discussed in more detail in Krewski and Van Ryzin,[20] and Kalbfleisch et al.[16]

The low dose risk estimate can be expressed either in the form of a point estimate or a confidence interval. Since overestimation of the VSD is the greatest concern in matters of public health, no attempt is generally made to infer an upper bound on the VSD. That is, the confidence interval contains all doses greater than a certain dose called the lower confidence limit. The confidence coefficient is the probability that the lower confidence limit does not exceed the true VSD.

The disadvantage of a point estimate is that it does not in any way reflect the uncertainty of the estimate. The lower confidence limit, on the other hand, has been criticized because it tends to underestimate the VSD and hence puts too much emphasis on safety as opposed to other considerations.

The chief difficulty with extrapolation procedures is that the estimates obtained depend highly on the model used. Since the mechanisms of carcinogenesis are not well enough understood to enable one to establish the correct model, the resulting estimates may appear to be rather arbitrary. Unfortunately, experimental data will not resolve the uncertainty as to the model, for diverse models could all provide good fits to the observed data, yet give very different estimates of the VSD or MFD.

As an example, consider the incidence of liver tumors induced in female mice following 24 months exposure to 2-acetylaminofluorene (2-AAF) shown in Figure 9.[29] In this unusually large experiment the number of animals ranged from 130 to 900 in each of the eight dose groups. While all of the models discussed provide a good fit to these data in the observable range, the divergence among these models in the low dose region is apparent. The ordering of these models is, however, consistent with that observed in a variety of other examples.[20]

A critical aspect of the dose response curve is its low dose behavior, which may be supralinear, linear, or sublinear (Figure 10). Other things being equal, a supralinear model will give lower estimates of the VSD than a linear model, which in turn will give lower estimates than a sublinear one. It is commonly believed (although without any firm justification) that supralinear dose response curves are not plausible from the biological point of view. For this reason, so called linear extrapolation procedures which impose low dose linearity are considered to provide estimates that are conservative in the sense that the true VSD will be higher than the extrapolated one if the dose response curve is actually sublinear.

Such procedures are sometimes criticized as being too conservative particularly if the dose response curve demonstrates strong sublinearity. However, Crump et al.[45] have shown that low dose linearity generally follows in the presence of additive background. Furthermore,

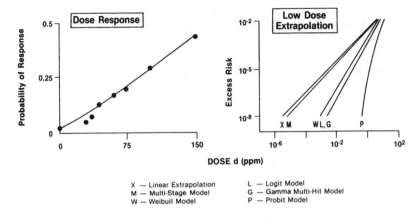

X — Linear Extrapolation
M — Multi-Stage Model
W — Weibull Model

L — Logit Model
G — Gamma Multi-Hit Model
P — Probit Model

FIGURE 9.   Low dose extrapolation for 2-AAF under several mathematical models.

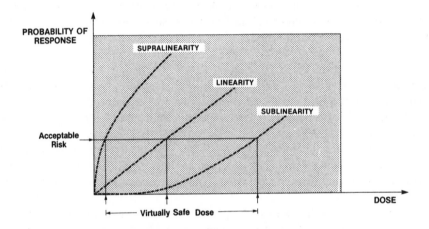

FIGURE 10.   Possible low dose behavior of dose response curves.

linear extrapolation provides conservative estimates only if the dose below which linearity is imposed is sufficiently low, and without knowledge of the true dose response curve this critical dose cannot be determined. One undesirable property of many models that suggest sublinearity is that the low dose behavior is largely inferred from the curvature in the high dose region. Since metabolic pathways and mode of action could well be different at high doses from those at low doses, such a property is probably best considered an artifact of the mathematical model without any true biological significance. For this reason, conclusions of low dose sublinearity based on empirical evidence are rather tenuous. Thus there is no support for the allegation that linear extrapolation is too conservative or even that it is conservative at all. Rather, it is an ad hoc procedure that provides a reasonable answer to a difficult question.

There are several ways in which low dose linearity can be imposed. The simplest way is to fit a straight line from the response at the lowest dose to the control responses.[25,46] An alternative procedure,[47,48] is to use the mathematical model to extrapolate to a moderate response level (say 1 to 10%) and then extrapolate linearly from this point. (Either procedure can be used for point estimates or confidence limits.) When the multi-stage model is used, lower confidence limits will automatically be linear at low doses.[49]

Low dose risk estimates are also possible where information on time to tumor is available. Ideally, one would like to know the ages at which the tumor appeared, and at which it caused death. More commonly, however, only the age when the tumor was noted is available, and in most cases this coincides with the age of necropsy. The cause of death may or may not be available. Methods for estimation have been proposed by Crump et al.,[49] Farmer et al.,[48] and Sielken.[43]

These and other procedures were tested empirically on a large simulated data base.[50] The advantage of simulated data is that the true dose response curve is known and thus the errors of the estimates can be determined. The study was designed to cover a range of plausible dose response models as well as assess the effects of competing risks, background response, latency, and experimental design on the performance of the different extrapolation procedures. It was found that point estimates of risk in the low dose region may differ from the actual risk by a factor of 1000 or more in certain situations even when precise information on the time to tumor is available. Although linearized upper confidence limits on risk were highly conservative when the underlying dose response curve is low dose sublinear, they were found not to exceed the actual risk in the low dose region by more than a factor of 10 in those cases where the underlying dose response curve was, in fact, linear at low doses. It also appeared that some confidence limit procedures were not valid in the sense that the 95% lower confidence limit on the VSD exceeded the true value in significantly more than 5% of the cases studied.

C. Mechanistic Studies

Statistical analysis of studies designed to examine certain hypotheses concerning the mechanisms of carcinogenesis will generally need to be tailored to the particular experiment at hand. Because the vast majority of past data has been collected for screening purposes, moreover, the statistical procedures required to adequately analyze mechanistic studies still remain largely to be developed. With studies of transplacental effects, synergism, reversibility, and other phenomena becoming more commonplace, however, the development of such statistical procedures satisfying the criteria of validity and efficiency becomes essential.

V. CONCLUSIONS

In this paper, we have considered the fundamental statistical principles involved in the design and analysis of chronic carcinogenicity bioassays. Statistical procedures must be valid in the sense of properly expressing the information contained in experimental data and they should be efficient in the sense of extracting the maximum amount of information possible. Sound experimental design is required for both the validity and efficiency of any subsequent analysis. Validity can only be achieved by proper randomization, and efficiency can be enhanced by manipulation of design parameters.

Although screening studies are most efficient with only two dose groups, a control and MTD, intermediate doses may be needed to protect against excessive early mortality in the high dose. Analysis of screening experiments will better satisfy the criteria of validity and efficiency if precise time to tumor information is available. Failing that, the time the tumors were observed along with an indication of tumor lethality should be given.

More research is required for determining optimal designs for low dose extrapolation, but it appears that designs having somewhat more animals in the intermediate doses are desirable. (It should be noted that screening and low dose extrapolation are at cross purposes, with designs that are optimal for low dose extrapolation being rather inefficient for screening.)

Although quite tractable statistically, low dose estimates of risk suffer from extreme dependency on the mathematical form of the postulated dose response curve. Since the correct form cannot be known with any certainty, linear extrapolation procedures which are somewhat conservative are recommended. Although these methods can greatly exaggerate the low dose risk when low dose linearity does not obtain, they tend to err on the side of safety.

ACKNOWLEDGMENTS

The authors would like to thank Charles Brown, Miles Clarke, Stephen Lagakos, and Leonard Ritter for helpful comments.

REFERENCES

1. Office of Technology Assessment, *Assessment of Technologies for Determining Cancer Risks from the Environment*, U.S. Govt. Printing Office, Washington, D.C., 1981.
2. **Krewski, D.**, Discussion: carcinogenic risk assessment, *J. Am. Stat. Assoc.*, 78, 308, 1983.
3. **Gart, J., Chu, K., and Tarone, R. E.**, Statistical issues in interpretation of chronic bioassay tests for carcinogeniaty, *J. Nat. Cancer Inst.*, 62, 957, 1979.
4. **Peto, R., Pike, M. C., Day, N. E., Gray, R. G., Lee, P. N., Parish, S., Peto, J., Richards, S., and Wahrendorf, J.**, Guidelines for simple, sensitive significance tests for carcinogenic effects in long-term animal experiments, in *IARC Monographs on the Evaluation of the Carcinogenic Risk in Humans*, Supplement 2, *Long-Term and Short-Term Screening Assays for Carcinogens: A Critical Appraisal*, Lyon, 1980, 311.
5. Environmental Protection Agency, Proposed health effects test standard for toxic substances control act test rules. GLP Standards for health effects, *Fed. Register*, 44, 27334, 1979.
6. Interagency Regulatory Liaison Group, Scientific bases for identification of potential carcinogens and estimation of risks, *J. Nat. Cancer Inst.*, 63, 241, 1979.
7. International Agency for Research on Cancer, *IARC Monographs on the Evaluation of the Carcinogenic Risk of Chemicals to Humans*, Supplement 2, *Long Term and Short Term Screening Assays for Carcinogens; a Critical Appraisal*, IARC, Lyon, 1980.
8. Organization for Economic and Cooperative Development, *Test Guidelines for Carcinogenicity Studies*, OECD, Geneva, 1980.
9. **Portier, C. and Hoel, D.**, Low dose rate extrapolation using the multistage model, unpublished manuscript.
10. **Fox, J. G., Thibert, P., Arnold, D. L., Krewski, D. R., and Grice, H. C.**, Toxicological studies II. The laboratory animal, *Food Cosmet. Toxicol.*, 17, 661, 1979.
11. **Grice, H. C., Munro, I. C., Krewski, D. R., and Blumental, H.**, *In utero* exposure in chronic toxicity/carcinogenicity studies, *Food Cosmet. Toxicol.*, 19, 373, 1981.
12. **Lagakos, S. and Mosteller, F.**, A case study of statistics in the regulatory process, *J. Nat. Cancer Inst.*, 66, 197, 1981.
13. **Fears, T. R. and Douglas, J. F.**, Suggested Procedures for reducing the pathology workload in a carcinogen bioassay program, part II; incorporating blind pathology techniques and analysis for animals with tumours, *J. Environ. Pathol. Toxicol.*, 1, 211, 1978.
14. **Berry, G.**, Design of carcinogenesis experiments using the Weibull distribution, *Biometrika*, 62, 32, 1975.
15. **Louis, T. A.**, Adaptive sacrifice plans for rodent bioassays. Technical report, Dept. of Biostatistics, Harvard School of Public Health, Boston, 1982.
16. **Kalbfleisch, J., Krewski, D., and Van Ryzin, J.**, Dose response models for time to response toxicity data (with discussion), *Can. J. Stat.*, 11, 25, 1983.
17. **Brittain, E. and Schlesselman, J. J.**, Optimal allocation for the comparison of proportions, *Biometrics*, 38, 1003, 1982.
18. **Krewski, D., Brennan, J., and Bickis, M.**, *The Power of The Fisher Randomization Test in $2 \times k$ Tables*, Carleton Mathematical Series No. 201, Dept. of Mathematics and Statistics, Carleton University, Ottawa, 1983.
19. **Munro, I. C. and Krewski, D.**, Risk assessment and regulatory decision making, *Food Cosmet. Toxicol.*, 19, 549, 1981.
20. **Krewski, D. and Van Ryzin, J.**, Dose response models for quantal response toxicity data, in *Statistics and Related Topics*, Csörgö, M., Dawson, D., Rao, J. N. K. and Saleh, E., Eds., North-Holland, Amsterdam, 1981, 201.
21. **Hoel, D. G.**, Incorporation of background in dose response models, *Fed. Proc. Fed. Am. Soc. Exp. Biol.*, 39, 67, 1980.

22. **Krewski, D., Kovar, J., and Bickis, M.,** Optimal experimental designs for low dose extrapolation II. The case of nonzero background, in *Topics in Applied Statistics,* Dwivedi, T. W., Ed., Marcel Dekker, New York, in press.

23. **Portier, C. J. and Hoel, D.,** Optimal design of the chronic animal bioassay, *J. Toxicol. Environ. Health,* in press, 1983.

24. **Portier, C. J.,** Optimal bioassay design under the Armitage-Doll multi-stage model. Institute of Statistics Mimeo series, Dept. of Biostatistics, University of North Carolina, Chapel Hill, 1981.

25. **Crump, K. S. and Langley, C. H.,** Experimental design in carcinogenicity extrapolations: selection of dose and sample size, unpublished manuscript, 1975.

26. **Chambers, E. A. and Cox, D. R.,** Discrimination between alternative binary response models, *Biometrika,* 54, 573, 1967.

27. **Crump, K. S.,** Designs for discriminating between binary dose response models with applications to animal carcinogenicity experiments, *Commun. Stat.,* 1981.

28. **Pilot, H. C. and Sirica, A. E.,** The stages of initiation and promotion in hepato-carcinogenesis, *Biochim. Biophys. Acta Rev. Cancer,* 605, 191, 1981.

29. **Littlefield, N. A., Farmer, J. H., Gaylor, D. W., and Sheldon, W. G.,** Effects of dose and time in a long-term, low-dose carcinogenic study, *J. Environ. Pathol. Toxicol.,* 3, 17, 1980.

30. **Abdelbasit, K. M. and Plackett, R. L.,** Experimental design for joint action, *Biometrics,* 38, 171, 1982.

31. **Fleiss, J.,** *Statistical Methods for Rates and Proportions,* Wiley, New York, 1975.

32. **Thomas, D. G., Breslow, N., and Gart, J. J.,** Trend and homogeneity analysis of proportions and life table data, *Comput. Biomed. Res.,* 10, 373, 1977.

33. **Barlow, R. E., Bartholomew, D. J., Bremner, J. M., and Brunk, H. D.,** *Statistical Inference Under Order Restrictions,* Wiley, New York, 1978.

34. **Tarone, R. E.,** The use of historical information in testing for a trend in proportions, *Biometrics,* 38, 215, 1981.

35. Task Force of Past Presidents, Society of Toxicology, Animal data in hazard evaluation: paths and pitfalls, *Fund. Appl. Toxicol.,* 2, 101, 1982.

36. **Dempster, A. P., Selwyn, M. R., and Weeks, B. J.,** Combining historical and randomized controls for assessing trends in proportions, *J. Am. Stat. Assoc.,* 78, 221, 1983.

37. **Peto, R.,** Guidelines on the analysis of tumour rates and death rates in experimental animals, *Br. J. Cancer,* 29, 1974.

38. **Cox, D. R.,** Regression models and life tables, *J. Roy. Stat. Soc.,* B34, 187, 1972.

39. **Breslow, N.,** Covariance analysis of censored survival data, *Biometrics,* 30, 89, 1974.

40. **Jonckheere, A. R.,** A distribution-free k-sample test against ordered alternatives, *Biometrika,* 41, 133, 1954.

41. **Fleming, T. R., O'Fallon, J. R., O'Brien, P. C., and Harrington, D. P.,** Modified Kolmogorov-Smirnov test procedures with application to arbitrarily right-censored data, *Biometrics,* 36, 607, 1980.

42. Environmental Protection Agency, Water Quality criteria availability, *Fed. Register,* 44, 56628, 1979.

43. **Sielken, R. L.,** Reexamination of the ED01 study: risk assessment using time, *Fundam. Appl. Toxicol.,* 1, 99, 1981.

44. **Crump, K. S.,** Dose response problems in carcinogenesis, *Biometrics,* 35, 157, 1979.

45. **Crump, K. S., Hoel, D., Langley, C., and Peto, R.,** Fundamental carcinogenic processes and their implication for low dose risk assessment, *Cancer Res.,* 36, 2973, 1976.

46. **Gaylor, D. W. and Shapiro, R. E.,** Extrapolation and risk estimation for carcinogenesis, in *Advances in Modern Toxicology,* Vol. 1, *New Concept In Safety Evaluation (Part 2),* Mehlman, M. A. Shapiro, R. E., and Blumenthal, H., Eds., Wiley, New York, 1979, 65.

47. **Van Ryzin, J.,** Quantitative risk assessment, *J. Occup. Med.,* 22, 321, 1980.

48. **Farmer, J. H., Kodell, R. L., and Gaylor, D. W.,** Estimation and interpolation of potential carcinogens and estimation of risks, *J. Nat. Cancer Inst.,* 63, 241, 1982.

49. **Crump, K. S., Howe, R. B., Masterman, M. D., and Watson, W. W.,** RANK81: a fortran program for risk assessment using time-to-occurrence dose-response data. Prepared under NIEHS Contract No. NIH-ES-77-22, 1981.

50. **Krewski, D., Crump, K. S., Gaylor, D. W., Howe, R., Portier, C., Salsburg, D., Sielken, R. L., and Van Ryzin, J.,** A comparison of statistical methods for low dose extrapolation utilizing time to tumour data, *Fundam. Appl. Toxicol.,* 3, 140, 1983.

Chapter 7

STATISTICAL ANALYSIS OF RODENT TUMORIGENICITY EXPERIMENTS

S. W. Lagakos and T. A. Louis

TABLE OF CONTENTS

I. INTRODUCTION AND OVERVIEW

In the absence of epidemiologic data, rodent tumorigenicity experiments are generally accepted as the best available means of assessing the safety of food additives, drugs, cosmetics, and pesticides. Although few, if any, scientists regard these experiments as foolproof, it appears as if they will continue to be the primary basis for safety evaluation for some time.

The typical rodent tumorigenicity experiment consists of a control group of rodents and two or three groups exposed to a test substance at varying concentrations in their diet throughout their lifetimes. Variations of this theme involve different routes of exposure, use of two strains of rodents, a different number of exposed groups, and multigenerational designs in which animals are exposed both in utero and during their lifetimes.

The first and often only goal of the tumorigenicity experiment is to determine whether the test substance is associated with an increase in tumor development. If there is an association, a second objective might be to estimate the risk at very low levels of exposure in order to predict human risk. This paper considers only the first of these objectives. We present and discuss what we believe to be the most appropriate and valid statistical procedures currently available for routine use in the analysis of these experiments. As the implementation of these procedures requires that decisions be made about the lethality of the tumor type in question, we also present guidelines and considerations for making these decisions. An attractive feature of the proposed approach is its simplicity. However, while routine use of this approach will be sufficient in many situations, it is not without pitfalls. Thus, we regard the proposed techniques as a first step in the analysis of a tumorigenicity study which may need to be followed-up with additional analyses. Hoel and Walburg,[1] Gart, Chu, and Tarone,[2] Peto et al.,[3] and Lagakos and Mosteller[4] discuss other important issues in the analysis of tumorigenicity experiments, including the multiple comparisons problem arising from the examination of numerous tumor types.

Section II of this report describes the construction of the statistical tests for tumorigenicity. The basic statistic used for making treatment comparisons has three components, two of which compare groups on the basis of their age-specific tumor prevalence rates, and the third with respect to the age-specific tumor mortality rates. For a given tumor type, one, two, or all three of the component statistics could be computed, depending on the type of data available and the lethality of the tumor.

Section III reviews the theoretical bases of the tests and discusses their general properties. In Section IV we discuss the assumptions underlying each test and present guidelines for determining which test to use in a given situation. This section also discusses the selection of time intervals for prevalence tests, the choice of dose metameter for trend tests, and stratification.

Section V gives a brief overview of our recommendations for presenting results, and Section VI discusses several extensions of the methods, including some which have advantages over those in Section II. Finally, we summarize our recommendations in Section VII.

II. STATISTICAL TESTS: CONSTRUCTION

A. General

Suppose a control group and K exposed groups are to be compared with respect to the development of a particular tumor type (e.g., bladder carcinomas). The K exposed groups usually correspond to different concentrations of the same test substance. However, they might also be K different durations of exposure to a fixed concentration, or even K distinct test substances. In any event, the K + 1 treatment groups are denoted as controls, dose 1, dose 2, . . . ,dose K, with the understanding that when an ordering is appropriate, ''controls'' refers to the lowest (often zero) exposure group, ''dose 1'' to the next lowest, and so on.

We assume throughout that the tumor type under consideration is not directly observable, but can be detected only after the animal dies naturally or is intentionally killed (i.e., 'sacrificed'). Observable tumor types such as skin or palpable mammary tumors can be analyzed using the same techniques as for the comparison of age-specific mortality rates, discussed in Section II, B. Also, the following discussion applies to the analysis of a single strain and sex; amalgamation of information over strains or sexes is considered later.

Two aspects of these data make their evaluation nontrivial and subject to misinterpretation. First, when a tumor is detected at death, we know for certain only that it developed sometime prior to death; how much sooner depends in part on the lethality of the tumor. Second, animals can die from causes other than their tumor, including toxic side-effects of exposure. Thus, a relatively nonlethal tumor might be observed sooner in the high-dose animals because of a greater death rate from toxic effects. On the other hand, greater toxicity in the exposed animals could cause them to die before their tumors develop, and thereby conceal a real tumorigenic effect. Hence, analyses based on simple proportions of tumor-bearing animals in the various treatment groups can be misleading.

The statistical techniques proposed in this section attempt to avoid the biases associated with the use of simple tumor rates by also using the time to death of each animal. Furthermore, even in circumstances when a test based on simple proportions is not biased, it is not as sensitive as one which utilizes time to death.[5] The appropriate way to utilize time to death, however, depends on several factors, including the lethality of the tumor type. As a result, the problem is one of deciding how best to incorporate age into the analysis. In general, the data contain information on both the age-specific tumor prevalence rates and the age-specific tumor mortality rates of the treatment groups.[6] A simple way of combining these different endpoints of a tumorigenic effect is to compute for each exposure group and each endpoint an observed-minus-expected number of tumor bearing animals[3] For each endpoint, these numbers form a vector (**O-E**) with rows corresponding to exposure groups. The mortality and prevalence **O-E**'s, denoted $\mathbf{O}^M\text{-}\mathbf{E}^M$ and $\mathbf{O}^P\text{-}\mathbf{E}^P$, can then be examined separately or combined. The prevalence counts themselves consist of two sources, based on naturally dying animals ($\mathbf{O}_N^P\text{-}\mathbf{E}_N^P$) and sacrificed animals ($\mathbf{O}_S^P\text{-}\mathbf{E}_S^P$), so that

$$\mathbf{O} = \mathbf{O}_N^P + \mathbf{O}_S^P + \mathbf{O}^M$$

and

$$\mathbf{E} = \mathbf{E}_N^P + \mathbf{E}_S^P + \mathbf{E}^M$$

In the remainder of this section, we describe the computation of these statistics and their covariance matrices. When each animal found to have the tumor at death is classified by the pathologist as either dying from the tumor or from other causes, **O-E** consists of three endpoints, However, in most tumorigenicity experiments, cause-of-death information is not determined on an animal-by-animal basis. In these circumstances, only one of ($\mathbf{O}^M\text{-}\mathbf{E}^M$) and ($\mathbf{O}_N^P\text{-}\mathbf{E}_N^P$) is usually computed, since the other will be taken to be zero by assumption. Which of these is taken to be zero depends on whether the tumor type is assumed to be more nearly rapidly lethal or nonlethal. If the tumor is assumed to be rapidly lethal, then every animal detected with the tumor at death is considered to have died as a result of the tumor. If the tumor type is assumed to be nonlethal, every animal found to have the tumor at death is considered to have died from causes other than the tumor of interest. Thus, whether or not a cause of death is actually determined on a case by case basis, we can proceed in our discussion as if the information available for each animal consists of (U,a,b), where U denotes age at death,

Table 1
DATA ORGANIZATION FOR COMPUTING O^M, E^M, AND V^M

Treatment group	Number of animals dying at t_j due to tumor	Number of animals not dying at t_j due to tumor	Number of animals alive just before t_j
Controls	n_0	$N_0 - n_0$	N_0
Dose 1	n_1	$N_1 - n_1$	N_1
Dose 2	n_2	$N_2 - n_2$	N_2
.	.	.	.
.	.	.	.
.	.	.	.
Dose K	n_K	$n_K - n_K$	N_K
Total	n_+	$N_+ - n_+$	N_+

$$a = \begin{cases} 0 = \text{tumor absent} \\ 1 = \text{tumor present} \end{cases}$$

denotes tumor status at death, and

$$b = \begin{cases} 0 \text{ tumor death} \\ 1 \text{ other natural death} \\ 2 \text{ sacrifice} \end{cases}$$

indicates cause of death.

B. Computing O^M, E^M and, V^M

Suppose that when the $K + 1$ groups are pooled together, $t_1 < t_2 < \ldots < t_j < \ldots t_j$ are the J distinct ages at which animals die due to the tumor. More than one tumor death can occur at each t_j. The relevant information for comparing groups at time t_j can be summarized in the $(K + 1) \times 2$ contingency table displayed in Table 1. For example, a total of N_O control animals are alive just before t_j, and n_0 of these die from their tumor at t_j. The ratio n_i/N_i estimates the age-specific tumor mortality rate at t_j for group i (i = 0,1,2, . . . ,K). Conditional on the marginal counts, the expected numbers of tumor deaths at time t_j in the exposed groups, if there were no exposure effect, are

$$\mathbf{e} = (e_1, e_2, \ldots, e_K)^T \tag{1}$$

where $e_i = n_+ N_i/N_+$. Letting $\mathbf{n} = (n_1, n_2, \ldots, n_K)^T$, the corresponding covariance matrix for $(\mathbf{n} \text{-} \mathbf{e})$ based on the hypergeometric distribution is

$$V = [V_{ii'}]$$

$$V_{ii'} = \begin{cases} \dfrac{N_i n_+ (N_+ - n_+)(N_+ - N_i)}{N_+^2 (N_+ - 1)} & \text{if } i = i' \\[2em] -\dfrac{N_i N_{i'} n_+ (N_+ - n_+)}{N_+^2 (N_+ - 1)} & \text{if } i \neq i' \end{cases} \tag{2}$$

Table 2

DATA ORGANIZATION FOR COMPUTING O_N^P, E_N^P, and V_N^P

Treatment group	Number of animals with tumor	Number of animals without tumor	Number of animals dying naturally from causes other than the tumor in interval j
Controls	m_0	$M_0 - m_0$	M_0
Dose 1	m_1	$M_1 - m_1$	M_1
Dose 2	m_2	$M_2 - m_2$	M_2
.	.	.	.
.	.	.	.
.	.	.	.
Dose K	m_K	$M_K - m_K$	M_K
Total	m_+	$M_+ - m_+$	M_+

Thus, the overall observed and expected counts and covariance matrix are obtained by summing the vectors **n**, **e** and matrices V over the times at which tumor deaths occurred to give

$$O^M = \Sigma_n \tag{3}$$

$$E^M = \Sigma_e \text{ and} \tag{4}$$

$$V^M = \Sigma V \tag{5}$$

C. Computing O_N^P, E_N^P, and V_N^P

For these statistics we use only those animals that die naturally from causes other than the tumor. Suppose that the time axis is partitioned into J intervals (guidelines for selecting intervals are discussed in Section IV). The data for the jth interval can be summarized in the $(K+1) \times 2$ contingency table displayed in Table 2. For example, there are M_O control animals that die naturally from non-tumor causes in interval j, and m_O of these are found to have the tumor at death. For reasons that will be made clear later, the ratio m_i/M_i estimates the age-specific tumor prevalence for group i. Note that this table has the same form as that for computing O^M-E^M. The expected counts and corresponding covariances for this section are obtained using formulas (1) to (5), but with n_+, n_i, N_+ and N_i replaced by m_+, m_i, M_+, and M_i. When summed over intervals, the analogs of O^M, E^M, and V^M are denoted O_N^P, E_N^P, and V_N^P.

D. Computing O_S^P, E_S^P, and V_S^P

The statistics O_S^P, E_S^P, and V_S^P are computed exactly the same way as O_N^P, E_N^P, and V_N^P, except that they are based on the sacrificial, rather than natural deaths. In many experiments, sacrifice occurs only at the end of the study, and only one interval is needed.

E. Test Statistics

We present an analysis that combines the prevalence and mortality O-E's. This analysis is appropriate if exposure elevates both tumor prevalence and mortality rates, but it can have very little power if exposure elevates one of these and decreases the other. While such an effect seems unlikely to us, it suggests that the separate O-E's always be examined, even when a combined analysis as described below is performed. Let

$$O = O^M + (O_N^P + O_S^P) = O^M + O^P$$

and

$$E = E^M + (E_N^P + E_S^P) = E^M + E^P$$

be the overall observed and expected numbers of tumor bearing animals. Approximate significance levels are obtained by regarding **O-E** as having a Gaussian distribution with zero mean vector and covariance matrix

$$V = V^M + (V_N^P + V_S^P) = V^M + V^P$$

1. Heterogeneity

A significance test for the hypothesis of no exposure effect on either prevalence or mortality can be obtained by comparing the statistic

$$Q = (O - E)^T V^{-1}(O - E)$$

to the upper percentage points of the χ_K^2 distribution. The chi-square approximation to Q should be accurate unless a large proportion of the E_i are small (e.g., less than 5). The statistic Q is not oriented to any particular alternative to the null hypothesis and, therefore, is not recommended for testing a dose-response relationship.

2. Trend

In situations where the K + 1 groups represent increasing exposure levels, it is more appropriate to use a test that will be sensitive to alternatives in the form of a monotone increasing dose-response. Suppose

$$\mathbf{c} = (c_1, c_2, ..., c_K)^T$$

is a vector of pre-specified constants such that $0 < c_1 < c_2 < ... < c_K$. The choice of c's is discussed in Section IV. If increased exposure increase tumor development, we would expect increasingly large values for $(O_i - E_i)$ as i increases, and therefore relatively large values for $\mathbf{c}^T(\mathbf{O}\text{-}\mathbf{E})$. Hence, an approximate test of the null hypothesis that is sensitive to a trend can be obtained by comparing the statistic

$$Z = \mathbf{c}^T(\mathbf{O} - \mathbf{E})/(\mathbf{c}^T V \mathbf{c})^{1/2} \tag{7}$$

to the upper percentage point of the N(0,1) distribution.

A test for deviation from trend can be made by comparing

$$Q - Z^2 \tag{8}$$

to the percentage points of the χ_{K-1}^2 distribution.[7] Deviations from trend signal that the null hypothesis of treatment equality does not hold, because either exposure effects exist but are non-increasing, or because they are increasing at a rate inconsistent with the weights c.

We note that these statistical tests have been based on data from a single strain and sex. If a single overall test is desired, similar techniques can be applied after first summing, over sex or strain, the vectors (**O-E**) and their corresponding covariances.

III. THEORETIC BASIS AND GENERAL PROPERTIES OF TESTS

The natural history of an animal can be represented as shown in Figure 1. After beginning in a normal state (N), the animal can next either develop a tumor (T) or die from other non-

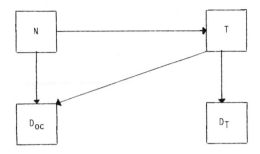

FIGURE 1.   Natural history of rodent.

tumor causes (D_{oc}). Animals that develop a tumor will either die from the tumor (D_T) or from other causes (D_{oc}). The analyses considered in this chapter assume that the process of death from other causes operates independently of the process of tumor development, and that no animals are misclassified with respect to cause of death. Together these assumptions imply that the tumor prevalence in rodents dying at a certain age of nontumor causes equals that for all animals alive at that age; this is the representativeness assumption described in Lagakos and Ryan.[8]

Suppose that $a(t)$ denotes a (living or dead) animal's tumor status at age t, with $a(t) = 1$ indicating that the tumor has developed by t and $a(t) = 0$ otherwise. The only estimable aspects of the tumor development process are functions of the tumor prevalence

$$p(t) = \Pr\{a(t) = 1|U>t\}$$

and the tumor-specific mortality function

$$\lambda(t) = \lim_{\Delta t \to 0} \frac{1}{\Delta t} \Pr\{t<U<t+\Delta t, b=0|U>t\}$$

(See Lagakos[6] and Louis et al.[9]

For the purposes of this discussion, let Z^M and Q^M be defined as in (7) and (6), but based only on O^M, E^M and V^M. Define Z^P and Q^P similarly. Then Z^M and Q^M are tests of the hypothesis

$$\lambda_0(t) = \lambda_1(t) = \ldots = \lambda_K(t)$$

where $\lambda_i(t)$ is the value of $\lambda(t)$ for dose group i. The tests Z^M and Q^M, which are just variations of the logrank test,[10] and also arise as the likelihood score tests from the proportional hazards regression model introduced by Cox.[11] Consequently, we know that both tests are particularly oriented to alternatives where the $\lambda_i(t)$ are proportional over time. Z^M is constructed to be especially sensitive to the alternative

$$\lambda_i(t) = c_i\lambda_0(t)$$

where $c_1, c_2, \ldots, c_K$ are the constants used in the trend test. Although oriented to proportional hazards alternatives, Z^M and Q^M maintain good efficiency for moderate departures from proportionality. Their power can be poor, however, when the hazard functions cross. When the hazards are proportional, Z^M will usually enjoy greater power than Q^M unless the weights used in Z^M differ markedly from the true hazard ratios.

Consider next Z^P and Q^P, which test the hypothesis of equal tumor prevalence across groups, i.e.,

$$p_0(t) = p_1(t) = \ldots = p_K(t)$$

for all t, where $p_i(t)$ denotes the prevalence in the ith dosage group. This type of test was first proposed by Hoel and Walburg.[1] It can be shown that Z^P and Q^P also arise as likelihood score tests based on a proportional-odds logistic regression model (see, for example, Dinse and Lagakos,).[12] Consequently, the tests are particularly oriented to alternatives in which the odds-function $p_i(t)/\{1 - p_i(t)\}$ are proportional over time.

IV. CONSIDERATIONS FOR SELECTING A TEST

In describing the general form of the recommended tests in Section II, we postponed discussion of several determinations that need to be made before a specific test statistic can be computed. This section presents some results relevant to these determinations and gives our recommendations on how to proceed in routine analyses.

A. The Use of Cause of Death Information

Recall that the statistics defined in Section II require that each animal found to have a tumor at death (a = 1) be further classified as either dying from the tumor (b = 0), from another natural cause (b = 1), or from a sacrifice (b = 2). This notion was originally proposed by Peto.[13] Although it is customary in tumorigenicity experiments to record whether animals died naturally (including moribund sacrifice) or were sacrificed, it is uncommon to have cause of death determined by the pathologist on an animal by animal basis for those that die naturally and were found to have the tumor. Many, if not most, veterinary pathologists are unaccustomed to this task and probably question whether it can be done with any degree of accuracy. When individual determinations of cause of death (i.e., b = 0 vs. 1) are not made, the proposed tests cannot be performed unless cause of death is defined in some other way.

There are two situations where individual determinations of cause of death are unnecessary. When the tumor type is rapidly lethal (i.e., kills its host immediately after onset), the state T in Figure 1 coincides with D_T, and there will be no transitions from T to D_{oc}. Hence, each animal found to have a tumor at (nonsacrificed) death (a = 1) must have died from the tumor. Accordingly, we can assign the value b = 0 to these animals. If the tumor type in question is nonlethal (i.e., cannot cause the death of the animal), on the other hand, then all transitions from T will be into the state D_{oc}. Thus, we can automatically set b = 1 whenever a tumor is detected at a natural death (a = 1).

Note that when the tumor of interest is rapidly lethal, O-E is determined entirely from ($O^M - E^M$) and ($O^{Ps} - E_S^P$). In theory $O_S^P - E_S^P$ will be zero if the tumor is truly rapidly lethal, but in practice this is not always the case. The component ($O^M - E^M$) is just the ordinary logrank test statistic. When the tumor is nonlethal, (O-E) is determined entirely by ($O_N^P - E_N^P$) and ($O_S^P - E_S^P$). This is essentially the Hoel-Walburg[1] prevalence test statistic, except for a stratification on the basis of type of death which we recommend as a partial hedge against violation of the representativeness assumption (see Lagakos and Ryan).[8]

In practice, no tumor type is strictly rapidly lethal, and few, if any, are entirely nonlethal. Rather, most tumor types lie somewhere between these extremes. However, since individual determinations of cause of death are usually not made, it has been customary to analyze these experiments using either a logrank or Hoel-Walburg test, depending on whether the tumor type in question is felt to be more nearly rapidly lethal or nonlethal, respectively. Note that this practice can be regarded as implicitly making, *a priori*, a determination of cause of death in each animal found to have the tumor at death.

When individual determinations of cause of death are not made, this approach is the only obvious course of action. When individual cause of death determinations are made, one must decide whether more accurate results are likely to emerge from using this information vs. *a priori* regarding the tumor as either rapidly lethal or nonlethal. The choice is not clear, and involves a tradeoff between incorrect assumptions about tumor lethality and misclassifications of cause of death. This problem has been studied analytically by Lagakos,[6] and several general results emerge. First, suppose that the tumor type is regarded as rapidly lethal, but in fact is only moderately lethal. Then if the rate of deaths from other causes (intercurrent death rate) does not vary much between dosage groups, there will be little distortion of the size and power of the logrank test. If, however, the intercurrent death rate varies substantially across dosage groups, serious distortions to both the size and power of the logrank test can occur. In particular, if the intercurrent death rate increases with dose, as is common for highly toxic test substances, then the resulting P-values will tend to be smaller (i.e., more significant) than they should be, and so the logrank test will tend to overstate the extent of the exposure effect. If the intercurrent death rate decreases with dose, just the opposite occurs, i.e., the logrank test will tend to understate the statistical significance.

Next, suppose that the tumor type is regarded as nonlethal when in fact it is somewhat lethal. Then there will be little distortion of the Hoel-Walburg test unless the intercurrent death rate varies considerably across dosage groups. If it increases with dose, serious biases can result, and will tend to dampen real carcinogenic effects. That is, the resulting Hoel-Walburg P-values will tend to be larger (less significant) than they should be. On the other hand, if the intercurrent death rate decreases with dose, the opposite tends to occur.

In general, the biases of the two tests are in the opposite direction. When one tends to overstate the extent of the exposure effect, the other tends to understate it. The degree to which a test is biased will depend on the extent to which the assumption on tumor lethality is violated and on the differences in intercurrent death rates between groups.

When cause of death is determined on an animal by animal basis and the combined test is used, the critical factor in potential distortions is the rate at which animals are misclassified with respect to cause of death. When misclassification rates are not dose-dependent, one would normally expect that using the cause of death information will be valid and better than assuming a priori that the tumor is either nonlethal or rapidly lethal. However, if misclassification error rates are dose dependent, the opposite might be true.

In our opinion, the added value in using cause of death information in tumorigenicity tests is still not fully understood. It depends on the accuracy with which cause is determined, and how uncertainty is incorporated into the analysis (a point we briefly discuss in Section VI). We urge that cause of death be determined in tumorigenicity experiments, at least in a few studies. The results from analyses which utilize cause can then be compared with analyses of the same experiments which do not use cause. If two approaches nearly always lead to the same conclusion, it would suggest that the added effort and cost associated with determining and analyzing cause of death is unnecessary. If they do not, it may be possible to determine when the use of cause of death is most important.

B. Selecting Intervals for the Computation of $O^p - E^p$ and V^p

The rationale for grouping non-tumor deaths into intervals for computing $O^p - E^p$, rather than using exact ages of death, is to insure that the M_i are sufficiently large for a meaningful treatment comparison. An interval should not be too wide, however, for then the tumor prevalence could vary substantially within it and result in bias.

To our knowledge, the only published recommendation on how to select intervals is given by Peto et al.,[3] who attempt to capitalize on the fact that for most tumor types, the prevalence function increases with age. The procedure proposed by Peto et al.[3] can be justified as the local score test under monotone prevalence. When the technique is applied in situations where the prevalence is not increasing, it can lead to intervals so broad that effectively no age adjustment is made. This is not a fault of the method, but one of misapplication. The

National Toxicology Program (NTP) of the U.S. Department of Health and Human Services sometimes uses four intervals for natural deaths in a standard 2 year experiment: 0 to 52 weeks, 53 to 78 weeks, 79 to 92 weeks, and 93 to 104 weeks.

When there are only small differences in intercurrent death rates across treatment groups and relatively small treatment effects, we suspect that these or similar intervals will perform satisfactorily. If intercurrent death rates differ, however, the choice of intervals can have a strong effect on results. This seems to us to be the main concern about any choice of intervals. If intervals are to be used, we prefer the use of more than four (say 6 to 8 for current sample sizes). Preferably, none should contain extremely few deaths and none should be excessively wide.

An alternative to the use of intervals which we endorse has recently been proposed by Dinse and Lagakos.[12] The method uses logistic regression techniques and, in so doing, avoids the arbitrariness of interval selection. This technique is described briefly in Section VI.

C. Choosing Weights for Trend Tests

As indicated in Section III, the best weights $\mathbf{c} = (c_1, c_2, \ldots, c_K)^T$ to use in the test of trend depend on the ratios of the age-specific tumor mortality functions $\lambda_i(t)$ and the ratios of the age-specific tumor prevalence odds functions $p_i(t)/\{1 - p_i(t)\}$. In practice, of course, these ratios are not known and so other criteria must be used for selecting weights. The three most commonly used weights are

$$\mathbf{c}^{(1)} = (1, 2, \ldots, K)$$

$$\mathbf{c}^{(2)} = (d_1, d_2, \ldots, d_K) \text{ and}$$

$$\mathbf{c}^{(3)} = (\ln d_1, \ln d_2, \ldots, \ln d_K)$$

where d_i is the dose for group i. A fourth choice for $\mathbf{c}$, which lies between $\mathbf{c}^{(1)}$ and $\mathbf{c}^{(3)}$, has been proposed by Mantel et al.[14]

For routine analyses of tumorigenicity studies, we favor $\mathbf{c}^{(1)}$. When the dosage groups are geometrically spaced, or nearly so, $\mathbf{c}^{(1)}$ will be nearly identical to $\mathbf{c}^{(3)}$. We prefer $\mathbf{c}^{(1)}$ to $\mathbf{c}^{(2)}$ because in some experiments d_K and other doses differ by more than an order of magnitude. Then the test based on $\mathbf{c}^{(2)}$ is essentially a comparison only of the high-dose groups to controls. However, as Mantel et al. point out, the various choices of $\mathbf{c}$ will give very similar results in many experiments.

D. Stratification

We indicated in Section II that analyses should routinely be stratified and reported by sex and strain. The separation of tables by age categories and type of death represent additional stratification, although we do not feel that these results routinely need to be reported separately. We also recommend stratification by any other baseline variables (e.g., cage position or initial body weight) that are strongly suspected to be correlates of tumor development, especially if they are unbalanced across treatment groups. One need only compute an $\mathbf{O} - \mathbf{E}$ and V for each stratum and then sum these over strata. Excessive stratification can be counterproductive, but the loss in efficiency produced by a few (e.g., <5) unnecessary strata is negligible.

V. REPORTING

Even under the limited goal of testing for an effect without estimating dose-response parameters or extrapolating to low doses, a tumorigenicity experiment provides the opportunity for a myriad of analyses. However, in selecting items for presentation, it is important to convey in as understandable and useful a way as possible what the data are saying and how strongly they are saying it. Thus any report ought to include information summarizing the data, defining the statistical significance of the experiment relative to unambiguous and stated null hypotheses, and assessing the validity of the findings.

Detailed guidelines on the presentation of results can be found in Peto et al.[3] and Gart, Chu, and Tarone.[2] The nature and amount of information that is presented is largely a matter of taste, and we do not in this section attempt to discuss all aspects of reporting. Rather we comment on a few ways in which reporting practices can be modified to be more informative to the reader.

A. Graphical Displays

Natural Longevity — It is important and customary to include in any report plots of natural longevity (from all causes except sacrifice), usually based on Kaplan-Meier[15] survival curves. For each sex and strain, the survival curves for the treatment groups should be displayed on a single graph. Each graph should be accompanied by the significance level based on the logrank test for treatment equality with respect to longevity. Also, it is sometimes useful to display error bars at two or three time points.

1. Cumulative Hazard Plots of Tumor Mortality

If there are deaths due to the tumor, either from individual determinations of cause of death, or from regarding the tumor as rapidly lethal, plots of the cumulative hazard $\Lambda(t) = \int_o^t \lambda(u)du$ should be presented. For the ith group, $\Lambda(t)$ can be estimated by

$$\sum_{tj<t} n_i^{(j)}/N_i^{(j)}$$

(See Section II), or as $-\ln[S(t)]$, where $S(t)$ is the Kaplan-Meier curve obtained by treating tumor deaths as uncensored observations and all others as censored observations. These two estimators will usually give very similar results.

For each sex and strain, all dose groups should be displayed on the same graph. The curves should be plotted on a logarithmic vertical axis. In this way, the proportional hazards assumption, against which Q^M and Z^M are particularly sensitive, corresponds to parallel curves (see, for example, Kalbfleisch and Prentice).[16] Curves which first move apart and then move together may signal crossing hazard functions, in which case the power of Q^M may be very low.

2. Cumulative Hazard Plots for Intercurrent Mortality

The validity and efficiency of many of the standard statistical tests for carcinogenic effects are adversely affected if the intercurrent death rates vary across dosage groups. This possibility can be examined graphically by plotting the cumulative hazard functions associated with nontumor deaths (D_{oc}). These plots can be formed in the same way as $\Lambda(t)$, except with (natural) non-tumor deaths playing the role of uncensored events. Significance levels based on the logrank statistic should accompany each graph.

3. Prevalence Rate Plots

If there are sufficient non-tumor deaths, a graph containing plots of the tumor prevalence rates of the treatment groups (for each sex and strain) should be reported. If the prevalence curves are assumed to be monotonic, they can be estimated using isotonic regression techniques. See, Barlow et al.[17] or Hoel and Walburg.[1] When the curves are plotted using a logit scale on the vertical axis, parallelism is evidence of proportional prevalence odds across treatments, the alternative for which $O^p - E^p$ is particularly sensitive. Deviations from parallelism, and in particular evidence of crossing odds functions, indicate that the power of Z^p and Q^p might be very poor. For many tumor types, however, there will be too few nontumor deaths for this type of plot to be meaningful. One alternative is to formally assess the proportional odds assumption by the logistic regression techniques given in Dinse and Lagakos.[12] The logistic model approach also provides a smooth estimate of the prevalence function.

B. Tabular Displays

Tabular summaries of the results of a tumorigenicity experiment may report, but should not in general focus on, lifetime tumor rates, since these may give a poor indication of rates of tumor development. Rather, methods based on observed minus expected counts, such as presented in Peto et al.[3] should be used and are easy to interpret.

1. Unevaluable Cases

Tabular displays should indicate how many animals in each dosage group have been excluded from the analysis as unevaluable. Animals that die before the first tumor death should not be discarded. In general, only animals that have not been (or could not be) grossly or microscopically examined should be excluded from evaluation.

2. Cause of Death

The tabulated results should indicate whether the $O - E$'s were computed using individual cause of death information for each tumor-bearing animal, or whether they were obtained by assuming the tumor to be either nonlethal or rapidly lethal.

3. Trend and Heterogeneity

It is sometimes suggested that the trend test (Z) and test for departure from trend $(Q - Z^2)$ should not be computed unless the overall test for heterogeneity (Q) is statistically significant. We disagree and feel that since trend is usually of primary scientific interest, it and Q should always be reported. If there is significant departure from trend, one might also choose to partition further its degrees of freedom (e.g., comparisons of individual dose groups with the controls).

VI. ADDITIONAL AND REPLACEMENT ANALYSES

Several extensions of the analyses in Section II can provide useful insights and possibly improved sensitivity. Some of these are especially important when standard analyses give equivocal results. We briefly describe a few alternatives to and modifications of the methods in Section II, some of which are still under development.

A. Regression Models for Tumor Mortality

We indicated in Section III that the logrank test arises as a likelihood score test from Cox's[11] proportional hazards regression model. The Cox model allows the analyses described in Section II to be refined in several ways, including the incorporation of several baseline variables (both continuous and categorical), formal tests of the proportional hazards assumption, and residual analyses. It also produces a slope estimate, relative to a specified dose metameter, and a corresponding confidence interval, which are useful descriptors of tumorigenic activity.

B. Regression Models for Tumor Prevalence

Dinse and Lagakos[12] show that the Hoel-Walburg test based on $O^p - E^p$ also arises as a likelihood score test from a proportional odds logistic regression model. This suggests a simple modification which avoids the need and problems with selecting intervals for grouping observations. The use of their proposed approach also allows incorporation of baseline covariates, formal tests of the proportional odds assumption, and a slope estimator (with a corresponding confidence interval) of the prevalence dose-response relationship.

C. Tests Oriented to Nonproportional Hazards or Odds Alternatives

Tarone and Ware[18] discuss a simple and useful generalization of the logrank test in which age-specific $\mathbf{n}^{(j)} - \mathbf{e}^{(j)}$ are weighted and then summed. Depending on the choice of weights, the resulting test is especially sensitive to alternatives other than proportional hazards. An important special case is the Generalized Wilcoxon test, obtained by weighting $\mathbf{n}^{(j)} - \mathbf{e}^{(j)}$ by the total number of animal at risk at t_j. This test is more sensitive to early differences in the treatment groups than the logrank test, which is customarily reported in NTP bioassays. The same ideas as in Tarone and Ware can also be applied to the Hoel-Walburg test (i.e., $\mathbf{O}^P - \mathbf{E}^P$), resulting in tests that place special emphasis on early or late-occurring differences.

Section III also indicates the basis for combining the prevalence and mortality $\mathbf{O} - \mathbf{E}$'s. These procedures are only one example of a class that can be generated by considering different alternatives. General structures are discussed by Louis[19] in the context of adaptive sacrifice plans for tumorigenicity studies.

D. Litter Effects

We have discussed (Section IV.D) the use of baseline variables as stratification factors in the calculation of $\mathbf{O} - \mathbf{E}$'s. Litters represent another baseline variable of possible importance. In little-matched designs in which littermates are assigned to different treatments, analyses which do not account for litters can understate the significance (i.e., produce too large a P-value) when testing for treatment equality. On the other hand, in multigenerational designs in which all littermates receive the same treatment, just the opposite is true. The extent to which time to tumor methods are likely to be distorted by not adjusting for litter effects is not well understood, and should be researched to determine whether more complicated analyses are appropriate. Mantel et al.[14] and Michalek and Mihalko[20] propose methods for litter adjustment.

E. Refining Cause of Death

We have discussed some of the difficulties associated with using information on cause of death. Peto et al.[3] proposed that pathologists report cause of death on a four-point scale: tumor definitely caused death, probably caused death, probably did not cause death, and definitely did not cause death. With this grading, different cutoff points can be tried as a means of checking sensitivity. Other strategies are considered in Kodell et al.[21] and Lagakos.[6] In addition, T. A. Louis and R. Kodell are currently investigating a formalization of uncertainty in cause of death, together with corresponding likelihood-based techniques for incorporating this extension into analyses.

VII. SUMMARY

We have described parts of those analyses recommended by the NTP, IARC, and NCI that are validated and contribute to an objective, preplanned analysis of the bioassay. To these we add reporting standards, modifications, and new procedures that should improve the analyses.

By structuring the data with unified statistical models, we show the relationship among the Hoel-Walburg, logrank, and Peto (cuase of death) analyses. Each is implicitly based on assumptions about tumor lethality, representativeness, the credibility of cause of death information, and the structure of alternatives to the null hypothesis. Making these assumptions explicit will help statisticians and other scientists to interpret the results of a bioassay and appreciate the limitations of the experiments.

We discuss graphics and other diagnostics that give clues to when a specific analysis is deceptive and recommend companion analyses. For example, in Section IV we state that when intercurrent death rates increase with dose, the logrank test based on a rapidly lethal tumor can overstate carcinogenic effect. On the other hand, the prevalence analysis (Hoel-Walburg) based on a nonlethal tumor tends to have the opposite effect (i.e., understate significance). In general, biases in the two types of tests are in opposite directions. Knowing this, one can informally combine the evidence from the two tests. For example, if the intercurrent death rate increases with dose, a significant Hoel-Walburg test can be believed since the true significance level, if different, will tend to be smaller.

Although we have identified some basic analyses, we cannot recommend a cookbook approach to assessing evidence from the experiments. Ultimately, these analyses can only report parameter estimates and statistical significance. Interpreting the scientific and policy significance of the results involves other experts.

ACKNOWLEDGMENTS

This work was supported by a contract with Health and Welfare Canada, and by grants from the National Cancer Institute (CA-33041) and the National Institute of Environmental Health Sciences (ES-02709). We are very grateful to David Amato, Edmund Crouch, Gregg Dinse, and Daniel Krewski for their comments and suggestions, and to Karen Abbett for her help in the preparation of this manuscript.

REFERENCES

1. **Hoel, D. G. and Walburg, H. E.,** Statistical analysis of survival experiments, *J. Natl. Cancer Inst.,* 49, 361, 1972.
2. **Gart, J. J., Chu, K. C., and Tarone, R. E.,** Statistical issues in the interpretation of chronic tests for carcinogenicity, *J. Natl. Cancer Inst.,* 62, 957, 1979.
3. **Peto, R., Pike, M. C., Day, N. E., et al.,** Guidelines for simple, sensitive, significance tests for carcinogenic effects in long-term animal experiments, in *IARC Monographs on the Evaluation of the Carcinogenic Risk of Chemicals to Humans, Supplement 2, Long-term and Short-term Screening Assays for Carcinogens: A Critical Appraisal,* IARC, Lyon, 1980, 311.
4. **Lagakos, S. W. and Mosteller, F.,** A case study of statistics in the regulatory process: the FDC Red No. 40 experiments, *J. Natl. Cancer Inst.,* 66, 197, 1981.
5. **Ryan, L. M.,** Efficiency of age-adjusted tests in animal carcinogenicity experiments. Technical Report 403 Z, Dana-Farber Cancer Institute, Biostatistics and Epidemiology Division, Boston, 1984.
6. **Lagakos, S. W.,** An evaluation of some two-sample tests used to analyze animal carcinogenicity experiments, *Utilitas Mathematica,* 21B, 239, 1982.
7. **Tarone, R.,** Tests for trend in life table analysis, *Biometrika,* 62, 679, 1975.
8. **Lagakos, S. W. and Ryan, L.,** On the representativeness assumption in prevalence tests for carcinogenicity, *J. Roy. Stat. Soc. Series C,* 33, 1985 (in press).
9. **Louis, T. A., Albert, A., and Heghinian, S.,** Screening for the early detection of cancer: estimation of disease natural history." *Math. Biosci.,* 40, 111, 1978.
10. **Mantel, N.,** Evaluation of survival data and two new rank order statistics arising in its consideration, *Ca. Chem. Rep.,* 50, 163, 1966.
11. **Cox, J. E.,** Regression model and life table, *J. Roy. Stat. Soc.,* 34, 187, 1972.
12. **Dinse, G. E. and Lagakos, S. W.,** Regression analysis of tumor prevalence data, *J. Roy. Stat. Soc. Series C,* 32, 236, 1984.
13. **Peto, R.,** Guidelines on the analysis of tumor rates and death rates in experimental animals, *Br. J. Cancer,* 29, 101, 1974.

14. **Mantel, N., Tukey, J. W., Ciminera, J. L., and Heyse, J. F.,** Tumorigenicity assays, including use of the jackknife, *Biometrical Journal* (to appear).
15. **Kaplan, E. L. and Meier, P.,** Nonparametric estimation from incomplete observations, *JASA.,* 53, 457, 1958.
16. **Kalbfleisch, J. D. and Prentice, R. L.,** *The Statistical Analysis of Failure Time Data,* John Wiley and Sons, New York, 1980.
17. **Barlow, R. E., Bartholomew, D. J., Bremner, J. M., and Brunk, H. D.,** *Statistical Inference Under Order Restrictions,* John Wiley and Sons, New York, 1972.
18. **Tarone, R. E. and Ware, J. H.,** On distribution-free tests for equality of survival distributions, *Biometrika,* 64, 156, 1977.
19. **Louis, T. A.,** Adaptive Sacrifice Plans for Rodent Bioassays, Technical Report, Dept. of Biostatistics, Harvard School of Public Health, Boston, Mass., 1982.
20. **Michalek, J. E. and Mihalko, D.,** On the use of logrank scores in the analysis of litter-matched data on time to tumor appearance, unpublished manuscript, 1982.
21. **Kodell, R. L., Farmer, J. H., Gaylor, D. W., and Cameron, A. M.,** The influence of cause-of-death assignment on time to tumor analyses in animal carcinogenesis studies, *J. Natl. Canc. Inst.,* 69, 659, 1982.

Chapter 8

USE OF THE HARTLEY-SIELKEN MODEL IN LOW DOSE EXTRAPOLATION

Robert L. Sielken, Jr.

TABLE OF CONTENTS

ABSTRACT

The Hartley-Sielken model is a statistical family of models for the probability, P(T; d), that an experimental unit at dose d will have a toxic response by time T. The model was originally developed under contracts with the Food and Drug Administration and the National Center for Toxicological Research as an extension of the quantal response multistage model to include the role of time. More recent research has shown that the model also arises quite naturally when response initiation is viewed in terms of either compartmental analysis and linear pharmacokinetics or simply as a result of attacks on the cells. Generalizations of the Hartley-Sielken model are indicated.

A maximum likelihood estimate of the model can be obtained when the experimental data contains either the observed time of the response or just the presence or absence of the response by observation time. That likelihood can incorporate competing risks and interim sacrifices as well as known or unknown causes of death. Some computer programs are available.

The estimated model can be used to describe the likelihood of a toxic response in terms of both dose and time. Such descriptions can include three-dimensional response surfaces, contour maps, graphs of how the risk at a particular time changes with dose, graphs of how the risk at a particular dose changes with time, etc. Some possible summary risk characterizations which emphasize the role of time are discussed. Real experimental data are used to illustrate these risk descriptions and summary characterizations.

The sensitivity of the estimation procedure to the elements of the experimental situation such as the observability of the time of the response, the availability of the cause of death, response lethality, the curvature in the low dose region, and errors are briefly discussed.

I. INTRODUCTION

This chapter focuses on the use of the Hartley-Sielken model to help quantify the probability of a specified toxic response in terms of both the chemical's dose level and the elapsed time since the exposure began. When several subjects are exposed at dose d, some subjects will respond by time T and some will not. Thus, it is the proportion P(T; d) of subjects developing a particular response by time T at dose d which is to be modeled, estimated, and characterized herein.

A very broad family of models for P(T; d) can be derived in general terms as follows: The chemical is conceptualized as being either comprised of or generating a number of units or packages which can attack the target cells and cause the specified response. An attacked cell has probability q(d) of failing to reach the response initiation stage. Either the cells have time to repair between attacks or there are sufficiently many cells so that the probability of more than one attack on the same cell is negligible. The experimental protocol generates a total number of attacks at time t for dose d equal to f(d,t). All the damage to the cell that is required to cause initiation is done at the time t of the attack. However, the initiation stage is not reached until $t + \tau_1$. This breakdown of a single cell may consist, for example, of a single stage process or may involve several stages. As soon as at least one cell reaches the initiation stage a response is apparent at time $T = t + \tau_1 + \tau_2$. (Although both τ_1 and τ_2 could be random times, they will both be treated as constants here.) The probability that a response is not apparent at time T is the probability that all attacks before time $T - \tau_1 - \tau_2$ failed to cause initiation; that is,

$$1 - P(T;d) = q(d)^{\int_0^{T-\tau_1-\tau_2} f(d,t)\, dt} \tag{1}$$

since $\int_0^{T-\tau_1-\tau_0} f(d,t) \, dt$ is the total number of attacks on the target cells before time $T - \tau_1 - \tau_2$. Let $q(d) = \exp[-w(d)]$, then

$$P(T;d) = 1 - \exp\left[-\int_0^{T-\tau_1-\tau_2} w(d) \, f(d,t) \, dt\right]. \tag{2}$$

Model 2 allows the dose level to influence the strength of the attacks (through $w(d)$) while both dose level and time influence the total number of attacks (through $f(d,t)$). Model 2 can also be extended to incorporate exposures where the dose level changes over time by replacing d in Equation 2 by a function of time, say $d(t)$.

Since the functions w and f in Equation 2 are not directly observable quantities, the role of Equation 2 is to serve as a framework upon which the available knowledge or lack thereof concerning a specific toxicological situation can be imposed. The more limited the knowledge is, the greater the need for flexibility in the functions chosen to approximate the unknowns in Equation 2.

II. THE HARTLEY-SIELKEN MODEL

In Hartley, Tolley, and Sielken[1] the following biological scenario is shown to lead to the Hartley-Sielken model for $P(T; d)$. The biological system is conceptualized as being comprised of compartments or as existing in different states. The chemical enters this system and follows a deterministic first order kinetic process as it flows between compartments. Within a compartment the probability of a transition from a normal state to the specified response state is proportional to the amount of the chemical in the compartment.

The Hartley-Sielken model is also a member of the general family of models (Equation 2). From the attack perspective, let $r(d)$ equal the relative number of attackers launched at dose d, and let $h(t)$ reflect the susceptibility of the target cells at time t and equal the fraction at time t of the launched attackers which are allowed to reach the target cells. Then, $f(d,t) = r(d) h(t)$ and Equation 2 simplifies to

$$P(T;d) = 1 - \exp\left[-g(d) \, H(T)\right] \tag{3}$$

where $g(d) = w(d) \, r(d)$ and $H(T) = \int_0^{T-\tau_1-\tau_0} h(t) \, dt$. Model 3 allows the dose level to influence

(1) the number of attackers, and
(2) the strength of the attacks

while the passage of time influences

(3) the percentage of the attackers which arrive at the target sites and hence the susceptibility of the target cells to attack.

If $\delta(d)$ is the minimum time to an observable response at dose d, then Model 3 is changed to

$$P(T;d) = 1 - \exp\left\{-g(d) \, [H(T) - \gamma(d)]\right\} \tag{4}$$

where $\gamma(d) = \int_0^{\delta(d)} h(t) \, dt$. In Equation 4 for time $t > \delta(d)$ the effect of t, namely $h(t)$, is independent of $\delta(d)$. If, on the other hand, the effect of time does not even start until after $\phi(d)$ units of time, then Equation 3 is changed to

$$P(T;d) = 1 - \exp\left\{-g(d)\int_{\phi(d)}^{T-\tau_1-\tau_2} h[t - \phi(d)] \, dt\right\} = 1 - \exp\{-g(d)H[T-\phi(d)]\} \tag{5}$$

Models 3, 4, and 5 are all referred to as the Hartley-Sielken model. The development of the model was supported by contracts with the Food and Drug Administration and the National Center for Toxicological Research as well as a NIH Biomedical Research Support Grant.

In Hartley and Sielken[2,3] the functions g(d) and H(T) were assumed to have the forms

$$g(d) = g(d;\alpha) = \alpha_0 + \alpha_1 d + \ldots, + \alpha_a d^a \tag{6}$$

and

$$H(T) = H(T;\beta) = \beta_1 T + \beta_2 T^2 + \ldots + \beta_b T^b \tag{7}$$

where a and b were maximum possible powers specified by the user of the model. The polynomial forms for g(d) and H(T) were chosen because of the general ability of low order polynomials to approximate many functions well. Since detailed knowledge of mechanistic processes involved in toxicology (especially carcinogenic processes) is currently limited, the authors did not want to be overly restrictive with respect to the forms of g and H.

Since $O \leq P(T; d) \leq 1$ and $P(T; d)$ is a nondecreasing function of T for each d, the parameters in the Hartley-Sielken model should be restricted so that the model for P(T; d) also has these characteristics. In particular α and β should be restricted so that $g(d;\alpha) \geq 0$, $H(T;\beta) \geq 0$, and $H(T;\beta)$ is nondecreasing in T. This is easily accomplished by requiring

$$\alpha_s \geq 0, \qquad s = 1, \ldots, a \tag{8}$$

and

$$\beta_r \geq 0, \qquad r = 1, \ldots, b. \tag{9}$$

Although the conditions in Equations 8 and 9 are sufficient to guarantee the desired characteristics, they are not necessary and in some instances may be too restrictive. A less restrictive alternative is to only require

$$g(d;\alpha) \geq 0 \quad \text{for a specified grid of d values} \tag{10}$$

and

$$H(T;\beta) \geq 0 \quad \text{and nondecreasing over a specified grid of T values.} \tag{11}$$

If Equation 8 is not required but it is desired to force P(T; d) to be nondecreasing in d, then an alternative to Equation 10 is

$$g(d;\alpha) \geq 0 \quad \begin{array}{l}\text{and nondecreasing over a specified}\\ \text{grid of d values.}\end{array} \tag{12}$$

The $H(T;\beta)$ contains no β_0 term since $P(0; d) = 0$. If $P(T; d) > 0$ for some d and T, then $H(T;\beta)$ is positive for all $T > 0$ and without loss of generality $H(1;\beta) = \sum_{r=1}^{b} \beta_r$ can be scaled so that

$$\sum_{r=1}^{b} \beta_r = 1 \tag{13}$$

since a common multiplier of the β_r's can be compensated for by a common divisor to the α_s's without altering the product.

The Hartley-Sielken model (Equation 3) has an age specific toxic response incidence rate (hazard rate) equal to g(d) h(t) which is a product form. When Equation 3 is derived from Equation 2, this product form arises because f(d,t) is assumed to be the product r(d) h(t). This assumption implies that the change in the susceptibility of the target cells over time is the same for all dose levels and that the role of time in determining the fraction of attackers reaching the target cells is the same for all dose levels. If, instead, the effect of time is allowed to differ slightly for slightly different dose levels, then a natural extension of the Hartley-Sielken model is to approximate

$\int_0^{T-\tau_0-\tau_2} w(d)\, f(d,t)\, dt$ in Equation 2 by the more general polynomial form $K(T,d) = \sum_{r=1}^{b}$ $\sum_{s=0}^{a} \kappa_{rs}\, d^s\, T^r$ and let

$$P(T;d) = 1 - \exp[-K(T,d)]. \qquad (14)$$

Naturally $K(T,d)$ would be restricted to being non-negative and nondecreasing in T for all relevant d.

Although the dose index d in the general model (Equation 2) could encompass a wide variety of exposure patterns such as

(1)   continuous dosing at a constant level d
(2)   a single exposure at level d at one point in time
(3)   a specified pattern of progressive or regressive dosing starting at level d
(4)   dosing at a specified level spaced d units of time apart, or
(5)   dosing at a specified level for d units of time,

the Hartley-Sielken model was derived with Patterns 1 and 2 in mind.

In the Hartley-Sielken model the definition of a response may specify a single site, a group of related sites, or simply refer to an occurrence anywhere in the body. The definition may or may not specify a degree of severity (e.g., the presence of a carcinoma, the presence of at least a moderately well differentiated carcinoma, death due to cancer).

III. INCORPORATING A BACKGROUND RISK

The spontaneous risk of a response is the probability of a response when $d=0$. Sometimes this risk implies that there is a background dose level d_0 which adds on to the increment d in the dose level so that the actual dose level is $d^* = d_0 + d$. In this case Equation 2 becomes

$$P(T;d) = 1 - \exp[\int_0^{T-\tau_1-\tau_2} - w(d_0 + d)\, f(d_0 + d,t)\, dt]$$

which for most representations of the functions w and f is just another member of the family characterized by Equation 2. Hence the presence of an additive background dose is encompassed by the same family of models (Equation 2).

If at least part of a non-zero background risk may be due to a process different from that associated with d, this part of the background risk is usually assumed to behave independently of d. Thus, if t_0 denotes the time to a response resulting from the independent portion of the background risk and t_1 denotes the time to response resulting from the process associated with

$$d^* = d_0 + d, \text{ then}$$

$$\text{Pr(no response by T;d)} = \text{Pr}(t_0 > T)\text{Pr}(t_1 > T;d^*) = \text{Pr}(t_0 > T) [1 - P(T;d^*)]$$

Without loss of generality $\text{Pr}(t_0 > T) = \exp[-H_0(T)]$ for some function $H_0(T)$. For a generalized non-product form model like Equation 14 a polynomial representation for $H_0(T)$ can be absorbed into the $K(T,d)$ term. For a product form model like Equation 3, $H_0(t)$ is easily incorporated if the susceptibility of the target cells changes with time t in the same manner for both the background process and the dose related process; i.e., if $H_0(T) = H(T)$.

In these ways an additive background risk or an independent background risk or both can be incorporated.

IV. ESTIMATING THE PARAMETERS IN THE HARTLEY-SIELKEN MODEL

The parameter estimation procedures select from a specified family of models the one model which maximizes the likelihood of obtaining the particular experimental outcomes observed. If, for example, the family of models under consideration is

$$P(T;d) = 1 - \exp[-g(d;\alpha) H(T;\beta)] \tag{15}$$

then the parameter estimation procedure determines the maximum likelihood estimate of the parameter vectors α and β say $\hat{\alpha}$ and $\hat{\beta}$. The best estimate of the dose-time-response model within this specified family is correspondingly

$$\hat{P}(T;d) = 1 - \exp[-g(d;\hat{\alpha}) H(T;\hat{\beta})] \tag{16}$$

The likelihood to be maximized by the parameter estimation procedures is the product of each experimental subject's individual contribution. This contribution depends on the subject's experimental dose level d, its observation time t, and what was observed. In order to clarify this contribution further let

T_1 = random time of response occurrence,
T_2 = random time from response to the time the response would cause death,
T_3 = random time of death due to competing risks, and
T_4 = sacrifice time.

Under the assumption that the random variables T_1, T_2, and T_3 are independent, the subject's likelihood contribution is either

(i) $\dfrac{dP(t;d)}{dt}$, if $t = T_1$

(ii) $\dfrac{d\text{Pr}}{dt} (T_1 + T_2 \leq t \mid \text{dose} = d)$, if $t = T_1 + T_2$

(iii) $\text{Pr}(T_1 \leq t \leq T_1 + T_2 \mid \text{dose} = d)$

$\quad$ if $t = T_3$ or T_4 and $T_1 \leq t$

(iv) $\Pr(T_1 > t)$,   if $t = T_3$ or T_4 and $T_1 > t$ or

(v) $\Pr(T_3 > t) \dfrac{d\Pr}{dt} (T_1 + T_2 \leqslant t \mid \text{dose} = d)$

$+ \Pr(T_1 \leqslant t \leqslant T_1 + T_2 \mid \text{dose} = d) \dfrac{d\Pr}{dt} (T_3 \leqslant t)$

if $T_1 \leqslant t$ and $t = \min(T_1 + T_2, T_3)$ but

the cause of death is not determined so that it is

not known whether $t = T_1 + T_2$ or $t = T_3$

The author has developed computer programs to determine the maximum likelihood estimate $\hat{P}(T; d)$ for some situations. The first program was completed and released to the public in 1978. Since the program provided "Statistical Methodology for Toxicological Research", the first letters SMTR were rearranged and the program nicknamed MRS. T. In 1981 an improved version of MRS. T called MRS. T81 was released. MRS. T81 can be used to determine the maximum likelihood estimates of the Hartley-Sielken models (Equations 3, 4, or 5) with g(d) as in Equation 6 and H(T) as in Equation 7 under the restrictions in Equations 9, 13, and either 8 or 10. MRS. T81 assumes that either T_1 is observable or the response does not cause death ($T_2 = \infty$). A new program is nearing completion for the situations where T_1 is not observable, the response can cause death, and the cause of death is determinable. In such situations $P(T; d)$ depends on the form of the distribution for T_2 but not that for T_3. The remaining situations where T_1 is not observable, the response can cause death, and the cause of death is not determinable are the only situations where likelihood contributions of type (v) arise and are the most difficult situations in that an exact determination of $\hat{P}(T; d)$ depends on the forms of the distributions for both T_2 and T_3.

V. UNDERSTANDING THE ESTIMATED MODEL

After the parameter estimation procedures have been used to obtain an estimate $\hat{P}(T; d)$ of the model, there are several things which can be examined to gain understanding of what $\hat{P}(T; d)$ implies. Basically these examinations should help in

(1)   evaluating the goodness of the fit of the estimated model to the observed experimental data
(2)   visualizing the way in which the probability of a response changes with the dose level and time and
(3)   summarizing and characterizing the probability of a response.

These three objectives will be considered in the following three subsections and will be illustrated in terms of the bladder cancer data from the recent ED_{01} study conducted by NCTR.

Briefly, the portion of the ED_{01} study considered involved 24,192 BALB/c female mice fed a known carcinogen, 2-acetylaminofluorene (2-AAF). The dose levels for these continuously dosed mice were 0, 30, 35, 45, 60, 75, 100, and 150 ppm in the diet. There were interim sacrifices scheduled at 9, 12, 14, 15, 16, 17, 18, and 24 months as well as a terminal sacrifice at 34 months. The only definitions of a response considered herein refer to the bladder, although other sites were also of interest in the ED_{01} study.

In the examples which follow time is measured in terms of 30-day months and all observations are recorded as the month in which they occurred; i.e., $t = 1, 2, \ldots, 34$. For small data sets it is not difficult to work with each individual observation time recorded to as fine a precision as available. However, for larger data sets, such as that from the ED_{01} study, it is more economical in terms of computer expense to partition the time scale (here almost 3 years) into time intervals (here 30-day months) and treat all observation times within an interval as the same time. This can be done with very little loss of information provided the intervals are not too large.

A. Evaluating the Goodness of the Fit

Usually it is impossible to observe the time to response for every experimental subject. This is because several subjects usually die before they respond and because many of the responses that do occur can not be detected until the subject is necropsied. Thus, there is usually no simple sample quantity which should be directly compared to $\hat{P}(T; d)$. The most straight-forward comparison is made as follows. Let

$$n_{t,d} = \text{the number of subjects at dose d which are observed at time t,}$$

$$p_{t,d} = \text{the observed proportion of these } n_{t,d} \text{ subjects which have responded by time t, and}$$

$$\hat{P}(t;d) = \text{the estimated or ``fitted'' proportion of subjects at dose d which would respond by time t}$$

Then

$$N_d = \sum_t n_{t,d} = \text{total number of subjects at dose d}$$

The proportion of subjects at dose d which have been observed at or before time T and which have responded is

$$Obs_{T,d} = \sum_{t \leq T} n_{t,d} p_{t,d} / N_d$$

The corresponding fitted proportion of subjects at dose d is

$$Fit_{T,d} = \sum_{t \leq T} n_{t,d} \hat{P}(t;d) / N_d$$

The values for $Obs_{T,d}$ and $Fit_{T,d}$ for the ED_{01} study mice are given in Table 1 when a response is defined to be the presence of a bladder hyperplasia or carcinoma. Naturally, since the $n_{t,d}$ values are not necessarily the same for each dose level, $Fit_{T,d2}$ may not necessarily exceed $Fit_{T,d1}$ even if $d_2 > d_1$ and $\hat{P}(T; d)$ is a non-decreasing function of d. Of course, $n_{t,d} p_{t,d}$ and $n_{t,d} \hat{P}(t; d)$ could also be tabled and compared instead of just the cumulative proportions $Obs_{T,d}$ and $Fit_{T,d}$.

It should be noted that $Obs_{T,d}$ would not equal $Fit_{T,d}$ exactly even if the postulated model were true and there were no statistical fluctuations. This follows since $Obs_{T,d}$ does not include responses occurring by time T but not observed by time T whereas $\hat{P}(T; d)$ and $Fit_{T,d}$ do.

The primary purpose of the above comparisons of observed and fitted proportions is to provide a rough ``feeling'' for the goodness of the fit and not the performance of a formal statistical hypothesis test for goodness of fit.

Table 1
CUMULATIVE OBSERVED AND FITTED PROPORTIONS OF MICE WITH A BLADDER HYPERPLASIA AND/OR CARCINOMA BY TIME T (MONTHS) AT DOSE (PPM)

T	Dose: 0		Dose: 30		Dose: 35		Dose: 45		Dose: 60		Dose: 75		Dose: 100		Dose: 150	
	Obs	Fit	Obs	Fit	Obs	Fit	Obs	Fit	Obs	Fit	Obs	Fit	Obs	Fit	Obs	Fit
10	.002	.001	.001	.000	.001	.000	.002	.000	.002	.003	.006	.006	.053	.026	.100	.099
12	.002	.001	.001	.000	.001	.000	.003	.000	.002	.004	.006	.006	.054	.028	.103	.104
14	.003	.002	.002	.000	.001	.000	.003	.000	.003	.011	.010	.019	.153	.084	.301	.296
16	.004	.003	.003	.001	.003	.001	.004	.001	.004	.016	.014	.027	.190	.120	.377	.375
18	.006	.006	.005	.001	.005	.004	.008	.009	.007	.028	.031	.052	.269	.179	.517	.519
20	.011	.011	.011	.010	.011	.012	.013	.017	.013	.036	.048	.077	.344	.239	.639	.645
22	.013	.012	.015	.012	.014	.014	.018	.019	.015	.039	.057	.086	.371	.261	.697	.707
24	.016	.014	.020	.015	.019	.018	.024	.024	.020	.046	.070	.099	.392	.286	.759	.771
26	.018	.021	.026	.024	.028	.027	.033	.037	.034	.063	.111	.140	.494	.372	.884	.899
28	.020	.022	.029	.026	.029	.029	.035	.039	.036	.065	.119	.146	.506	.384	.899	.915
30	.021	.023	.032	.028	.030	.031	.038	.040	.039	.067	.124	.150	.517	.393	.909	.925
32	.022	.023	.035	.030	.032	.032	.042	.042	.041	.068	.130	.154	.522	.397	.912	.929
34	.023	.024	.037	.032	.033	.033	.042	.043	.043	.070	.138	.158	.531	.405	.913	.929
Number of mice at risk:	2384		5024		3339		2243		2832		1982		1272		1272	

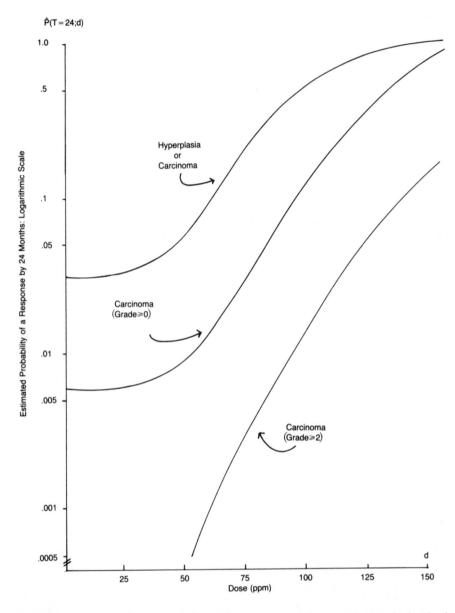

FIGURE 1. The estimated probability of a response by $T = 24$ months graphed versus the dose level d for three different definitions of a bladder response in the ED_{01} study.

B. Visualizing the Estimated Model

Although the model $\hat{P}(T; d)$ estimates the way in which the probability of a response changes with the dose level and time, it is often helpful to be able to visualize what $\hat{P}(T; d)$ implies. The simplest visual representations are graphs of

(1) the probability of a response by a fixed time T vs. the dose level d for one or more definitions of a "response" and hence one or more estimated models, say $\hat{P}_1(T; d)$, $\hat{P}_2(T; d)$, etc. (see, e.g., Figure 1),

(2) the probability of a response by time T vs. the dose level d for one or more fixed times, T, (see, e.g., Figure 2), and

(3) the probability of a response at dose d vs. the time T for one or more fixed dose levels, d, (see, e.g., Figure 3).

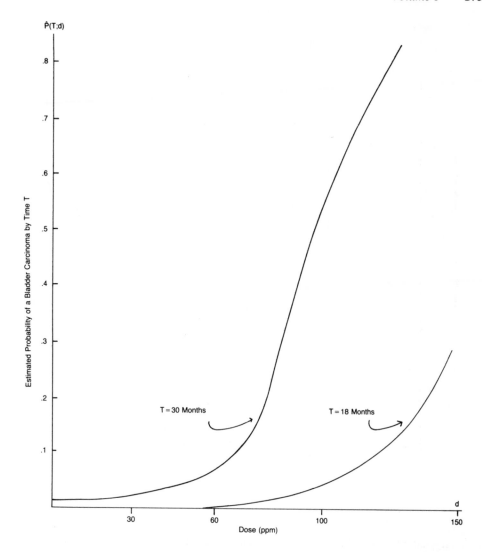

FIGURE 2.   The estimated probability of a bladder carcinoma by time T graphed versus the dose level d for T = 18 months and T = 30 months in the ED_{01} study.

The graphs of $\hat{P}(T; d)$ with T fixed and d varying and the graphs of $\hat{P}(T; d)$ with d fixed and T varying can be combined in a three-dimensional figure. Figures 2 and 3, for example, can be combined as in Figure 4. If enough such two-dimensional graphs are combined, a response surface emerges (see, e.g., Figure 5).

Another way of visualizing $\hat{P}(T; d)$ is a contour map (see, e.g., Figure 6). Here, the contours represent the combinations of dose and time which produce the same probability of a response.

C. Summarizing the Likelihood of a Response

Since the probability of a response depends on both the dose level and the time, virtually any representation of $\hat{P}(T; d)$ less than that in Figures 5 or 6 is going to omit some aspect of $\hat{P}(T; d)$ and be only an incomplete summary or characterization. However, simplified characterizations and summaries can be useful provided that they are regarded as only partial descriptions and not complete descriptions. The graphs of $\hat{P}(T; d)$ with either T or d fixed and the other component varying as in Figures 2 and 3 are examples of two-dimensional

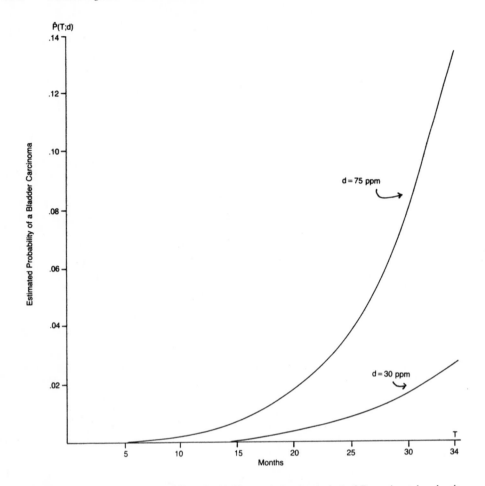

FIGURE 3. The estimated probability of a bladder carcinoma by the end of T months at dose levels 30 ppm and 75 ppm graphed versus T.

characterizations. Two other examples of such characterizations are described in the following two paragraphs.

The estimated time to reach a prescribed probability of a response can be graphed versus the dose level as exemplified in Figure 7. For a prescribed probability p of a response the equation $p = \hat{P}(T; d)$ is solved for T for each d, and the resulting T values graphed versus their corresponding d values.

The estimated mean time to response at dose d can depend very heavily upon $\hat{P}(T; d)$ at T values beyond the time range in the experiment and even beyond the normal lifespan of the subjects. Hence the estimated mean time to response may not be a particularly useful summary. An alternative summary is the estimated mean portion of a specified finite time interval that a subject at dose d is expected to be free from a response. This estimated "mean free period"(MFP) can be graphed versus d as in Figure 8. If, for example, the estimated MFP is 29.5 months out of the first 30 months following the onset of exposure to dose d, then this implies that on the average a subject will not have had a response until 29.5 months into the period or .5 months from the end of the period. In this example a MFP of 30 months would mean that no subject is expected to develop a response during the 30 month period. Obviously, the greater the mean free period the better. The estimated MFP for the interval from T=0 to T=T* is

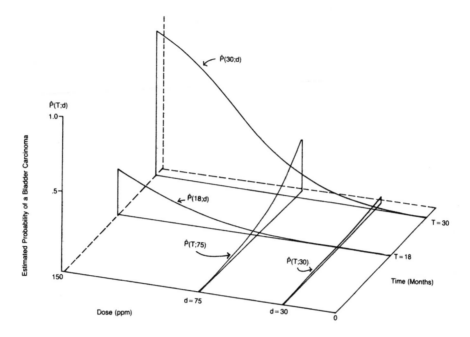

FIGURE 4. Building a three-dimensional representation of the estimated probability $\hat{P}(T; d)$ of a bladder carcinoma as a function of the time T and the dose level d from two-dimensional graphs of $\hat{P}(T; d)$ with T fixed and d varying and from two-dimensional graphs of $\hat{P}(T; d)$ with T varying and d fixed.

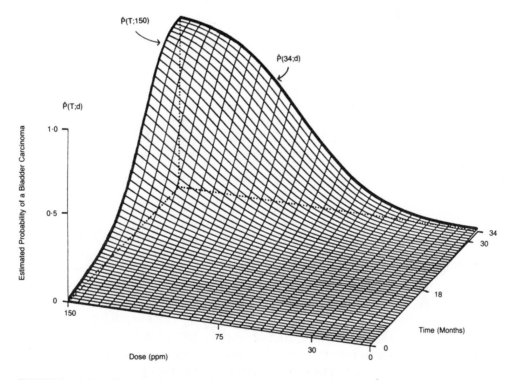

FIGURE 5. A three-dimensional representation of the way the estimated probability $\hat{P}(T; d)$ of a bladder carcinoma by time T at dose d changes with T and d (Modified from Society of Toxicology ED_{01} Task Force, *Fund. Appl. Toxicol.*, 1, 88, 1981. With permission.)

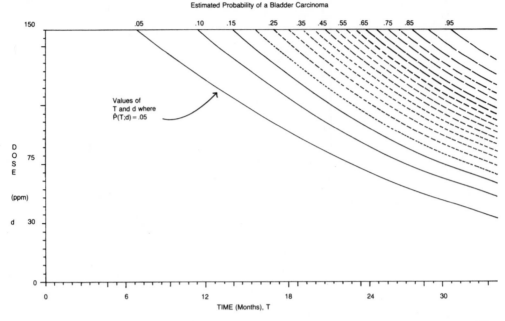

FIGURE 6. A contour map indicating the combinations of time T and dose d yielding the same estimated probability of a bladder carcinoma. (Modified from Society of Toxicology ED_{01} Task Force, *Fund. Appl. Toxicol.*, 1, 88, 1981. With permission.)

$$\widehat{MFP}(T^*,d) = T^* - \int_0^{T^*} (T^* - t) \left[\frac{d\hat{P}(T;d)}{dT}\right]_{T=t} dt$$

$$= T^* \left[1 - \hat{P}(T^*;d)\right] + \int_0^{T^*} t \left[\frac{d\hat{P}(T;d)}{dT}\right]_{T=t} dt.$$

It seems intuitively obvious that no single number can completely describe $\hat{P}(T; d)$. However, single number characterizations are often sought. The most common such characterization is the "virtually safe dose"(VSD). The definition of the VSD requires that a single point in time, say T', be specified and a maximum acceptable increment, say π, in the probability of a response by T' over that for $d = 0$ be specified. Then the estimated VSD is the dose level such that

$$\pi = \hat{P}(T';\widehat{VSD}) - \hat{P}(T';0).$$

This definition is also illustrated in Figure 9. Usually T' is near the expected lifetime of the subject and π is a positive number very near zero such as 0.00001.

Since the VSD ignores the way in which $\hat{P}(T; d)$ increases as T increases, an alternative characterization of the maximum acceptable dose level introduced in the re-examination of the ED_{01} study by a Society of Toxicology task force[4] is the "mean free dose" (MFD) defined as follows. For a specified time interval, say from $T=0$ to $T=T^*$, and a specified maximum acceptable fractional decrease ϵ in the MFP relative to the MFP for $d=0$, the MFD satisfies

$$MFP(T^*,MFD) = (1 - \epsilon) MFP(T^*;0)$$

This definition is illustrated in Figure 10. If $T^* = 25$ and $\epsilon = .00001$ or $1 - \epsilon = 0.99999$, then at the MFD the mean amount of time without a response having occurred is 99.999% of the mean amount of time without a response at the zero dose level.

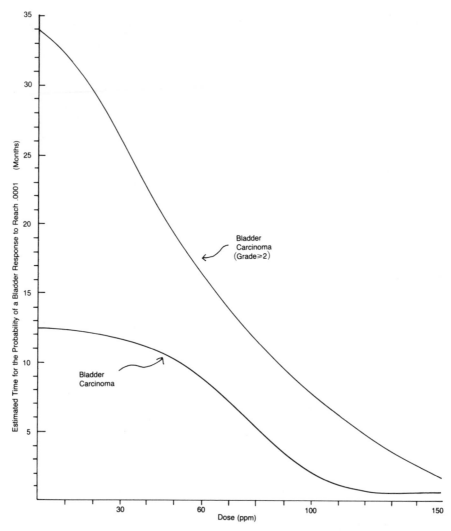

FIGURE 7. The estimated time for the probability of a bladder response to reach .0001 graphed versus the dose level.

If

$$P(T;d) = 1 - \exp[\alpha_k \, d^k \, T^j]$$

then the following approximations hold for small values of π and ϵ:

$$VSD \doteq [\pi/(T'^j \, \alpha_k)]^{1/k}$$
$$MFD \doteq [(j + 1)\epsilon/(T^{*j} \, \alpha_k)]^{1/k}$$

Hence the VSD decreases as either the permissible incremental risk π decreases or the time T' increases. Similarly the MFD decreases as the permissible relative reduction ϵ decreases or the time T^* increases. The powers j and k dictate the way both the VSD and MFD change with respect to (π, T') and (ϵ, T^*), respectively. If, for the sake of comparing the VSD and the MFD, both $\pi = \epsilon$ and $T' = T^*$, then

$$\frac{VSD}{MFD} \doteq \left[\frac{1}{j + 1}\right]^{1/k} \tag{17}$$

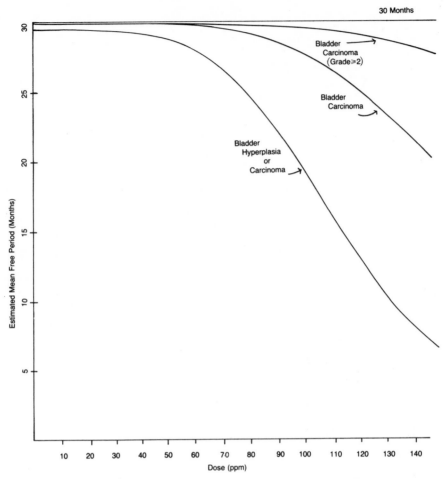

FIGURE 8. The mean number of months without a bladder response during the first 30 months of exposure graphed versus the dose level.

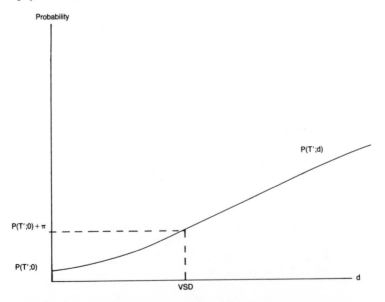

FIGURE 9. The definition of the virtually safe dose (VSD) in terms of the maximum acceptable increment π in the probability of a response by time T'.

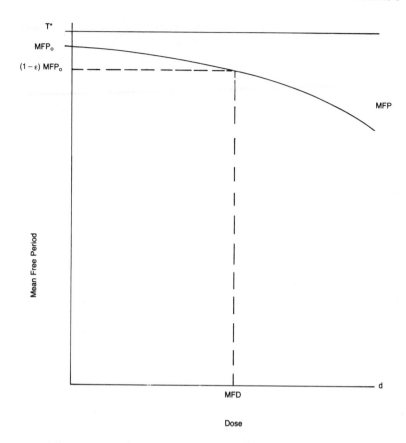

FIGURE 10. The definition of the mean free dose (MFD) in terms of the maximum acceptable fractional decrease ϵ in the mean free period (MFP) within the specified time interval from $T = 0$ to $T = T^*$.

From Equation 17 it is clear that the MFD will tend to exceed the VSD when $\pi = \epsilon$ and $T' = T^*$. Furthermore, Equation 17 implies that the relationship between the VSD and the MFD depends on how $P(T; d)$ changes with respect to both the dose and time (i.e., k and j in Equation 17).

VI. THE SENSITIVITY OF THE ESTIMATION PROCEDURES

The empirical behavior of the estimates of the virtually safe dose (VSD) and the mean free dose (MFD) is sensitive to many factors. Although several of these factors are beyond the control of the experimenter, it seems important for the experimenter to know which of the controllable factors will substantially affect the eventual estimates and also when the uncontrollable factors will make the risk estimates less reliable.

A recent study by Krewski et al.[5] considers the behavior of both the point estimates of the VSD and the lower confidence limits on the VSD for several time-to-response models (including the Hartley-Sielken model) and several quantal response models. In that study it was found that

(1) the availability of time-to-response data as opposed to quantal response data did not greatly alleviate the inherent difficulties of low dose risk extrapolation, and

(2) the shape of the underlying dose-time-response relationship (particularly with respect to dose) greatly affected the empirical behaviors with increased nonlinearity leading to a greater understatement in the lower confidence limits.

In another recent simulation study[6] Sabbagh reports on the influence of several factors on the empirical behavior of the estimated VSD and MFD using the Hartley-Sielken model (Equation 3) with Equations 6 to 9 and 13. In this study a response was defined as the onset of cancer as opposed to death due to cancer. The simulated experiment contained 250 subjects with 50 subjects at each of 5 doses d = 0.0, 0.3, 0.6, 1.0, and 1.5. The time to cancer was simulated from

$$P(T;d) = 1 - \exp[-g(d) T^2]$$

with either low dose linear behavior,

$$g(d) = 0.00001 + 0.5d$$

or low dose nonlinear (sublinear) behavior,

$$g(d) = 0.00001 + d^3$$

Figure 11 depicts the corresponding behaviors of P(T; d) for T = 1 which was the termination time for the experiment. The time from cancer onset to death due to cancer was assumed to be independent of the dose level and exponentially distributed with a median of either 0.1, 0.2, or 0.5. The time t' to death from a competing risk was assumed to be independent of the dose level and to have a Weibull distribution with $Pr(t' \leq T)$ being 0.0 for $T \leq .558$, 0.5 for T = .8, and 0.9 for T = .9. When $\hat{P}(T; d)$ was determined, the maximum possible powers a and b in Equations 6 and 7, respectively were the true powers plus one. A brief summary of the major findings of this study is given in the remainder of this section.

The distributions of the estimated VSD and MFD were heavily influenced by the low dose linearity or sublinearity of P(T; d). As illustrated in Table 2, when there was low dose linearity, the estimated VSD and MFD tended to be close to their true values (within a factor of 2 approximately 90% of the time). However, low dose sublinearity caused the VSD and MFD to often be underestimated (sometimes considerably so). The estimators of the VSD and MFD were also more variable under low dose sublinearity than under low dose linearity.

The simulation was repeated with the "pathologist" having either (1) a probability of 0.2 of falsely reporting the presence of a cancer when none was present, (2) a probability of 0.2 of falsely reporting the absence of a cancer when a cancer was present, or (3) both probabilities. When there was low dose linearity, the estimates of the VSD and MFD exceeded the true values much more often in situations (1) to (3) than they did without false reporting. On the other hand when there was low dose sublinearity, the underestimation of the true VSD and MFD got worse in situations (1) and (3) and didn't change much in situation (2).

The only other important factors identified were the values specified for the parameters (π, T') for the VSD and (ϵ, T^*) for the MFD when there was low dose sublinearity. When either the times T' and T^* increased or the allowable changes π and ϵ decreased, then the true VSD and MFD decreased and their underestimation increased.

As interesting as the factors which demonstrated their importance in determining the empirical behavior of the estimated VSD and MFD are the other factors which turned out to be relatively unimportant. In the Sabbagh study $\hat{P}(T; d)$ and the corresponding estimates of the VSD and MFD were determined under each of the following scenarios:

(a)   The time of the response was observed if it preceded the subject's death.

(b)   The time of the response was not observable. The presence or absence of the response at the subject's time of death could be observed (without error).

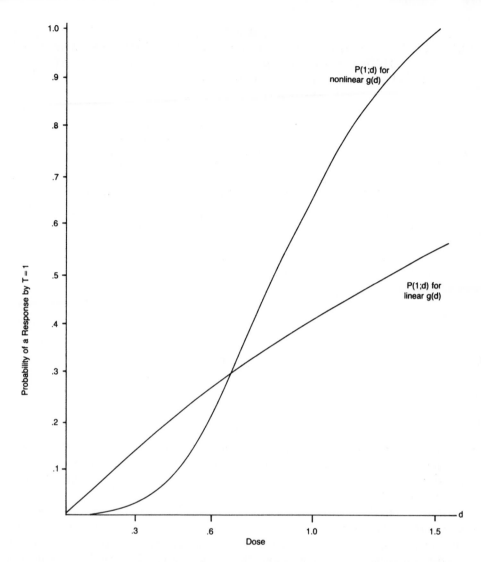

FIGURE 11. The graphs of the probability $P(T; d)$ of a response by time $T = 1$ in the simulation study where $P(T; d) = 1 - \exp[-g(d) T^2]$ and $g(d)$ was either linear or nonlinear.

The likelihood to be maximized is unaffected by the subject's assigned cause of death under (a) but is affected under (b). The estimation under (b) was repeated for each of the following methods of assigning the cause of death:

(1) The cause of death was always assigned correctly.
(2) Same as (1) but with a probability of 0.2 of falsely assigning cancer as the cause of death.
(3) Same as (1) but with a probability of 0.2 of falsely assigning competing risk as the cause of death.
(4) Same as (1) but with both probabilities of false assignment equal to 0.2.
(5) Cancer was assumed to never cause death ($T_2 = \infty$ in Section 4).

In studies where the objective is to demonstrate whether a chemical is or is not a carcinogen, it can be important to be able to determine the cause of a subject's death. However, in the

Table 2

FREQUENCY DISTRIBUTION OF RATIOS OF THE ESTIMATED VSD AND MFD TO THEIR CORRESPONDING TRUE VALUES: THE OBSERVED PERCENTAGE OF THE SIMULATIONS WITH THE RATIO IN THE INDICATED INTERVALS

Interval containing the ratio	Observed percentages			
	VSD $T'=1.0$, $\pi=.0001$		MFD $T^*=1.0$, $\epsilon=.0001$	
	Linear	Nonlinear	Linear	Nonlinear
[0, .0001]	0	0	0	0
[.0001, .001]	0	0	0	0
[.001, .01]	0	4	0	0
[.01, .1]	0	50	0	38
[.1, .5]	0	18	0	28
[.5, 2]	90	26	90	32
[2, 10]	10	2	10	2
[10, 100]	0	0	0	0
[100, 1000]	0	0	0	0
>1000	0	0	0	0
Number of simulations:	20	50	20	50
True value of risk characteristic:	.0002	.046	.0006	.067

Sabbagh study, where the objective was the quantification of the probability of a response, the distributions of the estimators of the VSD and MFD under (b) were nearly the same for (1) to (5); so that, the assignment of the cause of death was relatively unimportant. Similarly, these distributions were relatively the same for the three values of the median time from cancer onset to cancer caused death.

The distributions of the estimators for the VSD and MFD were also relatively the same under (a) and (b). That is, these distributions were essentially the same regardless of whether the time of the response was incorporated into the estimation or only the information that a response had occurred sometime before the subject's death. This conclusion should be tempered with the fact that in this study there were several subject deaths spread over most of the time range where responses occurred. Similar conclusions have been informally drawn in studies where there were several serial sacrifice times spread over the range of response times. No doubt, if there were no sacrifices or other deaths spread over the range of response times, then there would be a greater loss of information and a greater effect on the estimators of the VSD and MFD if the times to response were not observable.

Finally, there was little difference in the distributions of the estimators of the VSD and MFD between observing the times to response without error and observing the times to response plus an error when that error was normally distributed with mean zero and standard deviation $\sigma = .1$ (a fairly large standard deviation when the maximum possible time is 1.0).

VII. CONCLUDING REMARKS

Naturally not all aspects of the use of the Hartley-Sielken model in low dose extrapolation can be included in one short chapter. The two most important areas not discussed herein are the design of the experiment and the determination of informative confidence limits.

These areas are currently being intensely researched, and improved recommendations are continuing to emerge.

The dependence of risk on both the dose level and time has become evident. There are well-founded models for the probability of a response in terms of both dose and time. The computer software is available to fit many of these models to a wide variety of experimental data. The estimated risk can be characterized by three dimensional plots and contour maps or summarized in two-dimensional graphs and maximum acceptable doses. The empirical behavior of these estimated risk characteristics and summaries has been studied. Clearly, now is the time to meaningfully include time in risk assessment.

REFERENCES

1. **Hartley, H. O., Tolley, H. D., and Sielken, R. L., Jr.,** The product form of the hazard rate model in carcinogenic testing, *Curr. Top. Prob. Stat.,* 185, 1980.
2. **Hartley, H. O. and Sielken, R. L., Jr.,** Estimation of "safe doses" in carcinogenic experiments, *Biometrics,* 33, 1, 1977.
3. **Hartley, H. O., and Sielken, R. L., Jr.,** Development of Statistical Methodology for Risk Estimation: Final Report, National Center for Toxicological Research Contract No. 222-77-2001, Institute of Statistics, Texas A&M University, College Station, Texas, 1978.
4. **Society of Toxicology ED_{01} Task Force,** Re-examination of the ED_{01} study-risk assessment using time, *Fund. Appl. Toxicol.,* 1, 88, 1981.
5. **Krewski, D., Crump, K. S., Farmer, J., Gaylor, D. W., Howe, R., Portier, C., Salsburg, D., Sielken, R. L., Jr., and Van Ryzin, J.,** A comparison of statistical methods for low dose extrapolation utilizing time-to-tumor data, *Fund. Appl. Toxicol.,* 73, 140, 1983.
6. **Sabbagh, M.,** The Sensitivity of the Statistical Procedures Utilizing the Hartley-Sielken Models to Low Dose Cancer Risk Assessment, Master of Science Thesis, Institute of Statistics, Texas A&M University, College Station, Texas, 1982.

Chapter 9

A REVIEW OF METHODS FOR CALCULATING STATISTICAL CONFIDENCE LIMITS IN LOW DOSE EXTRAPOLATION

Kenny S. Crump and Richard B. Howe

TABLE OF CONTENTS

I. INTRODUCTION

Decisions regarding the control of environmental carcinogens should take into account the magnitude of the health effects, the effectiveness of controls in reducing health impairment, and economic, social, and political implications of regulatory options. To assist in such decisions, efforts have been made to estimate both the health effects of control alternatives and their effects upon the economy. Estimates in both areas are subject to considerable uncertainty. Thus, it is important that the nature and extent of this uncertainty be made clear to those using the analyses. A decision-maker concerned with setting an occupational exposure standard might justifiably reach a different decision if he were also presented some statement of the uncertainty rather than simply a single estimate of the health risk. Similarly, a realistic assessment of various energy alternatives requires that the uncertainties of both the health effects and the economic dislocations be accounted for.

Uncertainties in estimates of health effects of environmental carcinogens result from each of the following steps in carcinogenic risk assessment:

- extrapolation from high doses to low doses
- extrapolation of results observed in animal species to humans
- extrapolation of results from one route of exposure to another
- extrapolation of results from one temporal exposure pattern to another
- estimation of human exposure levels

The high to low dose extrapolation step has received a considerable amount of attention (Krewski and Van Ryzin).[1] This step is generally accomplished by fitting a mathematical dose response model to experimental carcinogenesis data collected at high doses and using the fitted model to estimate low dose responses. A number of dose response models have been proposed for this purpose. Often different models will describe dose response data about equally well and predict risks that differ considerably at low doses.[1] Even within a particular parametric family of dose response models, often there will be specific parameter values which are not clearly inconsistent with the data (e.g., the descriptions of the data determined by the parameter values cannot be rejected by statistical goodness of fit tests) and which likewise predict divergent risks at low doses. This latter type of uncertainty (roughly expressible as the range of risks consistent with the data within a particular parametric family) is generally quantified with the use of statistical confidence limits. Such confidence limits will be the focus of the present chapter.

The construction of confidence limits is a classical statistical problem and has been studied by many researchers. General methods for constructing confidence limits have been developed and are widely applied in data analysis. It might seem that there would be little controversy concerning the application of this previously developed theory to the low dose extrapolation problem. However, this has not been the case for several reasons. In some instances the regularity conditions required for applying a standard approach are not met. Because standard approaches have appeared not to be appropriate, ad hoc methods have been developed for measuring uncertainty whose interpretation is unclear. Further, the standard approaches yield confidence limits which are only asymptotically correct as the sample size approaches infinity. At sample sizes typically encountered in the low dose extrapolation problem, different asymptotically correct approaches sometimes yield considerably different results.

This chapter reviews and draws comparisons among the various proposals for constructing confidence limits related to the low dose extrapolation problem. Particular attention will be given to a method based upon the asymptotic distribution of likelihood ratios. Although this method has not been widely used in low dose extrapolation previously, we feel it has special merit. The emphasis of the chapter will be upon practical aspects; there will be little formal presentation of theory. Those readers interested in a more detailed and theoretical treatment should consult Krewski and Van Ryzin.[1] Also, Rai and Van Ryzin[2] give a theoretical development of an approach for constructing confidence limits for the gamma multihit model. Crump, Guess, and Deal[3] and Guess and Crump[4] give a similar development for the multistage model.

II. PRELIMINARIES

Extrapolation methods have been proposed which utilize either quantal data or time to occurrence data. We will focus mainly on those developed for quantal data. Quantal data from a carcinogenesis bioassay can be expressed as a group of triplets (N_i, X_i, d_i), $i = 1, \ldots, g$, where g is the number of treatment groups (including control groups), N_i is the number of animals in the ith treatment group, X_i is the number of those animals which are affected, and d_i is the dose to the animals in the ith group. Low dose extrapolation is accomplished through a mathematical dose response model $P(d; \underline{\Theta})$ representing the probability of an animal being affected when subject to a dose d, where $\underline{\Theta}$ represents a vector of free parameters. Frequently we will suppress the vector $\underline{\Theta}$ and write simply $P(d)$. Particular parametric forms for $P(d)$ which have been suggested include the multistage model[3,5]

$$P(d) = 1 - \exp(-q_0 - q_1 d - \ldots - q_k d^k) \tag{1}$$

$(q_i \geq 0$ for $i = 0,1,\ldots,k)$; the log-normal model[6]

$$P(d) = c + (1 - c)\Phi(a + b \log_{10} d) \tag{2}$$

$(0 \leq c \leq 1, b > 0)$

where Φ is the standard normal distribution function; the gamma multihit model[2]

$$P(d) = c + (1 - c)[(k - 1)!]^{-1} \int_0^{\lambda d} x^{k-1} e^{-x} dx \tag{3}$$

$(0 \leq c \leq 1, \lambda > 0, k > 0$ or $k \geq 1)$

and the Weibull or extreme value model[1]

$$P(d) = c + (1 - c)(1 - e^{-ad^k}) \tag{4}$$

$(0 \leq c \leq 1, a > 0, k > 0$ or $k \geq 1)$

The one-hit model is an important special case of the multistage, gamma multihit, and Weibull models obtained by fixing $k = 1$ in each of these models. In the application of the log-normal model recommended by Mantel et al.[6] the parameter b is fixed at $b = 1$. There has been considerable debate in recent years concerning the relative merits of these models in low dose extrapolation. A discussion of these models, and references to the attendant debate, may be found in Krewski and Van Ryzin.[1]

The outcome of a low dose extrapolation is usually expressed as estimates of the risk from a given environmental dose d_e or as "virtually safe doses" (VSDs). Both the "additional risk"

$$A(d_e) = P(d_e; \underline{\Theta}) - P(0, \underline{\Theta}) \tag{5}$$

and the "extra risk"

$$R(d_e) = [P(d_e; \underline{\Theta}) - P(0; \underline{\Theta})]/[1 - P(0; \underline{\Theta})] \tag{6}$$

have been suggested as appropriate measures of risk. The extra risk may be interpreted as the probability of a response at dose d_e conditional on the fact that no response would have resulted from zero dose. In the absence of background risk $(P(0) = 0)$, additional and extra risk are identical. A VSD represents the dose corresponding to a specific small level of risk and may be defined in terms of either extra or additional risk. Krewski and Van Ryzin[1] showed that for the Weibull, gamma multihit, and multistage models the difference between VSDs defined in terms of additional or extra risk is typically small, provided the background level of carcinogenesis is no greater than 25%.

III. REVIEW OF APPROACHES FOR SETTING CONFIDENCE LIMITS

A. Limits Based upon the Asymptotic Distribution of Maximum Likelihood Estimates

The asymptotic distribution of maximum likelihood estimators provides a general basis for constructing confidence intervals which has been specifically applied in the case of several models to the low dose extrapolation problem including the gamma multihit model and the multistage model.[2,3] By the asymptotic distribution of a statistic we mean a distribution which the true distribution of the statistic approaches as the sample size increases. At the fixed sample size used in a particular animal bioassay the asymptotic distribution is only an approximation to the true distribution and the closeness of the approximation is generally unknown. Confidence limits derived from asymptotic distributions will also be approximate and therefore subject to some doubt.

If animals respond independently and the probability that an animal in the ith group is a responder is $P(d_i; \underline{\Theta})$, then the likelihood of the quantal data from a bioassay is

$$\ell(\underline{\hat{\Theta}}) = \prod_{i=1}^{g} \binom{N_i}{X_i} P(d_i; \underline{\hat{\Theta}})^{X_i} [1 - P(d_i; \underline{\hat{\Theta}})]^{N_i - X_i} \tag{7}$$

The maximum likelihood estimate (MLE) $\hat{\Theta}$ of the parameter vector Θ is defined as the value for $\underline{\Theta}$ which maximizes the likelihood. Maximum likelihood estimates of functions of the parameter vector Θ are determined as the same function of the MLE $\underline{\hat{\Theta}}$. For example, the MLE of the extra risk is

$$[P(d; \underline{\Theta}) - P(0; \underline{\Theta})]/[1 - P(0; \underline{\hat{\Theta}})] \tag{8}$$

and the MLE $\hat{d}$ of the VSD corresponding to an extra risk of Π is given by the solution to the equation $R(\hat{d}) = \Pi$. Under certain regularity conditions[8] the vector $n^{1/2}(\underline{\hat{\Theta}} - \underline{\Theta})$ is asymptotically normally distributed with mean $\underline{0}$ and covariance matrix $\underline{\Sigma}$ where

$$n = \sum_{i=1}^{g} N_i, \qquad \underline{\Sigma}^{-1} = (\sigma_{rs}) \tag{9}$$

$$\sigma_{rs} = \sum_{i=1}^{g} c_i \frac{\partial P_i}{\partial \theta_r} \frac{\partial P_i}{\partial \theta_s} [P_i(1 - P_i)]^{-1} \tag{10}$$

$$P_i = P(d_i; \underline{\Theta}), \qquad c_i = \lim_{n \to \infty} N_i/n \tag{11}$$

These results can be used to obtain asymptotic distributions for parameters of interest in the low dose extrapolation problem which, in turn, can be used to determine approximate confidence limits for these parameters. Since others have already recorded the details of these calculations and our purpose is to examine the practical applications of these approaches, we will not present the explicit formulas here. Krewski and Van Ryzin[1] consider the asymptotic distribution of $\hat{A}(d_e)$, (the MLE of additional risk at a dose d_e) and of $\hat{d}$, $\log(\hat{d})$, and $1/\hat{d}$ where $\hat{d}$ is the MLE of the VSD corresponding to a given additional risk. They also derive sufficient conditions under which the asymptotic results hold and relate these conditions to the probit, logit, Weibull, gamma multi-hit, and multistage models. Guess and Crump[4] and Crump et al.[3] present similar results explicitly for the multistage model.

Both theoretical and practical difficulties arise when these methods are applied to the low dose extrapolation problem. If the true value of one of the parameters in the multistage model is zero, the MLEs are no longer asymptotically normal.[3] Also the choice made for k in this model strongly affects the confidence limits.

Crump and Masterman[9] observed that lower confidence limits on the VSD under the gamma multihit model, computed using asymptotic MLE theory, sometimes appear far too large. For example, for a carcinogenicity data set involving sodium saccharin exposure, a particular set of parameter values which was consistent with the data (the chi-square goodness of fit p-value being greater than 0.1) predicted a VSD which was a factor of 18,000 less than the lower 97.5% confidence limit for the VSD computed using asymptotic normal theory developed by Rai and Van Ryzin.[2,10] Similar observations have been made by Haseman and Hoel.[11]

Another disquieting feature of this approach is that the limits are not invariant under parameter transformations. For example, each of the asymptotic distributions of $\hat{d}$, log $\hat{d}$, and $1/\hat{d}$ can be used to develop confidence limits and these methods can give considerably different limits. Table 1 shows lower limits on the VSD for 14 data sets obtained from the asymptotic distributions of $\hat{d}$, log $\hat{d}$, and $1/\hat{d}$.[1] It should be noted that these limits differ considerably for almost every data set. The limits based upon $\hat{d}$, which, at first thought, might seem most appropriate, frequently assume negative values. The other two types of limits appear more reasonable, but even they differ by more than an order of magnitude in some instances. This is unsettling because there appears to be no clear reason for choosing one of these limits over another. Cox and Hinkley[12] discussed this difficulty in a general context and suggested as an alternative the approach we will discuss next.

B. Limits Based Upon the Asymptotic Distribution of the Likelihood Ratio

Denote by $L(\underline{\Theta})$ the logarithm of the likelihood $\ell(\Theta)$ defined in Equation 8, let $\hat{L} = \log \ell(\hat{\Theta})$ denote the logarithm of the likelihood evaluated at the MLE, and let $\hat{L}(\Theta_1)$ denote the constrained maximum of the log likelihood subject to the fixed value for a particular scalar parameter Θ_1. Then, under appropriate conditions, $2[\hat{L} - \hat{L}(\Theta_1)]$ has an asymptotic chi-square distribution with one degree of freedom whenever Θ_1 is the true parameter value.[8] This distribution can be used to construct approximate confidence limits for $\hat{\Theta}_1$. The value $\hat{\Theta}_u$ greater than the MLE Θ_1 which satisfies the equation

$$2[\hat{L} - \hat{L}(\hat{\Theta}_u)] = \chi^2_{1-2\alpha} \tag{12}$$

is a $100(1 - \alpha)\%$ upper confidence limit for Θ_1, where χ^2_p denotes the 100p percentage point of the chi-square distribution with one degree of freedom. Lower confidence limits are similarly constructed.

This approach can clearly be used to construct confidence intervals for a function of a single parameter. For monotone functions, the method is simple; if f is an increasing function

Table 1
LOWER CONFIDENCE LIMITS FOR VSDs CORRESPONDING TO AN ADDITIONAL RISK OF 10^{-5} DERIVED FROM WEIBULL MODEL USING ASYMPTOTIC NORMAL THEORY OF THREE MLEs

Substance	MLE	95% Lower limit obtained from asymptotic normality of		
		d*	log d*	1/d*
1. NTA	0.67	0.28	0.27	0.42
2. Aflatoxin	0.13	≤0	$9.5-3^a$	$3.5-2$
3. ETU	1.2	0.53	0.67	0.75
4. TCDD	$5.2-3$	≤0	$3.4-4$	$1.4-3$
5. DMN	$6.1-2$	≤0	$1.1-2$	$2.2-2$
6. Vinyl Chloride	$3.9-7$	≤0	$2.6-11$	$3.6-8$
7. HCB	$2.5-3$	≤0	$4.4-5$	$4.9-4$
8. Botulinum Toxin	$6.3-3$	$4.2-3$	$4.5-3$	$4.7-3$
9. Bischloromethyl Ether	0.12	≤0	$1.6-3$	$2.3-3$
10. Sodium Saccharin	0.86	≤0	0.13	0.29
11. ETU	12.	28.	5.6	6.9
12. Dieldrin	$4.6-3$	≤0	$4.4-4$	$1.4-3$
13. DDT	$8.3-4$	≤0	$7.2-3$	$2.4-2$
14. Span Oil	$5.9-3$	≤0	$2.3-7$	$5.2-4$
15. 2-AAF	32.	21.	23.	24.
16. 2-AAF	21.	17.	17.	18.
17. 2-AAF	12.	1.2	5.0	6.5
18. 2-AAF	0.17	≤0	$1.4-2$	$4.8-2$
19. 2-AAF	$9.1-2$	≤0	$3.3-2$	$4.3-2$
20. 2-AAF	0.13	≤0	$2.5-4$	$1.7-2$

Note: The first 14 data sets are listed in Table 3.

a   The notation $9.5-3$ means 9.5×10^{-3}, etc.

From Krewski, D. and Van Ryzin, J., *Statistics and Related Topics*, 1981, 201. With permission.

and Θ_u is an upper limit for a parameter Θ_1, then $f(\Theta_u)$ is an upper limit for $f(\Theta_1)$. Mantel et al.[6] used this method to obtain lower confidence limits for the VSD for extra risk under the probit model. Since they fixed $b = 1$, the extra risk is given by $\Phi(a + \log_{10}d)$, which is an increasing function of the parameter a and does not involve the background parameter c. Mantel et al. therefore used

$$\text{antilog}_{10}[\Phi^{-1}(\Pi) - a_u] \tag{13}$$

as a $100(1 - \alpha)\%$ upper confidence limit for the VSD corresponding to an extra risk of Π, where a_u is the corresponding upper confidence limit for the parameter a computed using the above approach.

Crump[5] developed a similar approach for the multistage model. For this model the extra risk is given by

$$1 - \exp(-q_1 d - \ldots - q_k d^k) \tag{14}$$

which is a function of the parameters $q_1 \ldots , q_k$. However, at low doses the extra risk can be approximated by $q_1 d$ whenever $q_1 > 0$. An approximate upper confidence limit for the extra risk at a small dose d_e is therefore estimated by $q_u d_e$, where q_u is upper limit for q_1 computed using the above approach. Similarly, Π/q_u represents an approximate lower limit for the VSD corresponding to an extra risk of Π.

This method will not be accurate for risk levels high enough so that the linearization is not a good approximation to the multistage dose response. For doses in the nonlinear region of the dose response curve, an upper limit on extra risk computed in this fashion can even lie below the MLE estimate. Further, it cannot be used without modification to compute two-sided confidence intervals because frequently (Equation 12) will not be satisfied even if q_1 is decreased to zero.[13]

There is a more general version of this approach which does not have either of these drawbacks. It can be shown that under appropriate regularity conditions

$$\max_{\underline{\Theta}} \; [R(d_e; \underline{\Theta}) : 2[1(\hat{\underline{\Theta}}) - 1(\underline{\Theta})] \leq \chi^2_{1-2\alpha}] \tag{15}$$

is an asymptotic $100(1 - \alpha)\%$ upper limit for the extra risk at an environmental dose d_e and

$$\min_{\underline{\Theta}} \; [d : R(d; \underline{\Theta}) = \Pi, \quad 2[1(\hat{\underline{\Theta}}) - 1(\underline{\Theta})] \leq \chi^2_{1-2\alpha}] \tag{16}$$

is an approximate $100(1 - \alpha)\%$ lower limit for the VSD corresponding to an extra risk of Π.[1,12] Similar confidence limits can of course be developed using the concept of additional risk.

C. Bootstrap Methods

Let $P^*(d)$ be some estimate of the dose response function and let $X_1^*, \ldots, X_g^*$ be independent random variables with X_i^* having a binomial distribution with parameters N_i and $P^*(d_i)$. Note that $X_1^*, \ldots, X_g^*$ may be thought of as the numbers of affected animals in the various dose groups of a hypothetical experiment with exactly the same design as the true experiment (i.e., same dose levels and numbers of animals on test); the only difference between the hypothetical experiment and the real experiment being that the response probability in the hypothetical experiment is $P^*(d)$ rather than $P(d)$. Given $P^*(d)$, the complete distribution of $X_1^*, \ldots, X_g^*$ is determined, as well as the distribution of "bootstrap estimators" such as the estimate of the VSD obtained by the method of maximum likelihood applied to $X_1^*, \ldots, X_g^*$ rather than to $X_1, \ldots, X_g$. These distributions may be used to estimate the accuracy of parameter estimates (i.e., their standard deviation) and to construct approximate confidence intervals for parameters. These methods, known as bootstrap procedures, have been discussed in general in a series of papers by Efron.[14-16] The distribution function of a bootstrap estimator given $P^*(d)$ is known as the bootstrap distribution function CDF$_*$.

Although these bootstrap distributions are completely known, at least in principle, they generally must be approximated by Monte Carlo methods. The hypothetical experiment producing the outcomes $X_1^*, \ldots, X_g^*$ is repeated N times by computer simulation and the resulting empirical distribution of the bootstrap estimator is used to approximate CDF$_*$. By the Law of Large Numbers, CDF$_*$ is approximated arbitrarily closely as N increases.

Crump et al.[3] proposed the use of "envelope curves" in connection with the multistage model as a substitute for confidence limits based upon asymptotic theory of MLEs. These curves are generated by computer simulation of 100 independent replications of the same experiment. Each of the 100 data sets involve the same set of test doses and the same number of animals tested at each dose as the actual experiment. The response probability at each test dose is the maximum likelihood estimate obtained from the experimental data. From each of the 100 simulated data sets a maximum likelihood dose response curve is calculated. The value of the upper 97.5% envelope curve for additional risk at a dose d, to use a specific example, is defined as the third largest of the 100 values of additional risk at dose d. Crump et al.[3] showed that these envelope curves sometimes agreed quite closely with confidence limits based upon asymptotic maximum likelihood theory. Although the limits depend upon the particular values simulated, they can be made as accurate as desired by increasing the number of simulated data sets.

These envelope curves represent approximations to the empirical distribution function CDF* of the bootstrap estimator of additional risk obtained by letting $P^*(d_i)$ be the maximum likelihood estimate of risk at dose d_i. The upper 97.5% envelope curve is what Efron[16] calls an upper 97.5% confidence bound computed by the percentile method. Efron[15,16] gives three general arguments supporting the use of the percentile method for constructing confidence limits. None of these arguments, to use Efron's terminology, is "overwhelming" and Efron recommends further investigation of the percentile method.

Hartley and Sielken[17] introduced the model

$$P(t,d) = 1 - \exp[-g(d)H(t)] \tag{17}$$

with

$$g(d) = \sum_{i=0}^{a} \alpha_i d^i, \quad H(t) = \sum_{j=1}^{b} \beta_j t^j \quad (\alpha_i, \beta_j \geq 0, \sum \beta_j = 1) \tag{18}$$

for low dose extrapolation using time to occurrence data. Hartley and Sielken interpret $P(t,d)$ as the probability of a tumor by time t when subject to a dose d. This model and related statistical methods can be applied to quantal data by fixing $H(t) = 1$. The parameters of the model are estimated by maximum likelihood.

Two methods have been suggested for constructing confidence limits for this model which are related to the bootstrap, although the first method is not strictly a bootstrap procedure. Under the method originally proposed[17] for calculating a lower limit for a VSD, the data are randomly divided into G smaller data sets (typically G = 6) containing roughly equal numbers of observations from each experimental dose group. A VSD is then estimated for each of the smaller data sets by maximum likelihood. The standard error of these estimates is used to define lower limits for the VSD through the use of a t-distribution. A drawback of this approach from a practical viewpoint is that the lower limit obtained depends upon the random division of the data, so that the approach defines not just a single lower limit but rather a distribution of limits. Apparently no formal investigation has been made of this distribution, although a report prepared for EPA showed that different divisions can result in lower limits for VSDs which differ by more than 2 orders of magnitude.[18] Unlike the bootstrap procedures, there is no procedure for reducing the spread of this distribution by increasing the number of samples. More general discussion of the Hartley-Sielken method and comparison with a similar approach for utilizing time to occurrence data[19] is also contained in this report. Mantel[20] made a critical review of the method proposed by Hartley and Sielken for computing confidence limits.

More recently Sielken has suggested, rather than subdividing the data, sampling the original data, with replacement, to form N − 1 additional data sets with the same doses and numbers of animals at each dose.[21] MLE estimates of the VSDs from these N − 1 sets of data plus the original data set are then used to estimate a standard error. This standard error is used with a t-distribution to estimate confidence limits in the usual way. This is similar to a bootstrap procedure in which the value used for $P^*(d_i)$ is the observed proportion $X_i/$

N_i rather than the MLE estimate of the response probability as used by Crump et al.[3] Efron[16] also suggested calculating confidence limits in this fashion. The standard error calculated by Sielken is what Efron[16] calls $\hat{\sigma}_{boot}$, except Efron used N sets of simulated data, and not the actual data, to calculate $\hat{\sigma}_{boot}$. This method produces symmetric confidence intervals and appears to assume an approximate t- or normal distribution for the MLE estimators. This may not be a reasonable approximation in this case because the MLE estimators often do not appear to have a normal distribution and can even have a bimodal distribution.[13] Krewski, et al.[21] compared the performance of this method with several others by applying them to sets of computer generated data.

D. Other Methods

It is plausible that a carcinogenesis dose response might be convex at low doses. If this is the case, a straight line joining the origin and a point on the additional or extra risk curve in the convex region will lie above the curve and therefore provide an upper limit on extra or additional risk. Gaylor and Kodell[22] and Van Ryzin[23] suggested using a fitted model to construct a statistical upper limit for the risk at some dose where the risk is large enough (e.g., $\geq 10^{-2}$) to be measured with at least some minimal precision in an experiment of moderate size, and then using a straight line to extrapolate to lower doses. It was thought that the particular model used should not greatly affect the outcome provided the take-off point for the linear extrapolation is within the experimental range. If the multistage model is used, this method will give very nearly the same extrapolated values as applying the model directly in the low dose range. This is because upper confidence limits computed from the multistage model are approximately linear at low doses. If the true dose response curve is convex throughout the region of extrapolation, then this method will yield conservative upper limits on extra risk and lower limits on VSDs.

If the quantity for which a confidence interval is required is a monotone function of each of the parameters, it is possible to obtain conservative limits from confidence limits on each of the parameters. Rai and Van Ryzin[10] suggested such an approach for the gamma multihit model which capitalizes on the fact that under this model the extra risk is a decreasing function of the parameter k and an increasing function of λ.

IV. NUMERICAL EXPERIENCE WITH CONFIDENCE LIMITS BASED UPON THE LIKELIHOOD METHOD

This section contains examples of confidence limits calculated using the "likelihood methods" as well as results of Monte Carlo studies of these models. The "likelihood method" refers to the method specified by Equations 15 and 16. Table 2 illustrates with a particular nonlinear data set the differences between the "linearized" multistage approach to confidence limits (Equations 14 and following) and the likelihood method applied to the multistage model. The linearized multistage approach was used by EPA in setting water quality criteria.[24] When the extra risk is small (e.g., 10^{-5}) the two methods coincide. However, for larger values of extra risk for which the linear approximation is inappropriate, the linearized lower limits are much too large, as they even exceed the MLEs. On the other hand, it is easy to see that, by their very definition, the likelihood lower limits will never exceed either the MLEs or the linearized lower limits.

Table 2 also illustrates an interesting behavior of likelihood lower limits when applied to nonlinear data. At the lowest levels of extra risk the only positive parameters other than possibly q_0 are q_1 and q_k. As the extra risk level is increased, lower order coefficients become zero and higher order coefficients become positive until, at the highest levels of extra risk, q_k is the only nonzero coefficient other than q_0.

Table 2
MULTISTAGE CONFIDENCE LIMITS FOR VSDs FOR EXTRA RISK USING THE LINEARIZED AND LIKELIHOOD METHODS[a]

		95% Lower Limits		Multistage coefficient values which determine lower limits using likelihood method
Extra risk	MLE[b]	Linearized method	Likelihood method	
1.0—5	0.200	2.04—3[c]	2.04—3	$q_0 = 3.92 - 3$
				$q_1 = 4.90 - 3$
				$q_2 = 0.0$
				$q_3 = 0.0$
				$q_4 = 6.44 - 3$
0.09	1.95	18.3	1.87	$q_0 = 3.72 - 3$
				$q_1 = 0.0$
				$q_2 = 9.24 - 4$
				$q_3 = 0.0$
				$q_4 = 7.41 - 3$
0.1	2.00	20.4	1.93	$q_0 = 3.26 - 3$
				$q_1 = 0.0$
				$q_2 = 0.0$
				$q_3 = 4.25 - 4$
				$q_4 = 7.44 - 3$
0.15	2.23	30.6	2.11	$q_0 = 3.25 - 3$
				$q_1 = 0.0$
				$q_2 = 0.0$
				$q_3 = 0.0$
				$q_4 = 7.66 - 3$

[a]   These calculations were made from the following data: Doses: # responders/# animals: 0 1/100 1 0/100 2 1/100 3 37/100 4 89/100.
[b]   MLE estimates of multistage parameters are: $q_0 = 3.44 - 3$, $q_1 = 0.0$, $q_2 = 0.0$, $q_3 = 0.0$, $q_4 = 6.55 - 3$.
[c]   2.04 − 3 means 2.04×10^{-3}.

The Food Safety Council[25] compiled data on 14 chemicals which was used by the Council, and subsequently by Krewski and Van Ryzin,[1] to illustrate low dose extrapolation techniques. The data from these studies is shown in Table 3. Additional information on these data sets, including references to the original studies, is provided by the Food Safety Council Report[25] and Krewski and Van Ryzin.[1] Tables 4 and 5 show lower and upper limits for VSDs corresponding to extra risks of 10^{-5} and 10^{-1} computed for these 14 data sets using the multistage, Weibull, and log-normal models. All of these confidence limits are computed using the likelihood method. (Unlike the method recommended by Mantel et al.[6] the parameter b in the log-normal model was allowed to vary.) Because of the similarities between the two models, results for the Weibull model should give a fair indication of what could be expected from the gamma multihit model.

At an extra risk of 10^{-5} multistage 95% upper and lower confidence limits differ by two orders of magnitude or more except for the data on vinyl chloride and hexachlorobenzene which exhibit a strong linear trend. The Weibull upper and lower limits show about the same degree of disparity.

There is much greater disparity between upper and lower limits, and among models, for 10^{-5} risk than for 10^{-1}. This is because a risk of 10^{-1} is near the "experimental range" where the dose response is known with greater certainty. However, even for an extra risk of 10^{-5}, except for span oil and vinyl chloride, the multistage and Weibull 95% lower limits differ by less than a factor of 1000 and are much closer than this in a number of instances.

Table 3
DATA SETS ANALYZED IN TABLES 4 AND 5[a]

Substance

NTA	D:[b]	0	0.02	0.20	0.75	1.50	2.00
	X/N:	0/127	0/48	0/48	1.91	2/91	12/48
Aflatoxin	D:	0	1	5	15	50	100
	X/N:	0/18	2/22	1/22	4/21	20/25	28/28
ETU	D:	0	5	10	20	40	80
	X/N:	0/167	0/132	1/138	14/81	142/178	24/24
TCDD	D:	0	0.125	0.25	0.50	1.00	
	X/N:	0/24	0/38	1/33	3/31	3/10	
DMN	D:	0	2	5	10	20	
	X/N:	0/29	0/18	4/62	2/5	15/23	
Vinyl	D:	0	50	250	500	2500	6000
chloride	X/N:	0/58	1/59	4/59	7/59	13/59	13/60
HCB	D:	0	10	20	40	60	
	X/N:	0/80	4/79	8/91	15/87	25/96	
Botulinum toxin	D:	0.010	0.015	0.020	0.024	0.027	0.030
	X/N:	0/30	0/30	0/30	0/30	0/30	4/30
	D:	0.034	0.037	0.040	0.045	0.050	
	X/N:	11/30	10/30	16/30	26/30	26/30	
Bischloromethyl ether	D:	10	20	40	60	80	100
	X/N:	1/41	3/46	4/18	4/18	15/34	12/20
Sodium saccharin	D:	0.01	0.10	1.0	5.0	7.5	
	X/N:	0/25	0/27	0/27	1/25	7/29	
ETU	D:	0	5	25	125	250	500
	X/N:	2/72	2/75	1/73	2/73	16/69	62/70
Dieldrin	D:	0	1.25	2.50	5.00		
	X/N:	17/156	11/60	25/58	44/60		
DDT	D:	0	2	10	50	250	
	X/N:	4/111	4/105	11/124	13/104	60/90	
Span Oil	D:	0	5	10	15	20	
	X/N:	1/10	1/10	4/10	4/10	5/10	

[a] See Krewski and Van Ryzin[1] and Food Safety Council[25] report for information on these data sets, including references to the original studies.

[b] D — experiment doses X/N — # responders/# animals at the respective experimental doses.

In the two exceptions, the parameter k in the Weibull model assumes values less than 1; if the biologically plausible restriction k ≥ 1 is imposed, these exceptions would disappear. Likewise, except for span oil and vinyl chloride, the lower limits from the log-normal model generally agree with those from the multistage model to within a factor of 1000. Although this cannot be considered close agreement, the discrepancies between the models are less than those previously reported.[25] This suggests that a considerable amount of the discrepancy among models noted in other studies is due to differences in approaches to confidence limits rather than differences among the models per se.

Upper limits appear to agree much more closely than lower limits. Except for vinyl chloride the upper limits computed using the multistage and Weibull models differ by no more than an order of magnitude. Upper limits on VSDs have not been given the attention that they possibly deserve. Although they probably are not appropriate for determining allowable human exposures, presentation of both upper and lower limits could give regulators and other decision makers a better understanding of the uncertainty of risk estimates.

Tables 6 to 9 give results of a Monte Carlo study of likelihood lower confidence limits for VSDs corresponding to specified values of extra risk for the multistage and one-hit models. The experimental design and dose response functions used in the Monte Carlo study

Table 4
95% UPPER AND LOWER LIMITS[a] ON VSDs CORRESPONDING TO AN EXTRA RISK OF 10^{-5}

DATA[b] (see Table 3)	Multistage			Weibull			Log-Normal	
	Lower	MLE	Upper	Lower	MLE	Upper	Lower	MLE
NTA	3.4 − 4[c]	1.9 − 3	2.9 − 1	1.9 − 1	6.7 − 1	1.8	5.9 − 1	9.6 − 1
Aflatoxin	3.5 − 4	2.0 − 3	1.9	6.0 −	1.2 − 1	2.5	8.0 − 1	2.5
ETU	8.6 − 3	9.1 − 1	2.0	6.4 − 1	1.2	2.0	3.9	5.2
TCDD	4.0 − 5	5.1 − 3	3.8 − 2	3.3 − 5	5.2 − 3	4.8 − 2	1.5 − 3	3.1 − 2
DMN	4.4 − 4	6.0 − 2	1.3 − 1	6.8 − 3	6.0 − 2	2.7 − 1	2.5 − 1	6.9 − 1
Vinyl chloride	1.3 − 1	1.9 − 1	3.4 − 1	1.8 − 12	3.8 − 7	4.2 − 4	1.2 − 6	4.8 − 3
HCB	1.6 − 3	2.1 − 3	5.1 − 3	4.2 − 6	2.5 − 3	5.1 − 2	3.2 − 3	1.2 − 1
Botulinum toxin	1.6 − 5	8.3 − 3	1.1 − 2	5.9 − 3	8.6 − 3	1.1 − 2	1.5 − 2	1.8 − 2
Bischloromethyl ether	1.6 − 3	4.0 − 3	2.5	4.2 − 3	1.2 − 1	3.2	2.9 − 1	2.4
Sodium saccharin	5.3 − 4	5.9 − 1	6.9 − 1	8.0 − 3	8.6 − 1	3.5	9.3 − 2	1.9
ETU	2.7 − 2	9.6	2.3 + 1	5.3	1.2 + 1	2.4 + 1	5.0 + 1	7.4 + 1
Dieldrin	5.5 − 5	1.9 − 4	1.8 − 2	2.4 − 4	4.3 − 3	8.0 − 2	3.8 − 2	1.4 − 1
DDT	2.7 − 3	4.9 − 3	6.1 − 1	2.6 − 3	8.1 − 2	1.4	9.7 − 1	4.0
Span Oil	2.0 − 4	5.2 − 4	1.5	1.0 − 31	5.5 − 3	2.1	9.2 − 12	2.8 − 1

[a]   All limits were calculated using the likelihood method.
[b]   Vertical comparisons are not valid because doses were not all in same units.
[c]   3.3—4 means 3.3×10^{-4}.

Table 5
95% UPPER AND LOWER LIMITS[a] ON VSDs CORRESPONDING TO AN EXTRA RISK OF 10^{-1}

DATA[b] (see Table 3)	Multistage			Weibull			Log-Normal
	Lower	MLE	Upper	Lower	MLE	Upper	MLE
NTA	1.6	1.7	1.9	1.6	1.8	2.0	1.8
Aflatoxin	4.2	1.1 + 1	2.8 + 1	6.4	1.3 + 1	2.6 + 1	1.4 + 1
ETU	1.6 + 1	1.8 + 1	2.0 + 1	1.6 + 1	1.8 + 1	2.0 + 1	1.7 + 1
TCDD	3.8 − 1[c]	5.3 − 1	7.9 − 1	3.7 − 1	5.3 − 1	7.7 − 1	4.9 − 1
DMN	4.4	6.2	9.0	4.3	6.2	8.4	5.9
Vinyl chloride	1.4 + 3	2.0 + 3	3.4 + 3	2.1 + 2	5.7 + 2	1.2 + 3	5.3 + 2
HCB	1.7 + 1	2.2 + 1	3.2 + 1	1.4 + 1	2.2 + 1	2.9 + 1	2.1 + 1
Botulinum toxin	2.8 − 2	3.0 − 2	3.2 − 2	2.8 − 2	3.0 − 2	3.2 − 2	3.0 − 2
Bischloromethyl ether	1.7 + 1	2.8 + 1	5.1 + 1	1.8 + 1	2.9 + 1	5.1 + 1	3.1 + 1
Sodium saccharin	4.3	6.0	7.0	4.3	6.1	7.0	6.0
ETU	1.6 + 2	2.0 + 2	2.3 + 2	1.7 + 2	2.0 + 2	2.3 + 2	
Dieldrin	5.3 − 1	1.1	1.7	6.7 − 1	1.1	1.7	1.3
DDT	2.9 + 1	5.1 + 1	1.1 + 2	2.7 + 1	5.1 + 1	9.0 + 1	5.7 + 1
Span oil	2.1	4.7	1.5 + 1	3.8 − 3	5.2	1.5 + 1	5.7

[a]   All limits were calculated using the likelihood method.
[b]   Vertical comparisons are not valid because doses were not all in same units.
[c]   3.8 − 1 means 3.8×10^{-1}

Table 6
EXPERIMENTAL DESIGN AND DOSE RESPONSE FUNCTIONS USED IN MONTE CARLO STUDIES

Doses:	0	0.5	1.0
# Animals:	50	50	50

Dose response functions
    One-hit (Tables 7 and 8)
    $P(d) = 1 - \exp(-0.0513 - 0.9163d)$
    Two-hit (Table 9)
    $P(d) = 1 - \exp(-0.0513 - 0.9163d^2)$

Note: Number in parentheses indicates number of animals.

Table 7
AVERAGE AND DISTRIBUTION OF MLEs AND LIKELIHOOD 95% LOWER CONFIDENCE LIMITS FOR VSD UNDER ONE-HIT MODEL WHEN TRUE MODEL IS ONE-HIT[a,b]

	MLE	95% Lower limit
[Extra Risk = $1.0-5^c$(VSD = $1.09-5$)]		
Average	**$1.1-5$**	**$8.6-6$**

Fraction of simulations
for which estimate was less
than VSD for extra risk of

$1.5-6$	0	0
$1.0-5$	0.496	0.959
$1.5-5$	0.990	1.0
$1.0-4$	1.0	1.0

[a] See Table 6 for experimental design and exact dose response function.
[b] All results based upon 2000 simulations.
[c] $1.0-5$ means 1.0×10^{-5}.

are listed in Table 6. The design is one frequently used in National Cancer Institute carcinogenesis bioassays, with a control and two treatment groups, and 50 animals per group. Tables 7 to 9 contain estimated average values and coverage probabilities for both MLEs and 95% lower limits. The coverage probability for a true 95% lower confidence limit should be 0.95 (i.e., a lower 95% limit should be exceeded by the true VSD 95% of the time).

A similar Monte Carlo study was recently carried out by Portier and Hoel;[13] the chief difference is that we present estimated coverage probabilities whereas they only provided average values. The two models studied were one-hit and two-hit models with background, both of which are special cases of the multistage model. Additional studies (not reported here) made with no background and twice the background level yielded very similar results to those reported here.

Table 8
AVERAGE AND DISTRIBUTION OF MLEs AND LIKELIHOOD 95% LOWER CONFIDENCE LIMITS FOR VSD UNDER MULTISTAGE MODEL WHEN TRUE MODEL IS ONE-HIT[a,b]

	MLE	95% Lower limit
[Extra Risk = 1.0 − 5[c](VSD = 1.09 − 5)]		
Average	**8.3 − 5**	**9.1 − 6**
Fraction of simulations for which estimate was less than VSD for extra risk of		
1.5 − 6	0	0
1.0 − 5	0.279	0.917
1.5 − 5	0.714	0.989
1.0 − 4	0.970	1.0
1.5 − 4	0.974	1.0
[Extra Risk = 1.0 − 1(VSD = 0.115)]		
Average	**0.149**	**0.0951**
Fraction of simulations for which estimate was less than VSD for extra risk of		
0.05	0	0
0.075	0.018	0.314
0.10	0.305	0.892
0.15	0.796	0.989
0.20	0.913	1.0
0.25	0.978	1.0

[a] See Table 6 for experimental design and exact dose response function.
[b] All results based upon 2000 simulations.
[c] $1.0 - 5$ means 1.0×10^{-5}.

Table 7 shows the performance of the likelihood estimates in the ideal setting in which the true model is one-hit and that model is also used to determine VSDs. The average MLE is almost exactly equal to the true VSD (1.1×10^{-5} vs. 1.09×10^{-5}). (It should be noted that the true mean of the MLE does not exist because there is a positive probability of no carcinogenic effect, which would result in an infinite MLE for the VSD. Our simulation study was constructed using a dose response trend strong enough so that this case never arose. However, it frequently arose when we attempted to duplicate the simulation study of Portier and Hoel.[13]) The simulated coverage probability of 0.959 is likewise very close to the nominal value of 0.95. The confidence limits are quite narrow, as the average 95% lower limit is only about 15% smaller than the true value. This is also exhibited by the fact that each of the 2000 lower limits for an extra risk of 10^{-5} was larger than the VSD corresponding to an extra risk of 1.5×10^{-6}. There was also little variability in the VSDs since all were less than the VSD corresponding to an extra risk of 1.5×10^{-5}.

Table 9
AVERAGE AND DISTRIBUTION OF MLEs AND LIKELIHOOD 95% LOWER CONFIDENCE LIMITS FOR VSD UNDER MULTISTAGE MODEL WHEN TRUE MODEL IS TWO-HIT[a,b]

	MLE	95% Lower limit
[Extra Risk = $1.0 - 5^c$(VSD = $1.04 - 3$)]		
Average	$1.8 - 3$	$1.8 - 5$
Fraction of simulations for which estimate was less than VSD for extra risk of		
$1.0 - 11$	0.0	0.0
$1.0 - 10$	0.002	0.131
$1.0 - 9$	0.204	0.923
$1.0 - 8$	0.387	1.0
$1.0 - 7$	0.457	1.0
$1.0 - 6$	0.471	1.0
$1.0 - 5$	0.743	1.0

[a]   See Table 6 for experimental design and exact dose response function.
[b]   All results based upon 2000 simulations.
[c] $1.0 - 5$ means 1.0×10^{-5}.

Table 8 shows the results of a similar Monte Carlo experiment in which the multistage model was used to fit the data. In this case the estimated coverage probabilities are 0.917 and 0.892 for extra risks of 10^{-5} and 10^{-1}, respectively, which are somewhat less than the nominal value of 0.95. However, the lower 95% limits were always fairly close to the true VSD; for an extra risk of 10^{-5} all 2000 VSDs were larger than the VSD for a risk of 1.5×10^{-6} and 98.9% were less than the VSD for a risk of 1.5×10^{-5}. The average 95% lower limit was about 10% less than the VSD.

Table 9 shows the performance of likelihood 95% lower limits under the multistage model when the true model has no linear component ($q_1 = 0$). In this case the 95% lower limits greatly underestimate the true VSD. Each of the 2000 estimated 95% lower limits corresponded to risks between 10^{-11} and 10^{-8}; this means that the lower limits were less than the true VSD by a factor of between $(10^{-5}/10^{-8})^{1/2} = 31.6$ and $(10^{-5}/10^{-11})^{1/2} = 1000$. This behavior of confidence limits under the multistage model has been pointed out by others[13,26] and seems impossible to avoid without running the risk that lower confidence limits might seriously overestimate the true VSD. The likelihood method selects as a lower confidence limit the lowest value of the VSD that is consistent with the data. At low levels of extra risk this lowest value will be defined by largest value for the multistage parameter q_1 consistent with the data. Of course, if one knew that the linear term q_1 was zero, it could be taken out of the model, thereby making the lower limits agree much more closely with the true VSD. However, this represents a change in the underlying model rather than the confidence limit method. Without making such a model change it is difficult to see how the confidence limits for the multistage model could reasonably be narrowed in this situation.

V. CONCLUSIONS

The principal methods which have been proposed for computing confidence limits in low dose extrapolation are MLE methods (those based upon the asymptotic normality of MLEs), likelihood methods (those based upon the asymptotic distribution of likelihood ratios), and bootstrap methods. Of these, the MLE method appears to be the least useful. Frequently, the limits obtained with this method do not appear sensible. The method is not invariant under the parameter transformations and different parameterization can give very disparate confidence limits.

The likelihood method has a number of features which we feel recommends it for use in setting confidence limits in low dose extrapolation. Unlike limits based upon the asymptotic distribution of MLEs, these limits are invariant under transformations; thus there is no ambiguity regarding which transformation is most appropriate. Unlike some of the ad hoc methods, this method has a firmly based theoretical justification (although the required regularity conditions may not be met in all instances). The method is usable with essentially any model and any data set; thus, it can provide a uniform basis for comparing results from different models. This property is particularly appealing because it appears that, to a considerable degree, the results obtained from different extrapolation methodologies are due to the approaches used for constructing confidence limits rather than to the properties of the extrapolation models themselves. Coverage probabilities for limits based upon the likelihood method have been shown to be close to their nominal values in some cases, and appear to be about as near to the nominal values as can reasonably be expected. Cox and Hinkley[12] argued that this method generally "can be expected to behave more sensibly than" those based upon asymptotic MLE theory and, based upon our experiences, we consider this to be true for the low dose extrapolation problem.

One practical drawback to the likelihood method is that it is computationally difficult. However, we believe that this is not a serious drawback. We have developed seemingly efficient computer programs for calculating these limits for several of the well known models including the multistage, probit, Weibull, and the multistage Weibull time-to-occurrence model.[21] (The program for the multistage is called GLOBAL 82;[27] programs for the other models are not yet ready for general distribution.)

Bootstrap methods share a number of the useful properties of the likelihood method. They too can be used in virtually any situation and are invariant under parameter transformations. However, they do not appear to be as firmly grounded in theory as likelihood methods, and there appears to be at least some doubt as to whether bootstrap confidence limits can be interpreted in the classical way in terms of coverage probabilities.[16] They generally require considerably more computation since their calculation requires a Monte Carlo approach. This makes it difficult to study their small sample properties because a Monte Carlo study of the bootstrap method requires nested Monte Carlo experiments and consequently very large amounts of computer time may be needed. This is one of the reasons we did not attempt such a study here. Another potential difficulty with the bootstrap is that different randomizations can produce different results. However, this is not a serious difficulty as results can be made as accurate as desired by using enough simulations. Overall we feel the bootstrap approach may be useful in low dose extrapolation, and further investigation into this method could be worthwhile.

REFERENCES

1. **Krewski, D. and Van Ryzin, J.,** Dose response models for quantal response toxicity data, in *Statistics and Related Topics,* Csörgö, M., Dawson, D. A., Rao, J. N. K., and Saleh, A. K. Md. E., Eds., North-Holland Publishing Company, Amsterdam, 1981, 201.
2. **Rai, K. and Van Ryzin, J.,** A generalized multi-hit dose response model for low-dose extrapolation, *Biometrics,* 37, 341, 1981.
3. **Crump, K. S., Guess, H. A., and Deal, K. L.,** Confidence intervals and tests of hypotheses inferred from animal carcinogenicity data, *Biometrics,* 33, 437, 1977.
4. **Guess, H. A. and Crump, K. S.,** Maximum likelihood estimation of dose-response functions subject to absolutely monotonic constraints, *Ann. Stat.,* 6, 101, 1978.
5. **Crump, K. S.,** An improved procedure for low-dose carcinogenic risk assessment from animal data, *J. Environ. Pathol. Toxicol.,* 5, 675, 1981.
6. **Mantel, N., Bohidar, N., Brown, C., Ciminera, J., and Tukey, J.,** An improved Mantel-Bryan procedure for safety testing of carcinogens, *Cancer Res.,* 34, 865, 1975.
7. **Rai, K. and Van Ryzin, J.,** Risk assessment of toxic environmental substances based on a generalized multi-hit model, in *Energy and Health,* Breslow, N. and Whittemore, A., Eds., Society for Industrial and Applied Mathematics, Philadelphia, 1979, 99.
8. **Rao, C. R.,** *Linear Statistical Inference and its Applications,* Wiley, New York, 1973.
9. **Crump, K. S. and Masterman, M. D.,** Review and evaluation of methods of determining risks from chronic low level carcinogenic insult, in *Environmental Contaminants in Food,* Congress of the United States OTA, Library of Congress Catalog Card No. 79-600207, 154, 1979.
10. **Rai, K. and Van Ryzin, J.,** MULTI80: a computer program for risk assessment of toxic substances, Technical Report No. N-1512-NIEHS, Rand Corporation, Santa Monica, California, 1980.
11. **Haseman, J. K. and Hoel, D. G.,** Some practical problems arising from use of the gamma multihit model for risk estimation, *J. Toxicol. Environ. Health,* 8, 379.
12. **Cox, D. R. and Hinkley, D. V.,** *Theoretical Statistics,* Chapman and Hall, London, 1974.
13. **Portier, C. and Hoel, D.,** Low dose rate extrapolation using the multistage model, *Biometrics,* 1983, to appear.
14. **Efron, B.,** Bootstrap methods: another look at the jackknife, *Ann. Stat.,* 71, 1, 1979a.
15. **Efron, B.,** Computers and the theory of statistics: thinking the unthinkable, *SIAM Rev.,* 21, 460, 1979b.
16. **Efron, B.,** Censored data and the bootstrap, *J. Am. Stat. Assn.,* 76, 312, 1981.
17. **Hartley, H. O. and Sielken, R. L.,** Estimation of safe doses in carcinogenic experiments, *Biometrics,* 33, 1, 1977.
18. **Science Research Systems, Inc.,** Investigation of Time-to-Tumor Risk Assessment Methodologies, Prepared for the USEPA, Contract 68-01-5975, 1980.
19. **Daffer, P. Z., Crump, K. S., and Masterman, M. D.,** Asymptotic theory for analyzing dose response survival data with application to the low-dose extrapolation problem, *Math. Biosci.,* 50, 207, 1980.
20. **Mantel, N.,** Aspects of the Hartley-Sielken approach for setting safe doses of carcinogens, in *Origins of Human Cancer Book C, Human Risk Assessment,* Hiatt, H. H., Watson, J. D., and Winsten, J. A., Eds., Cold Spring Harbor Laboratory, New York, 1397, 1977.
21. **Krewski, D., Crump, K. S., Farmer, J., Gaylor, D. W., Howe, R. B., Portier, C., Salsburg, D., Sielken, R. L., and Van Ryzin, J.,** A comparison of statistical methods for low-dose extrapolation utilizing time-to-tumour data, *Fundam. Appl. Toxicol.,* 3, 129, 1983.
22. **Gaylor, D. W. and Kodell, R. L.,** Linear interpolation algorithm for low dose risk assessment of toxic substances, *J. Toxicol. Environ. Health,* 4, 305, 1982.
23. **Van Ryzin, J.,** Quantitative risk assessment, *J. Occup. Med.,* 22, 321, 1980.
24. EPA Water quality criteria documents; availability, Federal Register 45, No. 231 (Friday, Nov. 28), 79317, 1980.
25. Food Safety Council, Quantitative risk assessment, *Food Cosmet. Toxicol.,* 18, 711, 1980.
26. **Guess, H., Crump, K., and Peto, R.,** Uncertainty estimates for low-dose-rate extrapolations of animal carcinogenicity data, *Cancer Res.,* 37, 3475, 1977.
27. **Howe, R. B. and Crump, K. S.,** GLOBAL 82. A computer Program to Extrapolate Quantal Animal Toxicity Data to Low Doses. Prepared for the Office of Carcinogen Standards, OSHA, U.S. Department of Labor, Contract 41USC252C3, 1982.

Chapter 10

INCORPORATION OF PHARMACOKINETICS IN LOW-DOSE RISK ESTIMATION

David G. Hoel

TABLE OF CONTENTS

I. INTRODUCTION

The problem of estimating the risk of cancer resulting from chronic exposure to low doses of a chemical carcinogen has been studied for many years, yet there still is not a wholly satisfactory means of calculating that risk.[1] There are many reasons why this issue has proven to be so problematic. The primary one is that data of the quality and quantity to support risk calculations and unquestioned conclusions are generally unavailable. Furthermore, there is no satisfactory mechanism for generating relevant human data. An alternative approach is to estimate low-dose response in laboratory animals, then to extrapolate the results to the human population. Most recent research has focused almost exclusively on the estimation of low-dose effects in laboratory animals, leaving the complex problem of species-to-species extrapolation largely unexplored.

The main difficulty in estimating low-dose response in laboratory animals is that the exposure levels of interest are so low that an impracticably large number of animals must be exposed to obtain a reliable estimate. The strategy for circumventing this problem has been to experiment at doses which are much higher than those generally encountered in the environment, but which produce tumors at a higher frequency. The results are then extrapolated to the dose levels of interest. This approach requires far fewer laboratory animals, but has been the object of controversy.[2,3]

Two aspects of this approach have been discussed at length by the scientific community. The first is a biological consideration. It is known that the biological processes of laboratory animals may be modified by the magnitude of the dose to which the animal is exposed. For example, it is possible that at high dose levels certain metabolic pathways for chemical carcinogens may become saturated; consequently the tumor yield in the test animals may not be indicative of what actually occurs at the low-dose level.[2] The second issue revolves around the low-dose extrapolation procedure.[3] It has received by far the greater amount of attention and the combination of these two issues is the main focus of this chapter.

The usual approach to low-dose extrapolation has been to assume a parametric model relating applied dose and tumor response, and to use the high-dose data to estimate model parameters. Historically speaking, three main types of parametric models have been used.[1] The earliest were tolerance models which include the probit and the logit. This type of model is primarily empirical without a good biological foundation. In addition, the probit, which was widely used in the 1960's is excessively "flat" in the low-dose region and is therefore a very non-conservative model. The second type of model is the multistage model proposed by Armitage and Doll. This model attempts to reflect the observation that cancer is a multistage process. The third type of model, more recently advocated, is the multi-hit model. This model assumes that a critical number of "hits" are necessary before a cell has the potential to generate a tumor. Although this model is useful in radiation biology, its biological relevance in chemical carcinogenesis is debatable.

For all of the foregoing models the statistical methodology has been worked out in great detail; hence, this aspect of the problem is not in question. The pressing issue is in deciding which model to use since the various models may all adequately fit the data in the experimental region but produce widely varying low-dose estimates. Since the data generally cannot be used to distinguish between models, the alternative is to judge them individually on their biological soundness. If it is agreed that the choice of model must be based on a biological foundation, the multistage model would fare best of the three types of models mentioned above. However this is also scientifically debatable, since a variety of biological mechanisms are no doubt involved in carcinogenesis; no single mathematical model is likely to describe accurately all the processes.[4]

II. SIMPLE KINETIC EQUATIONS

In order to understand the toxic effects of a compound, one must have an appreciation of the manner in which the material is handled pharmacologically by the organism. Species differences in the toxicity of a material are often explained by simple pharmacokinetic considerations. This also applies to the shape of dose-response relations in a given species. For a given exposure level or "administered dose", we need to determine quantitatively the amount of active chemical present at the tissue target site which we define as the "effective dose". This relationship depends upon the organism's ability to absorb the material and how it is distributed, metabolized, and excreted. In carcinogenesis, for example, we hope to be able to describe quantitatively the relationship between the exposure of a chemical and some measure of cellular activity such as the amount of a particular unrepaired DNA adduct formed in response to that exposure. If this relationship is linear and the tumor frequency is proportional to this effective dose, one would suspect that the frequency of tumor would then be proportional to the administered dose of the carcinogen. If, on the other hand, either the DNA repair process or a detoxification system is saturated, we would then expect to see a non-linear dose-response relationship.

In chemical kinetics the simplest reaction (i.e., first order) is the irreversible conversion of reactant chemical X into a product chemical P represented as

$$X \rightarrow P \tag{1}$$

From the law of mass action, the velocity of the reaction or rate of the formation of the product P is proportional to the concentration of X. Mathematically, this is written as

$$v = \frac{dP}{dt} = -\frac{dX}{dt} = kX$$

or $\qquad\qquad(2)$

$$X = X_0 e^{-kt}$$

where k is the rate constant of this first-order reaction. A second-order reaction would be

$$2X \rightarrow P$$

or $\qquad\qquad(3)$

$$v = \frac{dP}{dt} = kX^2$$

More complicated first-order reactions may be easily described by a set of linear differential equations. For example, the reaction

$$A \underset{k_2}{\overset{k_1}{\rightleftarrows}} B \overset{k_3}{\rightarrow} C \tag{4}$$

is written as

$$\frac{dA}{dt} = k_2 B - k_1 A$$

$$\frac{dB}{dt} = k_1 A - (k_2 + k_3)B$$

$$\frac{dC}{dt} = k_3 B$$

The reaction which is catalyzed by an enzyme is somewhat more complicated mathematically. Suppose the substrate S combines with the enzyme E forming an intermediate complex X which in turn forms the product P. Then we have

$$S + E \underset{k_2}{\overset{k_1}{\rightleftarrows}} X \overset{k_3}{\to} P + E \tag{5}$$

with kinetic equations

$$\frac{dS}{dt} = k_2 X - k_1 SE \tag{6}$$

$$\frac{dE}{dt} = (k_2 + k_3)X - k_1 SE$$

$$\frac{dX}{dt} = k_1 SE - (k_2 + k_3)X$$

$$\frac{dP}{dt} = k_3 X$$

This system would require a computer for solution and so a "steady-state" assumption is made which is equivalent to saying that

$$\frac{dE}{dt} = \frac{dX}{dt} = 0. \tag{7}$$

The idea here is that the concentrations of E and X vary only a slight amount until the end of the reaction is approached. By using Equation 7 and letting the total amount of enzyme be denoted by

$$E_{tot} = E + X$$

we have

$$X = \frac{k_1 S \cdot E_{tot}}{k_1 S + k_2 + k_3} \tag{8}$$

and thus

$$v = \frac{dP}{dt} = \frac{V \cdot S}{K + S} \tag{9}$$

$$\text{where } V = k_3 E_{tot} \text{ and } K = (k_2 + k_3)/k_1$$

Equation 9 is referred to as the Michaelis-Menten equation with V the maximum velocity of the reaction, and K the Michaelis constant, which is the concentration of S which will produce one-half the maximum velocity of the reaction.

From Equation 9 we observe that for large concentrations of the substrate S the reaction is saturated and so v is approximately equal to the constant maximum velocity V and thus becomes a zero-order reaction. On the other hand, for small amounts of substrate relative to enzyme, v is approximately equal to (V/K)S and the reaction is a simple first-order reaction.

III. CORNFIELD'S MODEL

Cornfield[5,6] considered the implication of simple kinetic models on the shape of dose-response functions. He began by proposing a system with a total dose D of a toxic substance that combined with S moles of free substrate forming X moles of an activated complex. Further he assumed that T moles of enzyme were available for detoxification. Schematically, Cornfield's model is described as

$$D + S \rightleftarrows X$$
$$+$$
$$T$$
$$\downarrow$$
$$DT$$

Also, he assumed that the probability P(D) of a toxic reaction in the organism is proportional to X. The first conclusion made by Cornfield is that if the detoxification is irreversible then steady-state considerations produce a threshold dose-response model, namely:

$$P(D) = 0 \qquad \text{if } D \leq T \tag{10}$$
$$P(D) = [D - S \cdot P(D) - T]/[D - S \cdot P(D) - T + K] \qquad \text{if } D > T$$

where K is the ratio of the rate constants associated with the complex X.

The threshold of P(D) = 0 if D ≤ T is not strictly correct since it is an asymptotic or steady-state result. Clearly some of the complex X will be formed before all of the toxic substance is bound to the detoxification enzyme T.

Cornfield[5] also considered a somewhat expanded version of this model by permitting a reversal of the detoxification pathway. If K* denotes the ratio of the rate constants for the detoxification pathway, then the dose-response equations become

$$P(D) = D/S + K(1 + T/K^*) \qquad \text{if } D \leq T \tag{11}$$
$$P(D) = [D - S \cdot P(D) - y]/[D - S \cdot P(D) - y + K] \qquad \text{if } D > T$$

where $y = K \cdot P(D) \cdot T/[K \cdot P(D) + K^*(1 - P(D))]$. For low doses we now have that P(D) is linear in the dose D instead of the result P(D) = 0.

Although Cornfield presented a flawed argument for the existence of a threshold, the general implications of his work for dose-response models are nonetheless pertinent. Using a very simple kinetic model, Cornfield has shown that abrupt changes in the mathematical dose-response curve can occur. These changes are associated with the saturation of a detoxification system. Because many chemicals go through pharmacological change before the active toxicant is at the target tissue, the kinetic models are very relevant to estimating risk.

IV. GEHRING'S MODEL

One of the first examples of an attempt to consider the effects of pharmacokinetic principles on risk estimation in carcinogenesis was carried out by Gehring and Blau.[2] They analyzed data of Maltoni and Lefemine[7] on the exposure of rats to vinyl chloride and the resulting hepatic angiosarcoma. They observed in the tumor data that the incidence of angiosarcoma plateaued at about 20%. In a separate study, Watanabe et al.[8] showed that the amount of metabolized vinyl chloride was non-linearly related to exposure and seemed to follow Michaelis-Menten kinetics, i.e.

$$v = V \cdot S/(K + S) \tag{12}$$

In this equation v and V are the velocity and the maximum velocity, respectively, for the transformation of vinyl chloride, S is the concentration of vinyl chloride inhaled, and K is the Michaelis constant. Using experimentally determined values of V and K to transform the administered dose to the effective dose of vinyl chloride, they were able to explain the plateauing effect of tumor incidence by the saturation of the activation of the vinyl chloride exposure.

Anderson et al.[9] have continued the study of the vinyl chloride example. They have shown that the parameters in the kinetic model could substantially influence low-dose cancer incidence estimates. This is demonstrated by using the kinetic model to transform the administered dose into an effective dose, then fitting a mathematical model to the observed tumor incidence data and the corresponding effective dose. Although the Michaelis-Menten transformation of the vinyl chloride exposure data eliminated the observed plateauing effect in the tumor data, one still must choose the mathematical model. Anderson et al.[9] found that the probit model and the multistage model gave different low-dose risk estimates, even after the kinetic information had been used to transform the exposure doses. For example, for the multistage model they found that the estimated dose for a lifetime risk of tumor of 10^{-7} was 162×10^{-4} µg/ℓ without applying the kinetic transformation to the exposure values and 6×10^{-4} µg/ℓ, using the Michaelis-Menten transformation. The corresponding dose estimates using the probit model were 0.5×10^{-4} µg/ℓ and 9657×10^{-4} µg/ℓ. Considering these four values, we see that the application of the kinetic transformation makes a substantial difference in the risk estimates, as does the choice of the mathematical model used to describe the relationship between transformed dose and tumor frequency.

Relating tumor response to the effective dose D* is important because the relationship between D* and the administered dose D may be dose-dependent. Hoel et al.[10] have studied the quantitative implications of the relationship between administered and effective dose from the standpoint of low-dose risk estimation. They followed the same approach as Gehring and Blau[2] in assuming a continuous exposure of the chemical as compared with the single dose model of Cornfield as previously described. The kinetic model studied was originally given by Gehring and Blau and is illustrated in Figure 1. In this model the chemical (C) is assumed to be converted to the reactive metabolite (RM) by Michaelis-Menten kinetics. This is also assumed to be the case for the detoxification of the active metabolite to its inactive form (IM). Other reactions, such as the binding of the reactive metabolite to both genetic (CBG) and non-genetic (CBM) material follow simple first order kinetics. The repair of the covalently bound genetic material is assumed to follow Michaelis-Menten kinetics and it is further assumed that the concentration of unrepaired genetic material is proportional to the tumor incidence. This model is fairly simplistic, however it does serve to illustrate the features of activation, detoxification, repair and binding of the administered chemical. Since the activation, detoxification and repair processes are enzymatically controlled, saturation is possible; hence non-linear relationships between D and D* are possible.

The kinetic model shown in Figure 1 can be described by a series of simple differential equations. Further, by appealing to steady state considerations the following two equations describe the relationship between D and D*.

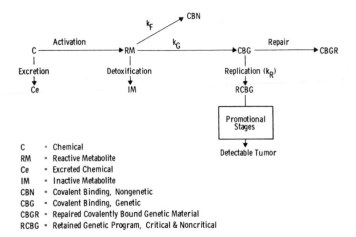

C = Chemical
RM = Reactive Metabolite
Ce = Excreted Chemical
IM = Inactive Metabolite
CBN = Covalent Binding, Nongenetic
CBG = Covalent Binding, Genetic
CBGR = Repaired Covalently Bound Genetic Material
RCBG = Retained Genetic Program, Critical & Noncritical

FIGURE 1.   Diagram of a simple pharmacokinetic model for the metabolic fate of some carcinogens. (From Hoel, D. G., Kaplan, N. L., and Anderson, M. W., *Science*, 219, 1032, 1983. Copyright 1983 by the AAAS. With permission.)

$$k_G[RM] - k_R D^* - \frac{V_M^R D^*}{k_M^R + D^*} = 0$$

$$(k_F + k_G)[RM] + \frac{V_M^D[RM]}{k_M^D + [RM]} - \frac{V_M^A D}{k_M^A + D} = 0$$

(13)

In this example we have equated the administered D with [C] and the effective dose D* with [RCBG]. Using both experimental and hypothetical values for the kinetic parameters in the above equations, Anderson et al.[9] obtained an excellent fit to the vinyl chloride data of Maltoni and Lefemine.[7] This vinyl chloride data has the feature of a concave dose-response relationship which the Equations 13 are able to describe.

In Equations 13, by modifying the Michaelis constant for the detoxification of the reactive metabolite in such a way that the detoxification process is saturated, the relationship between D and D* becomes nonlinear with a definite "hockey-stick" shape (See Figure 2 of Reference 10). This dose-response relationship has a threshold-like behavior in the low-dose region similar to what Cornfield described in his model while still retaining the concave shape at high dose levels. Assuming a carcinogenesis experiment was conducted with the true response following a "hockey-stick" shape, the experimenter would be unlikely to detect the nonlinear behavior in the low-dose region. Hoel et al.[10] showed that for the particular example seen in Figure 2 of Reference 10 that the low-dose risk would be statistically overestimated by a factor of 50 to 100.

At the present time there is very little experimental data illustrating the possible non-linearities between D and D*. Hoel et al.[10] present a few examples of dose response data associating particular DNA adducts with administered chemicals such as dimethylnitrosamine and benzo-a-pyrene. The actual measurement and determination of the metabolic pathways and the kinetic parameters is often extremely complicated. One approach for avoiding this problem for a given carcinogen would be to directly measure the effective dose D* and relate it quantitatively to the administered dose D. Simply conducting large scale animal experiments for purposes of estimating tumor frequency will not give us the shape of the dose-response curve in the low-dose region. What is required is knowledge or assumptions concerning the mechanisms of carcinogenesis and direct measurements of the effective chemical at the cellular level.

V. POPULATION VARIABILITY

The field of pharmacogenetics[11,12] attempts to define the effects of genetic variability on drug metabolism. The Ah gene complex regulates the induction of many enzyme systems including AHH and the associated cytochrome P-450 system. These enzyme systems are responsible for the metabolism of many environmental pollutants from fat-soluble to water-soluble products. Nebert et al.[13] have studied the inducibility of AHH activity in large numbers of various strains of rat and mouse. They observed considerable strain variability in both basal levels and the level of inducibility. In fact, six of twenty mouse strains were found to be noninducible using 3-methylcholanthrene. Since there is evidence that there is heritable variation in the Ah locus in man, the study of inbred strains of rodents is important in helping to understand human variability.

The form of the dose-response function for a population may be quite different from the individual dose-response functions for the members of the population. For example, suppose each individual in a population had the probability P(d) of a toxic effect from dose d of a chemical and that P(d) was quadratic, namely:

$$P_s(d) = 1 - \exp(-sd^2) \tag{14}$$

Here s represents the individual's sensitivity. If F(s) is the distribution function for sensitivities among individuals in the population, then the population response P(d) follows the form

$$P(d) = \int P_s(d)dF(s). \tag{15}$$

It is straightforward to show that, if F(s) is the distribution function for the reciprocal of a gamma distribution, then the population dose-response will be a linear or one-hit model, i.e.

$$P(d) = 1 - e^{-ad} \tag{16}$$

even though each individual has a quadratic dose-response (14). This somewhat contrived example illustrates the potential impact of genetic heterogeneity on dose-response models.

A different but related approach to including kinetics in toxicological dose-response functions has been used by Nordberg and his co-workers.[14,15] They have been especially concerned with heavy metal toxicities where response thresholds are likely to be present. They have developed a compartmental model which describes the metabolic processes controlling the distribution of the toxic substance in the body. They especially emphasize the variability of the kinetic parameters among individuals in the population. The metabolic model is then combined with a damage model to produce a total toxic response model. The damage function is generally assumed to be of the threshold type, although the critical level at which damage is likely to occur will vary among individuals. Nordberg is careful to differentiate this type of toxicity model from those toxic effects which are of a stochastic nature, i.e., no threshold for damage.

Nordberg and Strangert[14,15] use methylmercury to illustrate this approach. A single compartment model is appropriate when toxicity results from a peak concentration in brain tissue. Population variability for biological half-life of the methylmercury was estimated from high dietary levels observed in Iraq. The data followed a bimodal distribution with 10% of the population having twice the half-life as the remaining 90% This lower 90% group was itself normally distributed. Using paresthesia as the toxic endpoint, Nordberg and Strangert estimated the relationship between body burden and toxic effect to follow either a Weibull or a log-normal distribution.

The most important implication of this model is the recognition of population variability. Using a non-variable estimated threshold coupled with a safety factor, Kitamura[16] suggested that a safe long-term exposure of methylmercury would be 0.1 mg/day. The Nordberg-Strangert model, however, predicts 2% of the population being affected at a dose rate of 0.1 mg/day. For the more susceptible subpopulation with the higher half-life of methylmercury, 6% would be affected. Thus, even if thresholds are assumed, the use of safety factors may substantially underestimate possible effects on a population, especially with respect to susceptible subgroups in that population.

Nordberg and Strangert also mentioned the well-known fact that the choice of a mathematical model greatly affects low-dose estimates. Using the Weibull or the log-normal distribution for the interindividual variation in thresholds for symptoms, they found, for example, that at the dose rate of 0.1 mg/day the predicted probability of effect differed by a factor of 7 for the 2 distributions. At lower doses the difference increased even further.

VI. CONCLUSIONS

The concepts of pharmacokinetics are clearly a major component of risk estimation. The impact of the saturation of enzyme systems is perhaps the best recognized issue. This saturation and the resulting nonlinear kinetics can in some circumstances wreak havoc with the simple low-dose estimation methods currently in vogue in quantitative risk estimation. What is needed is the appropriate kinetic data along with the toxicology data prior to a hazard evaluation of a compound.

Although it has not been the subject of this chapter, species extrapolation is an equally difficult area in risk estimation. Currently the method used is to predict a toxic effect in man equal to the effect in the rodent using one of several possible dosage measures. Comparative pharmacology can at least improve the reliability of this process. This issue is related to the problem of population heterogeneity which was discussed. It was shown that variability in individual sensitivities can modify the dose-response relationships and therefore impact low-dose risk estimation. This variability in sensitivity may be partially ascribed to genetic variability in detoxification and repair systems. In addition to the impact on the population risk estimates, consideration should also be given to the susceptible subgroups in the population. All of these factors press us to place a greater emphasis on pharmacokinetics in human risk estimation.

REFERENCES

1. **Hogan, M. D. and Hoel, D. G.,** Extrapolation to man, in *Principles and Methods of Toxicology,* Hayes, A. W., Ed., Raven Press, New York, 1982, 711.
2. **Gehring, P. J. and Blau, G. E.,** Mechanisms of carcinogenesis: dose response, *J. Environ. Pathol. Toxicol.,* 1, 163, 1977.
3. **Hoel, D. G., Gaylor, D. W., Kirschstein, R. L., Saffiotti, U., and Schneiderman, M. A.,** Estimation of risks of irreversible, delayed toxicity, *J. Toxicol. Environ. Health,* 1, 133, 1975.
4. **Crump, K. S., Hoel, D. G., Langley, C. H., and Peto, R.,** Fundamental carcinogenic processes and their implications for low dose risk assessment, *Cancer Res.,* 36, 2973, 1976.
5. **Cornfield, J.,** Carcinogenic risk assessment, *Science,* 198, 693, 1977.
6. **Cornfield, J., Carlborg, F. W., and Van Ryzin, J.,** Setting tolerances on the basis of mathematical treatment of dose-response data extrapolated to low doses, in *Proceedings of the First International Congress on Toxicology,* Plaa, G. L. and Duncan, W. A. M., Eds., Academic Press, New York, 1978, 143.

7. **Maltoni, C. and Lefemine, G.,** Carcinogenicity assays of vinyl chloride: current results, *Ann. N.Y. Acad. Sci.*, 246, 195, 1975.

8. **Watanabe, P. G., Young, J. D., and Gehring, P. J.,** The importance of non-linear (dose-dependent) pharmacokinetics in hazard assessment, *J. Environ. Pathol. Toxicol.*, 1, 147, 1977.

9. **Anderson, M. W., Hoel, D. G., and Kaplan, N. L.,** A general scheme for the incorporation of pharmacokinetics in low-dose risk estimation for chemical carcinogenesis: example — vinyl chloride, *Toxicol. Appl. Pharmacol.*, 55, 154, 1980.

10. **Hoel, D. G., Kaplan, N. L., and Anderson, M. W.,** The implication of nonlinear kinetics on risk estimation in carcinogenesis, *Science*, 219, 1032, 1983.

11. **Nebert, D. W.,** Genetic differences in susceptibility to chemically induced myelotoxicity and leukemia, *Environ. Health Perspect.*, 39, 11, 1981.

12. **Nebert, D. W.,** Pharmacogenetics: an approach to understanding chemical and biologic aspects of cancer, *J. Natl. Cancer Inst.*, 64, 1279, 1980.

13. **Nebert, D. W., Jensen, N. M., Shinozuka, H., Kunz, H. W., and Gill, T. J., III,** The Ah phenotype. Survey of forty-eight rat strains and twenty inbred mouse strains, *Genetics*, 100, 79, 1982.

14. **Nordberg, G. F. and Strangert, P.,** Estimations of a dose response curve for long-term exposure to methylmercuric compounds in human beings taking into account variability of critical organ concentration and biological half-time: a preliminary communication, in *Effects and Dose Response Relationships of Toxic Metals*, Nordberg, G. F., Ed., Elsevier Scientific, Amsterdam, 1976, 273.

15. **Nordberg, G. F. and Strangert, P.,** Fundamental aspects of dose-response relationships and their extrapolation for noncarcinogenic effects of metals, *Environ. Health Perspect.*, 22, 97, 1978.

16. **Kitamura, S., Sumino, K., Hayakawa, K., and Shibata, T.,** Dose-response relationship of methylmercury, in *Effects and Dose Response Relationships of Toxic Metals*, Nordberg, G. F., Ed., Elsevier Scientific, Amsterdam, 1976, 262.

Index

INDEX

A

B

I

K

L

R

Rabbit, 108
Radiation, 15, 107—108
Random bred animals, 117
Randomization, 130—132, 202
Randomization test, 137
Randomized design, 132, 137
Randomized experiment, 132
Rapid lethality, 156—157
Rat, 108, 111, 117—118, 212
Reactive compounds, 61—62, 70, 210
Reactive metabolites, see Reactive compounds
Receptor site antagonists, 106
Reductase, 20
Reduction, 16
Regression models
    tumor mortality, 160
    tumor prevalence, 160—161
Relative efficiency, 129
Relatively unreactive compounds, 61—62
Renal tumorigenesis, 108
Repair, see DNA
Repair enzymes, 100
Replication, see DNA
Replicative cells, 26—28
Reporting
    graphical displays, 159—160
    rodent tumorigenicity, 158—160
    tabular displays, 160
Response, definitions of, 174
Response initiation stage, 166
Response lethality, see Lethality
Response surface, 175
Response thresholds, 212
Restorative hyperplasia, 101
Restricted parameter estimation, 168
Reversibility studies, 137
Risk analysis, 94
Risk assessment, steps in, 188
Risk characteristic, 184
Risk characterization, 175—176
Risk estimates, 54, 106, 181, 205—214
Risk summary, 175—176
RNA, 25, 114
Rodent test models, 5—6
Rodent tumorigenicity, 149—163
    baseline variables, 158
    bias, 157
    cause of death, 151, 155—157, 161
    considerations for selecting a test, 156—158
    covariance matrices, 151, 153
    death from other causes operating independently,
        155
    dose metameter, 150
    general properties of tests, 154—156
    goal, 150
    guidelines, 150
    hazard ratios, 155
    intercurrent death rates, 158

isotonic regression, 159
Kaplan-Meier survival curves, 159
lethality, 151, 157
litter effects, 161
local score test, 157
logistic regression, 156, 158, 160
logrank test, 155—157, 159
monotone prevalence, 157
mortality rates, 151—153
multigenerational designs, 161
natural death, 153, 156
natural longevity, 159
nonproportional hazards, 161
null hypothesis, 154
prevalence rates, 151, 153, 155
proportional hazards, 155
rapid lethality, 156—157
regression models
    mortality, 160
    prevalence, 160—161
reporting, 158—160
sacrificed animal, 151, 156
sacrificial deaths, 153
safety evaluation, 150
score tests, 156
side-effects, 151
significance level, 159
significance tests, 154
slope estimate, 160
statistical procedures, 150
statistical tests, 150—154
strains of rodents, 150
stratification, 156, 158
theoretic basis, 154—156
time to death, 151
treatment comparisons, 150
trend tests, 150
typical experiment, 150
weights for trend tests, 158
Rose Bengal, 45
Route dependence, 82—85
Route of administration, 45
Route of exposure, 85, 109
Rubella, 107

S

Saccharin, 15, 111
Sacrificed animals, 156
Sacrifice time, 170
Sacrificial deaths, 153
Safe dose, see Virtually safe dose
Safety evaluation, 150
Safety factors, 42, 213
Salicylic acid, 33, 65—66
Saturable processes, 46, 54—55, 57, 59—61
Schaafsma's test, 140
Score tests, 156
Screening studies, see also Carcinogenicity bioas-
    say, 133—134

T

U

V

W

X